Negotiating insanity in the southeast of Ireland, 1820–1900

D1338883

1824

Manchester University Press

Negotiating insanity in the southeast of Ireland, 1820–1900

Catherine Cox

Manchester University Press

Published by Manchester University Press
Altrincham Street, Manchester M1 7JA, UK
www.manchesteruniversitypress.co.uk

British Library Cataloguing-in-Publication Data is available

ISBN 978 0 7190 7503 2 *hardback*
ISBN 978 1 5261 4261 0 *paperback*

First published by Manchester University Press in hardback 2012

This edition first published 2019

Typeset by 4word Ltd, Bristol

Contents

Figures

Tables

Acknowledgements

In the preparation of this monograph I accumulated many debts. The book is based on my PhD dissertation and I am very grateful to my supervisor Professor Mary E. Daly, University College Dublin, for her support and encouragement. My former colleagues at the Department of History, University of Warwick, and current colleagues at the School of History and Archives, UCD, have provided rich intellectual environments, while I have benefitted from many stimulating conversations with graduate and post-doctoral scholars working in the field, especially those at the Centre for the History of Medicine in Ireland, UCD.

I would like to acknowledge the support and expertise of staff at the National Library of Ireland, the National Archives of Ireland, the Royal College of Physicians of Ireland, Carlow County Library, Dublin Diocesan Archives, the Wellcome Trust Library and the Wexford County Archives Service. Staff at St Dympna's Psychiatric Hospital, Carlow, and St Senan's Psychiatric Hospital, Enniscorthy, afforded me access to their records. In particular, I would like to thank Jim Hanley, Stephanie Lynch and Hugo Kelly. The team at Manchester University Press, including their expert reader, has been helpful and patient. I have also benefitted from funding from the Irish Research Council for the Humanities and Social Sciences and the Wellcome Trust.

At important junctures key practical support came from Catriona Crowe, Professor Greta Jones, Professor Maria Luddy and Dr Paul Rouse. I am immensely grateful to colleagues and friends who have enriched this study through conversation and comments. In particular, I would like to thank Professor Hilary Marland, Dr Leeann Lane, and Dr Lindsey Earner-Byrne. Finally, I would also like to thank my family for their support over the years, particularly my husband, William Murphy, and my brother, Damian Cox.

Abbreviations

CCA	Carlow County Library, Archives
CLA	Carlow Lunatic Asylum
CSO	Chief Secretary's Office
CRF	Criminal Reference Files
DJMS	*Dublin Journal of Medical Science*
DQJMS	*Dublin Quarterly Journal of Medical Science*
ELA	Enniscorthy Lunatic Asylum
IJMS	*Irish Journal of Medical Science*
JMS	*Journal of Mental Science*
KLA	Kildare Local Authority Archives
NAI	National Archives of Ireland
NLI	National Library of Ireland
DPH	St Dympna's Psychiatric Hospital, Carlow
SPH	St Senan's Psychiatric Hospital, Enniscorthy
WCA	Wexford County Archive Service

Introduction

As I cannot count on sufficient fair play according to my state of health and in every way my great need of fair play … I am badly in want of a powerfull [sic] friend so as to be able to work out much more good than usual – I feel sure he [John Redmond MP] will be able latter [sic] on to exercise his powerful influence over his own people for Ireland's best interest – when I was in Dublin some years ago I went in for a high tone [sic] I am still going in for the same as far as my state of health will permit – I am a lot better now than when I first came to Ireland – owing to the fact of having been driven into a state of dispair [sic] in England by means of going in for a low tone unconsciously, I have been driven into the extremes of it.[1]

However I see it is my duty to state that my present state of health and capacity for doing good is all due to the goodness of the government in the person of Dr Drapes because I was out of my right mind and incapable of doing good only from extremes of foul play so far as my health is concerned also because I was unable to follow the advice of a good soul when I was in England owing to overwhelming weakness … because so long as I am here in the country, if I have the name of being ill they can claim aright to come and distinguish themselves by a rare sort of kindness towards the sick patients …[2]

Between 1912 and 1914 Anastasia O'D., a patient in Wexford District Lunatic Asylum (Enniscorthy asylum), penned several letters to John Redmond, leader of the Irish Parliamentary Party and a local Waterford MP. In her correspondence, Anastasia provided her own narrative of her behaviour, of the events that contributed to her 'state of health' and of her future needs and requirements. Anastasia's letters never reached John Redmond. Dr Thomas Drapes, the Resident Medical Superintendent at Enniscorthy asylum from 1884 to 1919, withheld them.[3] Anastasia's narrative is sometimes confused and confusing, but it is useful in several respects. By her own account, Anastasia had been in and out of institutions in Dublin and in county Wexford. She believed the period she spent as an Irish migrant in England was crucial in precipitating her illness and identified her history of consumption as contributing to her mental decline. Throughout her correspondence, Anastasia displayed gratitude to Drapes as her carer, although this became more muted in later letters. She was acutely aware of her social status as someone who was 'ill', recognising that those outside the asylum distinguished themselves in relation to her: as kind but also as sane. She mapped her own behaviour and requirements onto contemporary national political debates. Her need for a 'powerful friend' reflected the Irish people's need for powerful advocates in a time of political turmoil and she claimed she abstained from religious services to ease national sectarian tensions.[4] She therefore inserted herself into the colonial relationship between Britain and Ireland. Anastasia was one of thousands of Irish people to enter asylums in the nineteenth and early twentieth centuries.

A state-funded system of district asylums was introduced to Ireland in July 1817.[5] The provision of welfare institutions bolstered the union between Britain and Ireland and was part of colonial endeavours 'to bring order to Ireland, to foster the conditions in which the transition to a prosperous, capitalist agricultural society might be effected.'[6] Central government retained high levels of control over the new Irish asylum system, and its administrative and bureaucratic structures were similar to those subsequently established in colonial contexts in Australasia. For example, lunacy inspectorates, which were less autonomous bodies than the English lunacy commission, oversaw both the Irish and the Australasian asylum systems. Also, legislation allowing the confinement of 'dangerous lunatics' was used extensively in both contexts, thereby ensuring the police fulfilled an important role in certification processes.[7] While Ireland's status as a colony has been contested, an assessment of the national governance of the asylum system indicates that it had colonial characteristics.[8]

Historians of asylums in India, South Africa and Australasia have stressed the importance of 'colonialism' as an analytic tool in the assessment of the activities of asylum officials and doctors. Catharine Coleborne, Shula Marks and Megan Vaughan have emphasised how asylum doctors and administrators educated in the metropolis transported European medical ideas and institutions to Africa, Australia and New Zealand.[9] As

Waltraud Ernst and Jim Mills identified, anxieties to assert ideas of racial superiority resulted in the provision of separate institutional spaces for European and non-European mentally ill patients. In her study, Coleborne locates a distinctive 'colonial family' and explores its engagement and negotiation with nineteenth-century asylums. In provincial Ireland, differentiating between 'the indigenous' and 'the settler' was no simple matter. The well-established nature of the colonial relationship and the waves of settlers moving into Ireland over several centuries meant that by the nineteenth century cultural cross-fertilisation ensured that there were 'varieties of Irishness'.[10] As the nineteenth century progressed, Irish-born doctors, often trained at universities in Dublin, Glasgow and Edinburgh, began to emerge from the ranks of the rising Catholic middle classes to join their Protestant Irish counterparts in the medical profession and the asylum system. The major determining factors that influenced asylum doctors' attitude towards patients were class and gender though racial stereotyping sometimes featured. As chapter two shows, occasionally the Irish lunacy inspectors and asylum doctors invoked the language of racial difference when talking about patients however, while racial theories were deployed to explain susceptibility to mental illness, such discourses were less explicit than in other colonial contexts. Though Anastasia inserted her own story within a colonial discourse, she was exceptional in doing so.

Taking as case studies the Carlow lunatic asylum district and Carlow and Enniscorthy asylums, this book explores the interactions and negotiations of local protagonists (such as Anastasia) with the Irish asylum system that Mark Finnane meticulously delineated. The selection of an individual asylum district has facilitated a detailed study of changes in the political, social and cultural history of several forms of nineteenth-century institutional provision for the mentally ill. The Carlow lunatic asylum district was the sixth of nine asylum districts created under the original lunacy legislation.[11] It initially served four counties – Carlow, Wexford, Kilkenny and Kildare – situated in the province of Leinster in the southeast of Ireland.[12] The first asylum to open in the district in February 1832 was in Carlow town. The selection of the sites of individual asylums depended on several factors. Generally, the chief town in the county was chosen as preference was given to towns with thriving markets and a sufficient number of physicians and local gentry to serve in the asylum.[13] Both Carlow town and Kilkenny city met these requirements. However, the cost of sites in Kilkenny city was higher and instead Carlow town was selected. Soon after opening, the new Carlow asylum became overcrowded and the original Carlow asylum district was divided. Two additional asylums were constructed: one in Kilkenny city to serve county Kilkenny (1852) and, from 1868, another in Enniscorthy town, serving patients from county Wexford. It was the largest of the three asylums in the original Carlow district.[14] The population of the four counties in the district was 543,000 in 1831.[15] By 1911, following the reduction of the Carlow asylum district to counties Carlow and Kildare, the population served by the original institution was 102,879.

The rationale for the selection of the southeast of Ireland for a detailed study of asylum provision rests on several factors. By 1911, counties Carlow, Wexford and Kilkenny exhibited particularly high rates of institutionalisation. Amongst Irish counties, the proportion of the population in asylums and workhouses was the sixth highest in county Carlow, and the eleventh highest in county Wexford.[16] By the twentieth century, there was a similarly high usage of dispensary and other medical services.[17] In addition, Carlow and Enniscorthy asylums are representative of a group of moderately sized asylums in provincial towns in Ireland that have been relatively absent from the literature. Neither asylum developed into monolithic institutional complexes. The region and asylums differed therefore in several respects from other institutions examined by historians to date. Connaught lunatic asylum in county Galway, explored by Oonagh Walsh, was one of the largest Irish asylums. It served a peculiarly expansive and mainly rural district that continued to exhibit the social and cultural traits of pre-Famine Ireland in the later nineteenth century.[18] Joseph Reynolds' and Elizabeth Malcolm's studies of individual asylums focused on the social role of the institutions in an urban context – Dublin – and highlighted the fortunes of public and charitable institutions in a city that exhibited extreme levels of poverty.[19]

The Carlow district is interesting in several other respects. It experienced many of the social, cultural and demographic adjustments that changed post-Famine Ireland. The main economic activities in the four counties were agricultural although there were pockets of industry. In the 1830s, there was a distillery on the outskirts of Wexford town as well as breweries, tan-yards and rope works.[20] Wexford was a maritime county with two steamers on the Wexford and Liverpool line. In county Kilkenny, the region north of Castlecomer was known for its collieries and, by the end of the century, the mining seams had been largely exhausted, resulting in

widespread poverty. In addition to the mines, there were some distill-
eries in the county. County Kildare, which possessed rich agricultural
lands, had almost no industries: it was renowned for its racing tracks
and, later, for the military camp on the Curragh.[21] There were pockets
of urban development and of affluence in the asylum district including
Kilkenny city with its imposing medieval castle, St Canice's Cathedral,
and the impressive courthouse and gaol. While not as badly hit as other
regions, the district suffered during the Great Famine (1845–51). Over
the course of the nineteenth century, the Carlow district also benefitted
from social and infrastructural developments. In the post-Famine period,
the population of the district had high levels of literacy, and from the
1840s there was significant development in railway and other communication and transport infrastructures.[22] Similar to the rest of Ireland,
the region suffered depopulation as a result of emigration: between 1861
and 1911 men formed approximately 54 per cent of the emigrant population from counties Carlow and Kildare. By 1911, 58.8 per cent of the
population was single, never having married and most were men (58.4
per cent).[23]

The sources used in this study will be discussed in more detail in
the relevant chapters; however, it is appropriate to make a few comments
here. In addition to official sources, newspapers and medical periodicals,
institutional and legal records were used extensively. Because Carlow
asylum was one of the first nineteenth-century Irish asylums, the records
from that institution lent themselves to a statistical analysis of patterns
of usage over an extended timeframe. The sources used in the analysis
were the Carlow admission, discharge and death registers, and through
nominal linkage these sources have been used to construct a social profile
of patients admitted between 1832 and 1922. This incorporates 5,517
admissions into Carlow asylum. The certification warrants for 340 individuals from counties Wexford, Kilkenny, Carlow and Kildare certified
as dangerous lunatics to Carlow asylum between 1838 and 1868 were
also used extensively. Surviving casebooks from Carlow and Enniscorthy
asylums provided the springboard for an in-depth exploration of late
Victorian asylum patients and doctors. The records of poor law institutions in counties Wexford and Carlow – workhouse and medical
dispensaries – ensured a more complete assessment of medical and
welfare provision for the mentally ill could be established. This brought
protagonists that have previously occupied a peripheral position in our

understanding of provision for the mentally ill in nineteenth-century
Ireland to centre stage.

*

The Carlow asylum district, and Enniscorthy and Carlow asylums, form
the basis for an exploration of how civil society and its local protagonists
– legal, medical and lay – negotiated and interacted with institutions of
the nineteenth-century state in Irish provincial towns. As Patrick Joyce
has demonstrated, the state can be interpreted 'as a neutral administrative
machine reacting to social and economic problems in terms of pragmatic
reform' and 'a centre from which power radiates' as well as a 'coordinating
entity'. In the latter incarnation, the state and its elaborations – asylums,
workhouses and legal courts – are more 'structureless'.[24] The less rigid
manifestation of the state, which Corrigan and Sayer have characterised
as the 'state as an effect', ensure that 'the boundaries between the state and
civil society – the family and the community' can be disrupted.[25] Robert
van Krieken has made similar observations in his work on child welfare
in Australia.[26] Similarly, this book will demonstrate how, in negotiating
the meanings of, and various responses to, mental illness in the southeast
of Ireland in the nineteenth century, the boundaries between the state
and civil society were porous. It therefore contributes to post-Foucauldian
debates on the governmentality of mental illness and the mentally ill, one
of the key concerns in histories of asylumdom and psychiatry. Foucault's
account of the rise of the asylum and of the dispersed nature of power
in society has been challenged and nuanced by subsequent scholarship,
which has studied the consumers of the asylum and mapped 'resistance
as well as the domination' of psychiatry and the asylum.[27] Therefore, this
study will assess how local actors and groups, in responding to and challenging state interventions, altered and negotiated the administrative,
legal and cultural structures of local asylums.

Chapters one and two build on Finnane's study of the origins and
subsequent development of the asylum system. His work has provided a
comprehensive assessment of the legal and administrative structures that
bound Irish asylums and remains the most important text on the history
of asylumdom in Ireland. Chapter one outlines the national context to
the introduction of asylum legislation and situates the Carlow asylum
district within the topography of institutional provision, while chapter

two considers the local debates that surrounded the division of asylum districts. Both chapters confirm Finnane's assertion that the governance of the Irish asylum system was centralised. Nonetheless, as will be argued local groups, including poor law guardians, magistrates and grand juries, fought over the control of asylums, partly in opposition to the centralised nature of Irish local governance and partly to align themselves as willing participants in the state's endeavours to transform, reform and pacify Ireland. Unlike other elements of local government in Ireland, throughout the nineteenth century, the governance of Carlow and Enniscorthy asylums continued to be dominated by landed elites who were politically loyal to British interests in Ireland. These governors were joined by local religious figures. Both chapters demonstrate that the individuals who provided the 'social leadership' in the 'promotion of the asylum'[28] – those who regularly attended asylum meetings and those who lobbied for new asylums – emerged from groups that were not only politically loyal but also committed to the vision of modernisation and improvement that the asylum represented in local contexts. The financial burden of the asylum would subsequently qualify this local enthusiasm. The politics of welfare is further examined in chapter six, which focuses on the national and local relationship between the poor law and the asylum system in Ireland, a subject that has received relatively little scholarly attention.[29] While the Irish asylum system remained formally separate from the poor law, asylum staff looked to workhouse facilities when managing the mentally ill throughout the nineteenth century. However, differing eligibility criteria limited the integration of the two systems.

The remaining chapters focus more explicitly on local actors in civil society – patients, families, poor law guardians, magistrates, police and doctors – and their interactions with asylums and with each other in responding to and managing the insane and insanity. What emerges from these chapters is that asylums and certification procedures were less prescriptive in form and structure than previously suggested. The role of the asylums and the certification procedures were repeatedly redefined through interactions with different groups in local contexts. This was in part facilitated by the patchy and faulty lunacy regulation and legislation as well as by informal manoeuvring and negotiations around legal and administrative structures.[30] The chapters also suggest that those who managed the asylums and the certification procedures could be flexible and responsive to pressures placed on them in local contexts. Chapter three delineates the evolution of various asylum certification procedures – 'ordinary', dangerous lunatic, and urgent certifications – identifying the lunacy inspectors' drive to publicly and practically place medical certification at the centre of the different procedures and establish medical rather than legal actors as asylum gatekeepers. Included here is a discussion of the structure and development of certification forms in Ireland. This allows an exploration of developments in medical definitions of mental illness and of the establishment of asylum doctors as expert in its treatment.

The existing literature on asylums in Ireland has emphasised the disciplinary function of the family, the asylum and certification procedures.[31] Forming a central part of these arguments are the accounts of the extensive use of the dangerous lunatic legislation to certify individuals in Ireland.[32] Finnane's 1985 article offers a revision to this argument.[33] In chapters four, five and seven these arguments are developed in relation to the politics of the Irish family and household. Irish families have been regularly portrayed as economic units that prioritised survival strategies at the expense of emotional satisfaction.[34] Here it is acknowledged that at times families invoked certification into an asylum to impose normative roles and to resolve conflict,[35] but this was complicated by individual and household poverty, distress and emotional disintegration. Gendered domestic roles among pauper households were disrupted when relatives negotiated with legal and medical authorities to access welfare. At times, these negotiations took place during petty session court hearings as part of the dangerous lunatic certification procedure. As chapter four will argue these legal procedures put 'insanity on display', publicly governing individuals' behaviour and manners, and also disseminating knowledge of certification procedures. This dispersed medical interpretations of aberrant behaviour among differing socio-economic groups in Irish society. The relationships between asylum doctors, patients and families within and outside the asylums are the focus of chapter seven. This includes an exploration of experiences within provincial asylums, utilising late nineteenth-century casebooks from Carlow and Enniscorthy. The now familiar tale of the demise of the optimism that first attended moral treatment and the advance of bleaker theories of degeneration and hereditary insanity that defined medical responses to mental illness is identifiable in Carlow and Enniscorthy asylums. However, while theories of degeneration were deployed to account for the apparent 'increase' in mental illness in the late nineteenth century, environmental factors such as poverty, class, fatigue, disappointment and difficult life circumstances continued to feature in psychiatric aetiologies explaining susceptibility to disease. This is in keeping with the evidence that has emerged in relation to the certification procedures and the complicated and multifaceted domestic reasons for committal, as outlined in chapter four and five. This book emphasises the degree to which the asylum 'was a contested site, subject to continual negotiation amongst different parties'.[36] It endeavours to place at the centre of the narrative individual protagonists and the various groups that navigated medical, legal and institutional provision and structures. The struggles and alignments between these groups reveal how asylums and the mentally ill were understood and defined in the nineteenth century by the forces pivotal to the processes of institutionalisation in Ireland.

Notes

1   St Senan's Psychiatric Hospital (hereafter SPH), Enniscorthy, File of miscellaneous letters, Anastasia O'D. to Mr [John] Redmond, 21 November 1912.

2   SPH, Enniscorthy, File of miscellaneous letters, Anastasia O'D. to Mr [John] Redmond, 29 July 1914.

3   Thomas Drapes, who had acted as visiting physician at Enniscorthy asylum from 1872, succeeded as Resident Medical Superintendent in 1884. He remained until 1919 and was succeeded by Dr Hugh Kennedy, see 'Notes and News', *JMS* 65:269 (April, 1919), 140.

4   SPH, Enniscorthy, File of miscellaneous letters, Anastasia O'D. to Mr [John] Redmond, 30 September 1914.

5   57 Geo. iii, c.106 (1817).

6   M. Finnane, *Insanity and the Insane in Post-Famine Ireland* (London: Croom Helm, 1981), p. 18. Alvin Jackson has argued that the relationship between Ireland and the English colonial state was not always coercive, see A. Jackson, 'The Survival of the Union', in J. Cleary and C. Connolly (eds), *The Cambridge Companion to Modern Irish Culture* (Cambridge: Cambridge University Press, 2005), pp. 25–41.

7   C. Coleborne and D. MacKinnon, '*Madness' in Australia: Histories, Heritage and the Asylum* (Queensland: University of Queensland Press, 2003); C. Coleborne, 'Passage to the Asylum: the Role of the Police in Committals of the Insane in Victoria, Australia, 1848–1900', in R. Porter and D. Wright (eds), *The Confinement of the Insane. International Perspectives, 1800–1965* (Cambridge: Cambridge University Press, 2003), pp. 129–148; S. Garton, *Medicine and Madness: A Social History of Insanity in New South Wales, 1880–1940* (Kensington: New South Wales University Press, 1988).

8   S. Howe, *Ireland and Empire: Colonial Legacies in Irish History and Culture* (Oxford: Oxford University Press, 2000), p. 37.

9   W. Ernst, 'European Madness and Gender in Nineteenth-Century British India', *Social History of Medicine*, 9:3 (1996), 357–382; W. Ernst, 'Out of Sight and Out of Mind: Insanity in Early-Nineteenth-Century British India', in J. Melling and B. Forsythe (eds), *Insanity, Institutions and Society, 1800–1914. A Social History of Madness in Comparative Perspective* (London and New York: Routledge, 1999), pp. 245–267; W. Ernst, 'Asylums in Alien Places: The Treatment of the European Insane in British India', in W.F. Bynum, R. Porter and M. Shepherd (eds), *Anatomy of Madness. Essays in the History of Psychiatry*, III (London: Tavistock, 1988), pp. 48–70; J. Mills, *Madness, Cannabis, and Colonialism: The Native Only Lunatic Asylum of British India, 1857–1990* (London: Macmillan, 2000); S. Marks, '"Every Facility that Modern Science and Enlightened Humanity have Devised": Race and Progress in a Colonial Hospital, Valkenberg Mental Asylum, Cape Colony, 1894–1910', in Melling and Forsythe (eds), *Insanity, Institutions and Society*, pp. 268–291; M. Vaughan, *Curing their Ills: Colonial Power and African Illness* (Cambridge: Cambridge University Press, 1991).

10   R. F. Foster, *Modern Ireland 1600–1972* (London: Penguin Books, 1989), p. 3; J. Leerssen, *Mere Irish and Fíor-Ghael. Studies in the Idea of Irish Nationality, its Development and Literary Expression prior to the Nineteenth Century* (Cork: Cork University Press, 2nd edn, 1996).

11   The three asylums opened after Carlow asylum were Ballinasloe (1833), Waterford (1835) and Clonmel (1834), see *Eleventh Report of the Inspectors General on the General State of the Prisons of Ireland (Report of Prison Inspectors)*, H. C. 1833 [67] xvii, p. 11.

12   *Eighth Report of Prison Inspectors*, H. C. 1830 [48] xxiv, pp. 18–19.

13   *Report of the Commissioners of Inquiry into the State of Lunatic Asylums and other Institutions for the Custody and Treatment of the Insane in Ireland*, H. C. 1857–1858 [2436] xxvii (hereafter *Inquiry into the State of Lunatic Asylums and other Institutions*), p. 23.

14   See chapter two.

15   *Returns Relating to District Lunatic Asylums in Ireland*, H. C. 1833 [695] xxxiv, p. 2. The population of each county in Carlow district was Carlow (81,988), Kilkenny county and city (169,945), Wexford (182,713), Kildare (108,424).

16   *Sixty-first Report on District, Local and Private Lunatic Asylums in Ireland* (hereafter *Report of Lunacy Inspectors*), H. C. 1912 [6386] xxxix, pp. xiii–xv.

17   *The Health Services and their further development* (Dublin: Stationery Office, January 1966), p. 28. Thanks to Professor Mary E. Daly for this reference.

18   O. Walsh, 'A Lightness of Mind: Gender and Insanity in Nineteenth Century Ireland', in M. Kelleher and J. H. Murphy (eds), *Gender Perspectives in Nineteenth-Century Ireland* (Dublin: Four Courts Press, 1997), pp. 159–167; O. Walsh, 'Gendering the Asylums: Ireland and Scotland, 1847–1877', in T. Brotherstone, D. Simonton and O. Walsh (eds), *The Gendering of Scottish History: An International Approach* (Glasgow: Cruithne Press, 1999), pp. 199–215; T. P. O'Neill, 'The Persistence of Famine in Ireland', in C. Póirtéir (ed.), *The Great Irish Famine* (Cork: Mercier Press, 1995), pp. 204–218.

19   J. Reynolds, *Grangegorman. Psychiatric Care in Dublin since 1815* (Dublin: Institute of Public Administration, 1992); E. Malcolm, *Swift's Hospital: A History of St Patrick's Hospital, Dublin, 1746–1989* (Dublin: Gill and Macmillan, 1989).

20 S. Lewis, *A Topographical Dictionary of Ireland*, II (London: S. Lewis and Co., 1837), pp. 707–711.

21 There was an informal military camp on the Curragh at the beginning of the nineteenth century. The permanent barracks were built in 1855, see C. Costello, *A Most Delightful Station: The British Army on the Curragh of Kildare, Ireland, 1855–1922* (Cork: Collins Press, 1999).

22 See chapter three.

23 W. E. Vaughan and A. J. Fitzpatrick (eds), *Irish Historical Statistics. Population, 1821–1971* (Dublin: Royal Irish Academy, 1978), pp. 274–275 and pp. 269–271.

24 P. Joyce, 'Postal Communication and the Making of the British Technostate', Centre for Research on Socio-Cultural Change, Working Paper Series, 54 (August 2008).

25 *Ibid.*, p.4.

26 R. van Krieken, *Children and the State: Social Control and the Formation of Australian Child Welfare* (North Sydney: Allen & Unwin, 1992), p. 7.

27 R. Porter, 'Introduction', in Porter and Wright (eds), *The Confinement of the Insane* pp. 1–19, p. 5. For responses to Foucauldian interpretations and accounts of other forms of engagement with the asylum, see essays in C. Jones and R. Porter (eds), *Reassessing Foucault. Power, Medicine and the Body* (London and New York: Routledge, 1994); J. Melling and B. Forsythe, 'Accommodating Madness: New Research in the Social History of Insanity and Institutions', in Melling and Forsythe (eds), *Insanity, Institutions and Society*, pp. 1–30; A. Scull, *The Most Solitary of Afflictions. Madness and Society in Britain, 1700–1900* (New Haven and London: Yale University Press, 1993); D. Wright, 'The Certification of Insanity in Nineteenth-Century England and Wales', *History of Psychiatry*, 9 (1998), 267–290; D. Wright, 'Getting Out of the Asylum: Understanding the Confinement of the Insane in the Nineteenth Century', *Social History of Medicine*, 10:1 (1997), 137–155; D. Wright, 'Family Strategies and the Institutional Confinement of "Idiot" Children in Victorian England', *Journal of Family History*, 23:2 (1998), 190–208; R. Adair, B. Forsythe and J. Melling, 'A Danger to the Public? Disposing of Pauper Lunatics in Late-Victorian and Edwardian England: Plympton St Mary Union and the Devon County Asylum, 1867–1914', *Medical History*, 42:1 (1998), 1–25; R. Adair, B. Forsythe and J. Melling, 'Families, Communities and the Legal Regulation of Lunacy in Victorian England: Assessments of Crime, Violence and Welfare in Admissions to the Devon Asylum, 1845–1914', in P. Bartlett and D. Wright (eds), *Outside the Walls of the Asylum. The History of Care in the Community* (London: The Athlone Press, 1999), pp. 153–180; J. K. Walton, 'Lunacy in the Industrial Revolution: A Study of Asylum Admissions in Lancashire 1848–50', *Journal of Social History*, 13:1 (1979), 1–22; J. E. Moran, 'Asylum in the Community: Managing the Insane in Antebellum America', *History of Psychiatry*, 9:34 (1998), 217–240; J. E. Moran, *Committed to the State Asylum. Insanity and Society in Nineteenth Century Quebec and Ontario* (Montreal and Kingston: McGill-Queen's University Press, 2000); N. Tomes, *A Generous Confidence: Thomas Story Kirkbride and the Art of Asylum-Keeping, 1840–1883* (Cambridge: Cambridge University Press, 1984); C. M. McGovern, 'The Myths of Social Control and Custodial Oppression: Patterns of Psychiatric Medicine in Late-Nineteenth-Century Institutions', *Journal of Social History*, 20:1 (1986), 3–23.

28 J. Melling and B. Forsythe, *The Politics of Madness. The State, Insanity and Society in England 1845–1914* (London and New York: Routledge, 2006), p. 6.

29 The exceptions are O. Walsh, 'Lunatic and Criminal Alliances in Nineteenth-Century Ireland', in Bartlett and Wright (eds), *Outside the Walls of the Asylum*, pp. 132–152 and H. Burke, *The People and the Poor Law in Nineteenth-Century Ireland* (Dublin: Women's Education Bureau, 1987), pp. 256–261. For studies of England see P. Bartlett, 'The Asylum and the Poor Law: The Productive Alliance', in Melling and Forsythe (eds), *Insanity, Institutions and Society*, pp. 48–67; P. Bartlett, *The Poor Law of Lunacy: The Administration of Pauper Lunatics in Mid-Nineteenth-Century England* (London: Leicester University Press, 1999); P. Bartlett, 'The Asylum, the Workhouse and the Voice of the Insane Poor in 19th Century England', *International Journal of Law and Psychiatry*, 21:4 (1998), 421–432; Adair, Forsythe and Melling, 'A Danger to the Public?'; B. Forsythe, J. Melling and R. Adair, 'The New Poor Law and the County Pauper Lunatic Asylum. The Devon Experience 1834–1884', *Social History of Medicine*, 9:3 (1996), 335–355; B. Forsythe, J. Melling and R. Adair, 'Politics of Lunacy: Central State Regulation and the Devon Pauper Lunatic Asylum, 1845–1914', in Melling and Forsythe (eds) *Insanity, Institutions and Society*, pp. 68–92; J. Melling and R. Turner, 'The Road to the Asylum: Institutions, Distance and the Administration of Pauper Lunacy in Devon, 1845–1914', *Journal of Historical Geography*, 25:3 (1999), 298–332; D. Wright, 'The Discharge of Pauper Lunatics from County Asylums in Mid-Victorian England: The Case of Buckinghamshire, 1853–1872', in Melling and Forsythe (eds) *Insanity, Institutions and Society*, pp. 93–112; J. Andrews, 'Raising the Tone of Asylumdom: Maintaining and Expelling Pauper Lunatics at the Glasgow Royal Asylum in the Nineteenth Century', in Melling and Forsythe (eds) *Insanity, Institutions and Society*, pp. 200–222; E. Murphy, 'The Lunacy Commissioners and the East London Guardians, 1845–1897', *Medical History*, 46:4 (2002), 495–524; E. Murphy, 'The New Poor Law Guardians and the Administration of Insanity in East London, 1834–1844', *Bulletin of the History of Medicine*, 77:1 (2003), 45–74; R. Ellis, 'The Asylum, the Poor Law and a Reassessment of the Four-Shilling Grant: Admissions to the County Asylums of Yorkshire in the Nineteenth Century', *Social History of Medicine*, 19:1 (2006), 55–73.

30 Melling and Forsythe make a similar point in the case of Devon Asylum, see Melling and Forsythe, *The Politics of Madness*, p. 6.

31 For examples, see E. Malcolm, '"The House of Strident Shadows": the Asylum, the Family and Emigration in Post-Famine Rural Ireland', in E. Malcolm and G. Jones (eds), *Medicine, Disease and the State in Ireland* (Cork: Cork University Press, 1999), pp. 183–185; E. Malcolm, '"Ireland's Crowded Madhouses": the Institutional Confinement of the Insane in Nineteenth- and Twentieth-Century Ireland', in Porter and Wright (eds), *The Confinement of the Insane*, pp. 315–334; Á. McCarthy, 'Hearths, Bodies and Minds: Gender Ideology and Women's Committal to Enniscorthy Lunatic Asylum, 1916–25', in A. Hayes and D. Urquhart (eds), *Irish Women's History* (Dublin: Irish Academic Press, 2004), pp. 115–136; O. Walsh, 'Gender and Insanity in Nineteenth-Century Ireland', in J. Andrews and A. Digby (eds), *Sex and Seclusion, Class and Custody. Perspectives on Gender and Class in the History of British and Irish Psychiatry* (Amsterdam and New York: Rodopi, 2004), pp. 69–94.

32   Finnane, *Insanity and the Insane*, pp. 87–128; P. M. Prior, 'Mad, Not Bad: Crime, Mental Disorder and Gender in Nineteenth-Century Ireland', *History of Psychiatry*, 8:32 (1997), 501–506; P. M. Prior, 'Prisoner or Patient? The Official Debate on the Criminal Lunatic in Nineteenth-Century Ireland', *History of Psychiatry*, 15:2 (2004), 177–192; P. M. Prior, 'Dangerous Lunacy: the Misuse of the Mental Health Law', *Journal of Forensic Psychiatry and Psychology*, 14:3 (2003), 525–541; Walsh, 'Lunatic and Criminal Alliances', pp. 132–152. It was not used as frequently in England, see J. F. Saunders, 'Institutionalised Offenders: a Study of the Victorian Institution and its Inmates, with special reference to Late Nineteenth-Century Warwickshire' (PhD dissertation, University of Warwick, 1983).

33   M. Finnane, 'Asylums, Families and the State', *History Workshop*, 20 (1985), 134–148.

34   D. Fitzpatrick, 'Irish Farming Families before the First World War', *Comparative Studies in Society and History*, 25:2 (1983), 339–374; P. P. Boyle and C. Ó Gráda, 'Fertility Trends, Excess Mortality and the Great Irish Famine', *Demography*, 23:4 (1986), 543–562; R. Breen, 'Dowry Payments and the Irish Case', *Comparative Studies in Society and History*, 26:2 (1984), 280–296; T. Inglis, *Moral Monopoly: The Rise and Fall of the Catholic Church in Ireland* (Dublin: University College Dublin Press, 1998).

35   P. E. Prestwich, 'Family Strategies and Medical Power: Voluntary Committal in a Parisian Asylum, 1876–1914', *Journal of Social History*, 27 (1993–1994), 799–818.

36   Porter, 'Introduction', in Porter and Wright (eds), *The Confinement of the Insane*, p. 4.

1

Shaping the Irish asylum system

The frequent outbreaks of epidemic diseases in Ireland during the early decades of the nineteenth century brought into sharp relief the limits of existing philanthropic medical and welfare institutions for the poor.[1] Legislation was introduced to promote both the establishment of institutions and to halt the spread of diseases and fevers. This resulted in a precociously high level of state provision of medical facilities for the sick poor in Ireland,[2] which has led historians to conclude that by the early nineteenth century Ireland had 'one of the most advanced health services in Europe'.[3] The existence of enabling legislation did not necessarily result in the establishment of institutions. Funding difficulties hampered development, and the founding of institutions depended on local initiative and subscriptions. In certain regions, poverty and the absence of proactive landlords ensured that legislation was not acted upon. Consequently, the distribution of medical institutions across the country was uneven.[4] The provision of specialist medical facilities was even less widespread and in the first decade of the nineteenth century there were few institutional facilities for the mentally ill. St Patrick's Hospital in Dublin, a charitable asylum known as Swift's Hospital, was the largest specialist hospital to provide care for pauper lunatics. By the beginning of the nineteenth century, Swift's Hospital was experiencing severe financial difficulties, which resulted in the admission of fee-paying patients.[5] Described by government bodies as a 'partly charitable' hospital,[6] in practice Swift's was a model of a 'mixed economy of care' and financial contributions were elicited from the state, the private sector and charity.[7] There were other small charitable asylums, including a Quaker asylum at Bloomfield in Donnybrook (1812).

Among those with financial resources, there were relatively few private madhouses and they were predominately situated in counties Dublin and Cork. As discretion was important to the success of private asylums, their existence may not have been recorded in official sources despite the introduction of legislation in 1787, 1810 and 1826 that required the prison inspectorate to report on institutions with mentally ill inmates.[8] By 1825 there were at least five private asylums in Ireland, in addition to charitable asylums in Dublin, and the county asylums.[9] Three private asylums in Finglas, county Dublin, were managed by Dr Harty, by Dr Alexander Jackson, the first physician at the Richmond asylum,[10] and by Mr Gregory. There was a small institution in Downpatrick, county Down, run by a Mr Reed, while the influential alientist William S. Hallaran established the Cittadella in Cork in 1799.[11] Following the foundation of the public asylum system in 1817, the number of private institutions increased and by 1850 there were fourteen institutions, accommodating 446 patients.[12] This pattern of expansion diverges from England where the number of private asylums decreased during the century though they continued to provide a significant portion of asylum accommodation.[13] In England and Wales, the old poor law provided additional provision for the mentally ill as parish overseers assisted in the cost of domestic or institutional accommodation.[14] The absence of a poor law prior to 1838 in Ireland ensured that an important source of relief was not available and would suggest that an Irish equivalent of the English 'trade in lunacy' was not particularly significant.[15]

These somewhat meagre facilities were inaccessible to the poor, ensuring that most pauper lunatics were consigned to houses of industry, gaols and bridewells. Introduced in 1772, houses of industry in Ireland were mainly, though not exclusively, concerned with the relief of the destitute poor, usually within the institutional context of a workhouse. Again, the establishment of houses of industry was not mandatory and implementation of the legislation was patchy.[16] In the years immediately following their establishment, large numbers of pauper lunatics were accommodated within these institutions.[17] Legislation passed in 1787 empowered grand juries to attach separate lunatic wards to individual institutions.[18] Conditions in these wards were very basic. The prison inspectors, Majors James Palmer and B. B. Woodward, frequently criticised the insanitary conditions, the 'want of accommodation' and the need for 'adequate means' of treatment.[19] The largest ward outside the capital was

attached to the Cork house of industry, which was managed by William
S. Hallaran.[20] The prison inspectors' annual reports also testify to large
numbers of pauper lunatics confined in gaols and bridewells throughout
the country, a practise they frequently censured.[21]

Finnane has suggested that 'the scarcity of specialist institutions'
in addition to 'the absence of a poor law' and 'the state of rural Ireland
itself' prompted the introduction of legislation to establish a system of
asylums in Ireland in 1817.[22] The paucity of specialist provision for the
mentally ill ensured that Ireland was deemed to be in particular need of
a 'national' system. In the two decades following the Act of Union, there
were several attempts to introduce provision.[23] For example, in 1805 Sir
John Newport, MP for Waterford, proposed a bill to establish four asylums
dispersed throughout the country.[24] The bill was defeated, but Newport
continued to lobby for the introduction of public asylums. These initiatives were not 'an indigenous development'.[25] The architects of different
bills were influenced by the contemporary agitation for lunacy reform
occurring throughout Europe and England.[26] There was, however, an
important distinction between the deliberations in England and Ireland.
The agitation in England was focused on reforming private, charity and
public lunatic asylums following the disclosure of a series of scandals in
asylums.[27] In Ireland, the focus of reform agitation was less concerned
with the type and regulation of existing provision, private or otherwise,
than with the limited nature of provision per se.

The events at the Dublin house of industry during the first decades
of the nineteenth century served to reinforce the perception that there
was an urgent need for lunatic asylums in Ireland. As in other houses of
industry, several lunatic wards had been attached to the original institution. In 1810, the governors were provided with a grant to establish a
separate hospital for lunatics, subsequently named the Richmond Lunatic
Asylum after Charles Gordon Lennox, the Duke of Richmond, Lord
Lieutenant of Ireland, who had been instrumental in securing the grant.[28]
The new asylum received its first patients in 1814 and quickly became
the major centre for the care of the mentally ill in Ireland. Patients
were sent from all parts of the country to the capital city. Although the
Richmond asylum became overcrowded and lacked sufficient funds to
remedy the problem,[29] its establishment created 'expectations for the care
of lunatics'.[30] This, coupled with Newport's persistent 'calls for legislative provision', and the conclusions of the Committee on Madhouses in

England that 'the necessity of making some further provision for Insane Persons appeared to be more urgent in Ireland than England',[31] brought the question of asylum provision in Ireland to prominence. In October 1816, Robert Peel, Chief Secretary for Ireland, ordered an investigation into the Richmond asylum's management.[32] The subsequent report concluded that the asylum had become the repository of the country's mentally ill population and endorsed the view, expressed by the Richmond's governors, that asylum facilities outside the capital city were required to alleviate the pressure. The cities of Cork and Belfast were identified as being especially in need.[33] In December 1816, Peel established a parliamentary committee to inquire into the 'relief of the lunatic poor in Ireland.'[34] Irish members who had already indicated their support for a form of legislative initiative dominated the committee. These included John Leslie Foster, who was governor of Richmond Lunatic Asylum, Thomas Spring Rice, Lord Monteagle, governor of Limerick house of industry and a campaigner for lunacy reform, and Sir John Newport.[35]

Foster and Spring Rice supported the construction of separate, specialist institutions, which would facilitate the introduction of moral treatment and the classification of patients. As discussed in chapter seven, by the end of the eighteenth century, moral treatment, a regime of care associated with the York Retreat in England and based on moral discipline, was believed to offer the greatest hope for curing mental illness. The construction of specialist asylums was central to the regime of relief and cure while classification was part of the orthodoxy of nineteenth-century institutional management.[36] Foster and Spring Rice had been impressed by the work of Dr Alexander Jackson, governor of the Richmond asylum, who had already introduced a form of moral treatment in his institution.[37] Foster was also opposed to the establishment of separate institutions for 'incurable lunatics' along the lines proposed by Thomas Bakewell in his vision of an asylum system for England.[38] Such was Foster's faith in the proposed new system, he maintained that most patients would be cured and the separation of 'incurables' within the proposed public asylums would be sufficient.[39] This decision would have a long-term impact on the asylum system.

The final report of the 1817 Select Committee recommended the establishment of separate district asylums with sole responsibility for 'pauper lunatics'. This was a relatively predictable recommendation given that most committee members had previously indicated their support for such a measure. These recommendations were the basis of the act 'to provide for the establishment of asylums for the lunatic poor in Ireland', passed in July 1817.[40] Under its terms the Lord Lieutenant was empowered to 'direct and order that any number of Asylums for the Lunatic Poor in *Ireland* shall be erected and established in and for Districts in *Ireland*'. Significantly, the power was not given to local grand juries, generally regarded as the 'most important local body' in early nineteenth-century Ireland. They were 'empowered to raise money' for a range of purposes including road construction and repair, and the establishment of local hospitals.[41] Under the 1817 act, the grand juries' powers were limited to raising necessary funds, while the authority over construction of institutions lay with the Lord Lieutenant and his office. Central government's retention of these powers reflected the state's frustration with Irish landlords who were generally regarded as corrupt and incompetent.[42] As Colonel Thomas Larcom, Under-Secretary for Ireland, subsequently argued the establishment of asylums was 'in advance of public opinion' and 'if the grand juries had been left to erect them or not as they pleased few if any would have been erected'.[43] The lunacy legislation was part of the trend towards the centralisation of powers away from local government and landlords and to Dublin Castle.

Under the 1817 act, Ireland was divided into separate asylum districts comprising one or more counties, towns and cities. The 1817 Select Committee had estimated that, in addition to Richmond Lunatic Asylum, four or five district asylums would be required. After deliberations, it was decided that approximately twice that number would be established. It was also determined that the Cork asylum would be amalgamated into the district asylum system. Early on, the 1817 act required a series of amending and re-enforcing laws passed in 1820, 1821, 1825, 1826 and 1845.[44] As a result of the mandatory nature of the legislation, public asylums became a common feature of the Irish landscape. Nine asylums were constructed before 1835 (Armagh, Limerick, Belfast, Derry, Carlow, Maryborough, Connaught, Waterford and Clonmel), complementing the existing Richmond asylum in Dublin and the Cork asylum. A further six were commenced in 1846 and completed before 1853 (Cork, Killarney, Kilkenny, Mullingar, Armagh and Sligo). In 1859 and 1860 the construction of six more asylums was authorised and by 1904 there were twenty-five district asylums operating in Ireland, including the Portrane asylum within the Richmond district, Belfast asylum within the

Antrim district, and the Youghal auxiliary asylum in the Cork district.[45]
Nineteenth-century Ireland shared the remarkable growth in the number
and size of lunatic asylums and the expansion of the asylum population
witnessed throughout the Anglo-American and western worlds.[46]

The Carlow asylum district

The new Carlow asylum district, established under the act, expanded
the medical and welfare institutional marketplace in counties Wexford,
Kilkenny, Kildare and Carlow. By the mid-1830s there were several general
medical institutions located in the four counties. There was an infirmary,
seven dispensaries and two fever hospitals dispersed throughout county
Carlow, while in county Kilkenny there were sixteen dispensaries and
three fever hospitals in addition to a county infirmary. A county infirmary,
five combined fever hospitals and dispensaries, four fever hospitals, thirteen dispensaries and a house of industry (1816) were located in county
Wexford. In contrast there was only one dispensary in county Kildare,
which was opened in Athy by 1830.[47] The introduction of the poor law to
Ireland in 1838 and the subsequent construction of workhouses, discussed
in chapter five, expanded this institutional marketplace. By the 1850s there
were thirteen workhouses in the Carlow district.[48] In spite of the expansion of welfare institutions, at the time of the 1817 Select Committee,
most lunatic paupers in counties Kildare, Wexford, Carlow and Kilkenny
were confined in various gaols, scattered across four counties. In addition, there were lunatic wards attached to the Wexford house of industry,
a former gaol, which was opened in the town in January 1816,[49] and
further wards attached to the house of industry in nearby Kilkenny city,
which housed ten patients. There was also a small purpose-built asylum
in Kilkenny city. It could accommodate twenty persons – twelve 'enraged'
and eight convalescent patients – and its construction was influenced by
contemporary theories concerning the care of insanity.[50] The asylum in
Kilkenny remained separate from the asylum system established under the
1817 legislation and, as discussed in chapter two, by 1847 it was regarded
as inadequate.

In keeping with early nineteenth-century theories on asylum architecture, the buildings were small; the 1817 act limited their size to 100
to 150 patients.[51] Carlow asylum was initially intended to accommodate

104 patients in separate cells. The government architect, William Murray, was responsible for the design of the new asylums.[52] In 1825, Murray had succeeded Francis Johnston as architect to the board of works, and although Murray retired from the board in 1832, he remained as the asylum architect.[53] The contractor on Carlow asylum was a Dublin builder, Arthur Williams, who also worked on the asylums at Ballinasloe, Derry and Limerick.[54] Carlow asylum was built on ten acres of land, situated on the edge of the town. The architectural plans included one central block and four radiating arms or wings. Patient accommodation comprised mainly of single cells and there were relatively few larger rooms.[55] Reuber has suggested that this design was influenced by a combination of radial and panoptical elements identifiable in the West Riding Asylum at Wakefield built between 1815 and 1817.[56] These were in part based on Samuel Tuke's instructions that patients should be accommodated in single cells allowing for privacy.[57] The cost of the site, completion of the building and supply of basic furniture was estimated at £322 10s 4d.[58] On 3 May 1832, the board of governors, comprising magistrates, influential merchants and traders, and members of the local landed elite, received the first request for patient admissions. In common with most asylums opened under the 1817 and 1821 legislation, admissions to Carlow asylum quickly exceeded its original capacity.[59]

Asylum governance

In the early decades of the nineteenth century, numerous inspectorates and boards of commissioners were established as organs of centralising policy and soon became a familiar feature of administration in Ireland.[60] The original lunacy legislation and subsequent amendments ensured central government retained a large degree of control over the establishment and administration of the asylum system in Ireland. The 1821 act established the board of control and correspondence, and in 1845 a separate lunacy inspectorate was introduced, relieving the prison inspectorate of that task. The enabling legislation also vested a significant amount of authority in the office of the Lord Lieutenant. Technically this was the most senior position in the Irish administration, though it was not necessarily the most important. The Lord Lieutenant was assisted in his duties by the Chief Secretary, a position which, by the late nineteenth century, carried far more 'political weight than that of the Lord Lieutenant.' As Virginia Crossman has demonstrated 'the Chief Secretary acted as main exponent of government policy' and 'supervised the running of his office, the hub from which the spokes of government radiated.' By the end of the century the Chief Secretary's office was responsible for twenty-nine government departments, including the board of control and correspondence and the lunacy inspectorate.[61]

The board of control and correspondence was the body responsible for implementing the asylum acts and its duties were confined to 'superintending and directing the Erection, Establishment and Regulation' of the new asylums.[62] Comprised of government appointments, the 1817 act stipulated that the board was not to exceed eight in number. Along with John Leslie Foster, members of Dublin's influential medical and social elite were nominated to it.[63] The significance and duties of the board fluctuated over the years, reflecting changes in Dublin Castle's involvement in, and policy towards, local government during the nineteenth century.[64] In March 1835, on completion of the initial phase of asylum construction, the original board of control resigned and the Irish board of works assumed responsibility for asylum building.[65] This was in accordance with a general move to place more control over local building schemes under the auspices of the board of works. By 1831 most funds for public works were managed by that body.[66] It was responsible for the asylums constructed between 1835 and 1854.[67]

In addition to the board of control, a lunacy inspectorate was appointed to oversee the asylum system. The equivalent of the English and Scottish lunacy commission was not established in Ireland.[68] The roots of the Irish lunacy inspectorate lay with the inspectors general of the prisons who had assumed responsibility for the inspection of all institutions that accommodated the insane in 1787.[69] This arrangement was criticised by the editors of the *Dublin Journal of Medical Science* as contributing to the 'vulgar notion that asylums were neither more or less than a species of gaol, and that "madness" was, by consequence, if not a crime, at least a disease of degradation.'[70] Francis White, who had served as secretary to the board of health and was surgeon to Richmond Lunatic Asylum since 1835, also questioned the competence of prison inspectors to fulfil this role.[71] White's lobbying resulted in his appointment to the prison inspectorate in 1841. In 1842 legislation was passed that formally appointed the prison inspectors as inspectors of lunatic asylums.[72] While not creating a separate body, this represented a first attempt to distinguish the function of the inspection of asylums from that of inspection of prisons.

White used his position of influence to lobby for the establishment of a separate lunacy inspectorate and three year later, in August 1845, a separate inspectorate for district, local and private lunatic asylums in Ireland came into being.[73] The lunacy inspectorate comprised two medical appointments only. This differed from the English lunacy commission, established in the same year, which comprised six appointees with medical and legal backgrounds.[74] In Ireland, the office of the Lord Lieutenant and the board of control retained many of the duties and powers held by the English lunacy commission and, consequently, a large inspectorate was not regarded as necessary. The first appointee to the Irish inspectorate was White, who was subsequently joined by John Nugent. Travelling physician to Daniel O'Connell, Nugent did not have any previous experience in managing the mentally ill.[75] The Irish inspectorate was responsible for overseeing the management of lunatic asylums, the admission and discharge of patients, and ensuring that the treatment of patients was adequate. Their workload was quite extensive: they annually assessed and visited institutions that housed the mentally ill, including private and public lunatic asylums, houses of industry, gaols and workhouses.[76] By 1915, there were twenty-four district asylums with a daily average of 21,539 resident patients.[77] Under these circumstances it is hardly surprising that the effectiveness of the inspectorate was limited.

The relationship between the board of control and the inspectorate was fractious and generally unsatisfactory. Larcom, commenting in the 1850s, characterised the 1835 decision to incorporate the activities of the board of control into the board of works 'as a mistake'. While the board of works was responsible for the maintenance of existing asylums and the erection of new institutions, the 'internal management of the patients' was left 'without any central or general control save inspection by the inspectors general of prisons and a committee of the grand juries'.[78] The appointment of a separate lunacy inspectorate had failed to resolve the problem 'as there was no communication and indeed but little harmony between the co-equal parties [the board of works and the lunacy inspectors].'[79] The board of control, operating through the board of works, was never a popular body particularly with local authorities. It was considered to have excessive power over expenditure on the construction of new asylums.[80] By 1855, following a scandal over the cost of asylums constructed by the board of works, which resulted in a Treasury Inquiry, it was thought expedient to reconstruct a separate board of control. This was included in a draft of a primarily financial bill entitled the 'Lunatic Asylums Repayment of Advances (Ireland) Act (August 1855)'. The bill proposed that the Lord Lieutenant appoint four commissioners to sit on a new, revitalised board of control. It did not specifically name the lunacy inspectors as members of the board of control whereas John Radcliffe and Richard Griffith, commissioners of the board of works, were identified. The bill quickly became a cause of tension between the inspectors and the legislature. White was horrified at the omission of the inspectors and in a memorandum he claimed they were 'practically the legitimate commissioners of Control and Correspondence'. White went on to insist that every 'communication whether governmental or upon matters relating to the management of various asylums, questions for the decision of the Privy Council, communications with the Audit Office, Military constabulary Prisons and workhouses are effected through the inspectors [sic].'[81] The inspectors were acutely conscious that they did not enjoy the more extensive powers of English and Scottish commissioners in lunacy and were concerned that the re-creation of the board would result in interference with their powers. John Bucknill (1817–97), editor of the *Journal of Mental Science*, supported them criticising the unequal position of the Irish inspectors in comparison with the English and Scottish commissioners.[82] The lunacy reformer, Lord Naas, was less indulgent of White, correctly characterising his complaints as an attempt to expand the inspectors' influence.[83] John Radcliffe, one of the formulators of the bill and board of works commissioner, also dismissed White's fears as 'rest[ing] entirely on a delusion'.[84]

In the event the bill was referred to a Treasury Select Committee in May 1855, and following several amendments it was enacted in August 1855. The act specified that the membership of the re-constituted board of control was to include representatives from the board of works while the Lord Lieutenant nominated the remaining members. The lunacy inspectors were not specifically mentioned in the legislation though by 1860 they were appointed, but at the Lord Lieutenant's discretion. The resuscitated board of control was responsible for asylum structural alterations, 'superintending and directing the Erection, Establishment, and Regulation of Asylums for the Lunatic Poor' and their approval was required before funding was made available.[85] The board considered applications from asylum governors and the lunacy inspectors for building extensions and they made recommendations for the formation of new asylum districts.[86] Larcom opined that the board acted as a counterweight to growing demands from 'county gentlemen' who sought control over the asylums through the grand jury system. Larcom claimed that the 'local system was the soundest [form of government] when the country was fit for it', however, Ireland in the 1850s was clearly not deemed 'fit'.[87] While the 1855 act gave the board of control a distinct identity, in the late nineteenth century a series of parliamentary commissions recommended that a single central board with more extensive powers be appointed.[88] It was also suggested that the administration of lunacy be placed under the control of the Local Government Board.[89] These recommendations were not carried out, and while there were changes to its membership, the board of control remained in place throughout the expansion of the asylum system in the late Victorian period. It was finally disbanded under the 1898 Local Government Act.[90]

Locally, the governance and administration of individual institutions was the responsibility of two sets of governors nominated by the Lord Lieutenant and known as the board of directors and the board of governors.[91] Boards of directors were the larger of the two bodies and answered to the board of control in matters concerning asylum regulations, finance and building programmes.[92] The financial records were subsequently forwarded to the Treasury and the relevant grand juries. The close management of asylums was the responsibility of a subsidiary board of governors, which met once a month.[93] In addition to supervising the staff, governors were obliged to inspect the asylum and inmates regularly, and to 'keep a watchful eye over the accounts' which they were required to submit for an annual audit.[94] They were also responsible for the allocation of asylum contracts, ensuring that they were an important source of patronage in a community. Nonetheless, due to the lack of clarity and legal ambiguity surrounding their powers, the governors were often hampered in fulfilling their duties and this could lead to disputes with other bodies. The powers of Irish boards of governors were more limited than English visiting committees. For example, magistrates on the asylum committees in England had the power to dismiss asylum officers, whereas in Ireland, it was unclear with whom such authority rested and this became an area of contention.[95] The original legislation, and the 1843 privy council rules, implied that appointments came within the remit of

the Lord Lieutenant.[96] In March 1852 Clonmel asylum circulated a memorandum to all asylums demanding a change to this system of appointment
while, in 1853, a high court ruling on an incident at Belfast asylum found
that Lord Lieutenant appointments were illegal as they lacked 'statutory
authority'.[97] The situation remained unclear, a point noted in the 1857–58
Report of the Commission of Inquiry into the State of Lunatic Asylums.[98]
There was no definitive resolution of the situation until the 1898 Local
Government Act, when local asylum committees were finally granted the
power to appoint officers.

Asylum boards of governors comprised members of the rural landed
gentry, local magistrates, influential merchants and traders, representatives of the Church of Ireland and the Roman Catholic Church, and after
1838, poor law guardians. In 1852 the lunacy inspectors were appointed
ex-officio governors of all asylums. Larcom insisted that the inspectors were
'a medium of communication' between local asylum boards and parliament
while 'the real control of each asylum rests in its board of governors.'[99]
However, it is clear that the inspectors took part in proceedings of ordinary business at meetings and this caused tension.[100] The arrangement
was later altered and the inspectors only sat on boards as observers. The
Irish asylum boards therefore differed in composition from the committees of visitors of English asylums which were comprised of justices of
the peace, 'directly appointed by, and answerable to, the County Quarter
Sessions each year'.[101]

The composition of Carlow and Enniscorthy boards reflected
the dominant social and political hierarchies of the region. At Carlow,
the governors appointed during the first three decades were generally
politically conservative. A significant proportion were *ex-officio* poor
law guardians, who were regarded as essentially loyal to the interests of
Dublin Castle while others were involved in the management of the local
gaols. Approximately thirty governors were appointed to the first board.
While county Carlow appointments dominated, each of the four counties was represented. A similar number, twenty-seven, were appointed
to the Wexford asylum at Enniscorthy in November 1867.[102] Governors'
poor attendance at meetings hindered and, at times, neutered the boards.
Once the initial enthusiasm that greeted the opening of Carlow asylum
subsided, the numbers in attendance rapidly declined although the
presence of a lunacy inspector usually ensured a high attendance.[103] In
some instances, meetings were adjourned due to the failure to muster a

quorum.[104] In other cases, when just one or two board members appeared, only 'ordinary' administrative asylum business was conducted. By the 1880s, only three Carlow governors attended eight or more meetings in the year and there were no board meetings from May to December of 1893 and for several consecutive months in 1894.[105] In a bid to curb what was a national problem, the lunacy inspectors introduced an appendix to their annual reports that detailed governors' attendance at the meetings but this had little effect.

The non-attendance of governors at meetings not only crippled the business of the asylum, it also ensured a small number of governors – three or four regular attendees – exercised greater influence. From the 1830s to c.1850, the most active Carlow governors were poor law guardians, often *ex-officio* who represented conservative interests in the Carlow district. Colonel Henry Bruen was one of the most influential members of Carlow board, frequently acting as chairman.[106] He was a dominant figure in the county.[107] A magistrate, an *ex-officio* member of Carlow poor law union, a member of the board of superintendence of Carlow gaol, he was also the leading Tory landowner in the town.[108] His son, the right honourable Henry Bruen, also an *ex-officio* poor law guardian, succeeded him. The Faulkners of Castletown estate in county Carlow were also influential in asylum business. Henry Faulkner regularly attended meetings in the 1830s and 1840s, although later in the century, his descendant, Hugh, was less punctilious.[109] Henry Faulkner was an *ex-officio* poor law guardian. In the 1850s, another scion of the landed class, Robert Clayton Browne, became a regular attendee and he continued to participate until 1886.[110] He was an *ex-officio* poor law guardian and a member of the board of superintendence of Carlow gaol.[111] He was related to William Browne, who owned a substantial property, Browne's Hill in county Carlow, and had attended meetings regularly in the 1830s. Samuel and Thomas Haughton represented Carlow's merchant community on the board. Samuel Haughton was an elected member of the Carlow poor law union, but was described as 'conservative' in outlook while Thomas was an *ex-officio* member.[112] They were joined by the incumbents in the Catholic See of Kildare and Leighlin, including bishops Francis Haly[113] and James Walshe.[114] Other members of the clergy to participate in asylum business were Dean Bernard of the Church of Ireland Diocese of Leighlin and James Maher, the controversial Catholic parish priest of Graigue. Maher was an ardent supporter of the poor, of the Catholic interest, and a critic of the Irish poor law.[115] He attended asylum meetings intermittently until his death. Consequently, until the end of the 1860s, the main business of the asylum was pursued by a combination of representatives of the old ruling elite, influential traders and a representative of the clergy. These men were poor law guardians and those that were magistrates frequently signed certification warrants.[116] The Irish boards of governors cannot be characterised as a 'magisterial fiefdom', nor can it be argued that the poor law unions and the asylum were 'administrated by the same people' though as discussed in greater depth in chapter six, there was overlap.[117]

The composition of asylum boards remained relatively unaffected by the democratisation of, and the rise of nationalism within local government politics in nineteenth-century Ireland. The most important organ of local politics in Ireland were the poor law union boards of guardians, and by the 1870s, they were no longer exclusively dominated by members of the aristocracy, magistrates and landowning elites. As Crossman observed: 'the only administrative body in rural areas with a popularly elected element, poor law boards provided tenant farmers and rural businessmen with a rare opportunity to participate in local government'.[118] The greater participation of this group in the administration of local affairs ensured that their political priorities shaped the activities of poor law boards. A combination of demands for self-government and a 'sustained assault' on poor law boards 'under the auspices of the Land League, and its successor, the National League' after the 1880s ensured that the poor law boards were becoming 'nationalised'.[119] The centrality of the poor law boards in the campaign for self-government was made explicit in 1881 when Charles Stewart Parnell, future leader of the Irish National League, 'called on tenant candidates to contest poor law elections'. The aim was to 'wrestle the local government of the country from the landlord classes'.[120] This produced a series of conflicts between the older representatives of local government – the magistracy and the landed elite – and those elected poor law guardians.

Demands for greater representation of ratepayers on asylum boards did emerge from local grand jurists, feeling excluded from asylum management and seeking greater representation. In 1858, the commissioners inquiring into the state of lunatic asylums, recommended that two-thirds of individual asylum boards should be nominated by local grand juries and the final third selected by the executive.[121] However these demands were resisted, angering local grand juries. In the 1880s at Richmond and

Cork asylums, grand juries and corporations were invited by the Lord Lieutenant to nominate new board members. While this was successful in Dublin, it became a source of friction for the Cork asylum board, where the Lord Lieutenant refused to appoint the nominees on receipt of information that they were nationalists.[122] Thus, until there was a fundamental reform of the appointment procedures, nationalists struggled to exert much influence among asylum governors.

While the asylum boards remained relatively immune to the rise of nationalism in the nineteenth century, they also continued to be dominated by politically conservative interests and remained the preserve of three or four governors. From the 1870s to the 1890s, the most active Carlow governors continued to be members of local landed elites, and *ex-officio* poor law guardians. This included Sir Charles Burton, Colonel Henry Bruen, John Frederick Lecky, and later Thomas Anderson and William Clayton Browne who joined the board in the 1890s. Joseph Caulfield was an exception. The Carlow nationalist, Patrick Hanlon, was a governor from 1898, but he was not active until a decade later.[123] The conservative interest also dominated Wexford asylum board at Enniscorthy. The governors appointed in 1867 included magistrates and significant landlords such as the fifth Earl of Courtown, James George Henry Stopford, the second Baron Carew, Robert Shapland, Sir Thomas Esmonde, Thomas Braddell, Patrick Walter Redmond and Henry Bruen who had served on Carlow asylum board. By 1876 the Esmonde family owned approximately 8,000 acres in counties Wexford, Wicklow, Queen's, Tipperary, Longford, Kilkenny and Waterford.[124] While Esmonde and Redmond were from Catholic families, they had demonstrated loyalty to the crown interests in Ireland.[125] Redmond was dubbed an 'Orange Catholic'.[126] Thomas Esmonde was an inspector-general of the Royal Irish Constabulary and won the Victoria Cross in the Crimean War.[127]

There is also evidence that members of the landed elite, who were excluded or absented themselves from increasingly nationalised, poor law boards, became more active in asylum business. This allowed them to retain influence over aspects of local government and patronage. For example, several *ex-officio* guardians on Athy poor law board were 'systematically insulted' and 'eventually driven from the boardroom'.[128] At least one of these members, Thomas Anderson, became a frequent attendee at Carlow asylum board meetings from 1890. Although Carlow poor law board was not as 'nationalised' as others,[129] and may not have been as hostile towards *ex-officio* poor law guardians, governors such as Bruen, Burton, Lecky and Clayton Browne became more involved in asylum business during the final decades of the nineteenth century. They were all *ex-officio* members of Carlow board of guardians while Lecky, Bruen and Clayton Browne explicitly represented unionist interests. The participation of the merchant, middle-classes in asylum business was reduced considerably in the 1890s.

Clerical participation in asylum business expanded in the late nineteenth century, reflecting the developing influence of both churches in Ireland, particularly the Catholic Church, which went through a process of reorganisation. Initiated in the early decades of the century and consolidated in the decades after the Famine, a reformed Roman Catholic Church emerged as a powerful influence and, by the final decades of the century, it had established a dominant position within a variety of welfare and educational institutions.[130] Due to the proximity of St Patrick's College in Carlow town, the influence of the Catholic clergy was particularly evident on the Carlow board. From the 1860s, the College's Professor of Moral Philosophy, John Dunne, attended meetings. From the 1890s, the Roman Catholic Bishop of Kildare and Leighlin, Reverend Patrick Foley, Reverend Mathew Lalor from St. Patrick's College and the parish priests for Athy and Castledermot, Reverends Canon Germaine and Martin Walsh were Carlow governors.[131] The clergy were also members of the Enniscorthy asylum board including the Bishops of Ossory and the Bishop of Ferns, Thomas Furlong (1802–75).

Major reform of the composition and duties of local boards of governors was introduced in August 1898 by the Local Government Act.[132] The act restructured local government, which after 1898 was administered by county councils, urban and rural district councils, and the poor law boards of guardians. *Ex-officio* poor law guardians were abolished and the distinction between county cess and poor rates was removed. Subsequently, local government was funded from a single local taxation that was collected by county councils and paid in full by occupiers of land. The act stipulated that every county council provide 'sufficient accommodation for the lunatic poor in the county in accordance with the Lunatic Asylum Acts'.[133] Where a district lunatic asylum served several counties, individual county councils were responsible for their respective patient cohort. A local management committee, appointed by county councils, replaced the older local board of governors and the board of control was abolished. Although county councillors were entitled to be members of the new committees, they could not exceed a quarter of the membership.

In reality, county councillors controlled almost every aspect of the management of asylums through the local committees. The council appointed asylum staff, regulated finance and had jurisdiction over asylum buildings and land. However, elements of the old influences were still apparent. Among the twenty-three Carlow appointees to the new asylum management committee in February 1900, seven were members of the old board of governors including the unionist landlords Henry Bruen and William Clayton Browne.[134] Eleven members were elected county councillors some of whom were nationalists. Several members were elected members of the poor law boards for counties Kildare and Carlow and the remainder were either magistrates or clergymen. During the first decade of the twentieth century, the most active members of the committee were members of the clergy, particularly the Catholic priest, Martin Walshe,[135] in addition to local county councillors such as Edward Hayden and Michael Governey, a mineral water and boot manufacturer. Governey was a leading figure locally, a magistrate and a nationalist.[136] Therefore, the asylum committees appointed after 1898 reflected the more democratised and nationalist character of local government generally. Also, sympathy for the nationalist cause emerged among staff and board members following the alteration of the political landscape during the Irish revolutionary period (1912–23).[137] In contrast to the governors' indifference to asylum business in the 1890s, initially the members of the new committees were active and during the first decade of the twentieth century, the number of patients certified by the committee rose: this was, however, short-lived.[138]

The governance of asylums was hampered by the delay in introducing regulations for day-to-day management. The original 1817 act specified that the Lord Lieutenant and the privy council were responsible for the formulation of asylum regulations. These were not compiled until 1843 and in their absence, most of the country's asylums adopted the rules governing Armagh lunatic asylum.[139] Armagh asylum, which opened in July 1825,[140] was the first institution built under the original legislation and its superintendent, Thomas Jackson, devised a set of regulations based on those in operation at the Richmond asylum, which his board formalised into a code and adopted in December 1824.[141] Thomas Jackson was a firm advocate of moral management, as was Alexander

Jackson, who had developed the regime of care in the Richmond asylum. The similarities with the system of management at the influential York Retreat in England are abundant.[142]

Eventually, in 1843 the Armagh rules were replaced by the privy council regulations. Francis White was central to their compilation and, as Finnane has shown, he used the opportunity to press home the need to place asylums firmly under the management of the medical profession.[143] The rules outlined the responsibilities and duties of the governors and staff members, provided detail on admission procedures and on regulations that shaped patients' lives in the asylum. They were amended on several occasions; the most significant changes were introduced in January 1862, August 1870, May 1897 and October 1898.[144] Under the 1898 Local Government Act, county councils were made responsible for the formulation of asylum regulations and had power to appoint staff, including the resident medical superintendent and an assistant medical officer.

A range of difficulties therefore dogged the governance of Irish asylums. These were caused not only by the failure to clearly delineate regulations but also to define the boundaries of responsibilities and powers within the hierarchy of bodies responsible for asylum management. As a result, local asylum staff and governors managed the institutions without adequate regulations, and there was significant tension between and within national and local administrative bodies. While some of the tensions were a product of resistance to the centralised nature of government in Ireland, others were caused by medical and political ambitions.

Finance

The district asylum system became a very significant drain on local and national financial resources. Under the 1817 legislation and the subsequent 1826 amendment, the capital required for the initial phase of asylum building was issued by the exchequer in the form of a loan from the consolidated fund, which was then to be repaid within fourteen years through county grand jury presentments. In addition, the asylums were to repay maintenance costs advanced at the time of construction.[145] The asylums day-to-day costs were funded from local taxation – the county cess. County grand juries within asylum districts contributed annually to loan repayments and to the maintenance of patients. Repayments were estimated according to the number of patients from each county in receipt of treatment in the asylum. It was therefore necessary to keep records of the chargeability of each patient. The repayment of the initial outlay of capital and the management of the finances was a cause of unease, particularly at a local level and governors were generally anxious to reduce the local taxation burden. These concerns became more acute as the financial burden of asylums rose during the century. In addition, the curative regime of moral management necessitated the provision of good food and an engaging and stimulating atmosphere. This was relatively expensive when compared with maintenance cost of inmates in other institutions. While local ratepayers paid the taxes, the centralised nature of the asylum system, particularly in relation to the expensive programmes of expansion, meant that the privy council and the Lord Lieutenant held the 'purse strings';[146] they were advised by the board of works on matters relating to asylum building and by the inspectors in relation to asylum expenditure. Consequently, local agencies were not party to decisions that incurred additional local taxation and this was a source of considerable resentment. This antipathy was particularly acute during the 1850s when individual counties alleged that asylums constructed by the board of works were both extravagant and of inferior quality. The 1855 Treasury Inquiry concluded that there had been 'irregularities in the issuing of advances from the Treasury' and legislative intervention was required to resolve the situation.[147] This was the background to the 1855 Repayment of Advances (Ireland) Act, which normalised the repayment process.[148] As discussed in chapter two, this was just one of several disputes over the expanding cost of the asylums to the local ratepayers.

Expenditure on the asylums rose significantly over the course of the century. In 1871, the annual maintenance cost nationally was estimated at £162,249 16s 11d. This rose to £174,345 4s 2d in 1872.[149] The inspectors, anxious to defend the expansion of the asylum system, blamed this increase on inflationary conditions in the 1870s. Ireland had experienced a crisis in industry and craft production that was followed by an increase in inflation, which the inspectors identified as the source of the problem.[150] In 1874, in a bid to alleviate the burden on local taxation, the Treasury introduced a grant-in-aid of four shillings per week per head, which reduced the cost of patient maintenance to the local tax payers.[151] A complementary act passed a few years later halted further Treasury advances from the consolidated funds to individual asylums.[152]

The intention behind the 1874 act was to allow local authorities to focus their funding on other activities such as road improvements and housing. The Irish lunacy inspectors, however, interpreted the grant as the government's 'contribution to the improvement of the asylums' and used it for these purposes.[153] Subsequently, the cost to the Treasury continued to rise and, unsurprisingly, the lunacy inspectors were sharply criticised in the 1880s when they initiated another phase of expansion. The inspectors defended themselves against accusations of extravagance in their 1881 report, insisting that there was 'little room for extravagance when the object attaining justifies the mode of securing it'.[154] The cost to the exchequer was not reduced until after the 1890s, when the Treasury re-established central control of the 1874 grant. As we will see in chapter two, the transfer of financial powers to the county council after 1898 resulted in county councils delaying expenditure to the detriment of the asylums.

Patients

The Irish lunatic asylums were specifically intended to accommodate the pauper classes and as demonstrated in chapter five, the poor comprised the largest patient group. Nonetheless, relatively small numbers of non-paupers were admitted. This produced a more diverse patient population that had the potential to disrupt class barriers within the asylum. Some asylum patients were shopkeepers, clerks and skilled craftsmen and approximately one fifth (17 per cent) of patients, whose occupation was recorded between 1838 and 1868, were described as 'farmers'. In addition, sons of farmers may have been included as 'labourers' reflecting their activities on family farms rather than economic category. They were of course economically less vulnerable than most male patients who were described as 'labourers'.[155] Non-pauper patients were also admitted into asylums under the 1838 and 1867 dangerous lunatic acts, which, in contrast to alternative forms of certification, did not require proof of poverty. This was reinforced by police guidelines, which specifically stated that anyone could be certified as a dangerous lunatic.[156] Non-paupers were also admitted into Irish asylums as paying patients and the appropriateness and legality of this became a cause of some debate and concern during the nineteenth century.

In 1835 the prison inspectors initiated a discussion on the admission of paying patients. Those in favour argued that it provided relief to the respectable poor who could not afford to pay for private asylums.[157] The lunacy inspectors feared that without some form of provision, 'respectable' families would be forced to maintain mentally ill relatives at home or lodge them with an individual paid to care for them thereby reducing opportunities for recovery and leaving the mentally ill open to abuse.[158] Similar arguments were made in favour of developing provision for different classes of patients in Australia and New Zealand, resulting in the construction of separate asylums for paying patients by the late 1880s.[159] However, there was ambivalence about the proposals in Ireland. The scandals surrounding English private lunatic asylums that emerged in the early nineteenth century tainted the reputation of private madhouse-keepers and of institutions that accepted payment for patient care.[160] The Irish medical community felt a system of payment was open to wholesale abuse and asylum boards were ambivalent.[161] The lunacy inspectors stressed that asylum governors would not be permitted to exploit the system for monetary gain.[162]

When the Carlow governors were advised by the prison inspectors to accept paying patients in 1836, several argued that it was against the ethos of district asylums.[163] They were also concerned about the legality of accepting money. Consequently, in January 1836, on receipt of a request from the commissioners of public works for opinions on a proposed amendment to the laws relating to district asylums, the Carlow board requested the inclusion of a clause that allowed the admission of a limited number of paying patients into district asylums.[164] Although the clause was not included, the admission of patients who contributed, in one form or another, to maintenance costs was permitted. By the 1840s paying patients were accepted into Richmond, Carlow and Maryborough asylums. There continued to be confusion as to the legality of the practice. The Carlow governors sought the advice of the crown's law officers in one case[165] and, while awaiting a decision, the governors accepted payment in April 1844 but told the manager 'not to enter the same to the credit of the Institution, until the opinion of the Law Officers be made known'. Eventually, in February 1845, the year's payment for this patient's maintenance was accepted. Carlow asylum accepted small numbers of paying patients with the payments coming from diverse sources.[166]

By 1858 governors from several asylums, including Carlow, were requesting the introduction of a regulated system for the admission of paying patients. The 1856 draft bill to amend the lunacy legislation included a clause to legalise the admission of paying patients but by the time of its passage, in July 1856, the relevant clause had been omitted, having fallen foul of a broader controversy surrounding the Lord Lieutenant's power to appoint asylum staff.[167] The confusion over the admission of paying patients continued. In July 1862, during a Cork asylum board meeting, which Nugent attended, there was a detailed discussion of the case of a mother of a male patient who had failed to pay the agreed sum of £17. Nugent informed the asylum board that accepting the stipend was contrary to the law. In addition, having accepted the patient, the asylum was obliged to care for him and could not force his removal as entitlement to relief in the asylums was determined by his mental condition not the ability to pay a fee. While Nugent argued that patients' friends could be requested to contribute, he expressed concern that family members did not always adhere to financial agreements made with asylum officials.[168] Regulations were eventually included in the 1870 revision to the privy council rules and regulations. These stipulated that 'patients who have not sufficient available means of their own for payment of their maintenance in a private lunatic asylum, but whose friends are willing to pay wholly or in part for their care and maintenance, may be admitted into District Lunatic Asylums'. Preference was, however, always to be given to paupers, and applications for the admission of paying patients were to be accompanied by statements signed by magistrates and clergymen that confirmed the patient was unable or unwilling to pay for a private asylum. These patients were not to be admitted without previous approval from the lunacy inspectors and payments from family or friends were not to 'exceed the average of the general cost, nor be less than one half of the average cost, for the care and maintenance of patients in the District Asylum'.[169] The asylum system was thereby protected from allegations of profiteering.

Once the admission of paying patients was regulated, the lunacy inspectors decried its limited uptake, interpreting its unpopularity among the 'respectable poor' and the farming classes as evidence of a sense of entitlement. The inspectors claimed that families were opposed to paying, as they felt they already contributed to the cost of the establishment and maintenance of the asylums through taxation.[170] The failure to maintain class boundaries within the asylum through the separation of paupers from paying patients was likewise regarded by families as problematic.[171] The difficulties in admitting paying patients must also have been an obstacle. The asylums were overcrowded and in the event of a vacancy, precedence was given to pauper patients. Consequently, the admission of paying patients was a slow process and the numbers remained small. In October 1885, it was estimated that there were only thirteen paying patients in Enniscorthy asylum.[172] For such a small number of patients, they created significant additional management problems. As Nugent suggested in the 1880s, asylum authorities spent considerable time pursuing payments and they were obliged to contact the lunacy inspectors on each application.[173] Nor did paying patients become a significant source of income. In 1882 the inspectors received £1,165 7s 10d from paying patients accommodated throughout the country while in 1890 the receipts from paying patients admitted to Carlow asylum amounted to only £165 11s 0d.[174]

Conclusion

The Irish asylum system formed part of a broader pattern of precipitate state intervention in social, medical and welfare services in Ireland. Its establishment was informed by a general trend towards the institutionalisation of mental illness within allegedly 'humane' curative asylums that was evident throughout Europe in the early nineteenth century. The system that emerged also represented particular Irish concerns. There was a high level of centralised control, which was resented at local level and demands were repeatedly made to allow local grand juries to select board appointments. As James McConnel has observed, nineteenth-century landlords shared a deeply engrained belief that they were entitled to 'political influence and representation.'[175] The retention of central control over board membership ensured that governors, who were loyal to the crown and relatively politically conservative in outlook, particularly in relation to local taxation, dominated the asylum boards. While pockets of nationalism emerged on boards, this was rare until the early twentieth century. Nonetheless, as subsequent chapters will argue, the centralised governance of Irish asylums was in several respects more apparent than real. The original lunacy legislation was deficient in many respects and despite the introduction of numerous amendments, the initial provision of relatively few asylums, alongside the failure to devise clear regulations to provide a more robust inspectorate and to incorporate the asylums into other forms of welfare provision, ensured that legal frameworks were negotiated at a local level. Consequently, as we shall see, local protagonists – magistrates, county officials, families and doctors – altered the workings of the asylum system.

Notes

1 V. Crossman, *The Poor Law in Ireland 1838–1948* (Dundalk: Irish Economic and Social History Society, 2006), p. 5.
2 T. P. O'Neill, 'Fever and Public Health in Pre-Famine Ireland', *Journal of the Royal Society of Antiquaries of Ireland*, 103 (1973), 1–34.
3 O. MacDonagh, 'Ideas and Institutions, 1830–45', in W. E. Vaughan (ed.), *A New History of Ireland V: Ireland Under the Union, 1801–1870* (Oxford: Clarendon Press, 1989), pp. 193–217; 210; O. MacDonagh, *Ireland* (New York: Prentice-Hall, 1968), p. 27; G. O'Tuathaigh, *Ireland before the Famine 1798–1848* (Dublin: Gill and Macmillan, 1972), p. 95; C. Ó Gráda, *Ireland: A New Economic History 1780–1939* (Oxford: Oxford University Press, 1994), p. 97.
4 MacDonagh, 'Ideas and Institutions', p. 208; O'Neill, 'Fever and Public Health in Pre-Famine Ireland', p. 5.
5 Malcolm, *Swift's Hospital*, pp. 73–83.
6 *Twelfth Report of Lunacy Inspectors*, H. C. 1863 [3209] xx, p. 48.
7 L. D. Smith, 'The County Asylum and the Mixed Economy of Care', in Melling and Forsythe (eds), *Insanity, Institutions and Society 1800–1914*, pp. 33–47.
8 27 Geo. iii, c.39 s.12 (1787); 50 Geo. iii, c.103 (1810) amended by 7 Geo. iv, c.74 s.55 (1826).
9 The county asylums were attached to houses of industry.
10 A. Williamson, 'The Beginnings of State Care of the Mentally Ill in Ireland', *Economic and Social Review*, 1 (1970), 281–290, 285.
11 T. P. C. Kirkpatrick, *A Note on the History of the Care of the Insane in Ireland up to the end of the Nineteenth century* (Dublin: University Press, 1931), p. 17; Finnane, *Insanity and the Insane*, p. 21; Williamson, 'The Beginnings of State Care of the Mentally Ill in Ireland', 285. For a biography of William S. Hallaran see B. Kelly, 'Dr William Saunders Hallaran and Psychiatric Practice in Nineteenth-Century Ireland', *IJMS*, 177:1 (2008), 79–84.
12 *Fifth Report of Lunacy Inspectors*, H. C. 1851 [1387] xxiv, p. 16; 'Insanity and Hospitals for the Insane', *DJMS*, 12 (1851), 391; A. Mauger, '"Confinement of the Higher Orders"? The Significance of Private Lunatic Asylums in Ireland, 1820–1860' (MA dissertation, University College Dublin, 2009).
13 W. L. I. Parry-Jones, *The Trade in Lunacy: A Study of Private Asylums in England in the Eighteenth and Nineteenth Centuries* (London: Routledge & Kegan Paul, 1972), pp. 31, 55.

14 E. G. Thomas, 'The Old Poor Law and Medicine', *Medical History*, 24:1 (1980), 1–19.

15 Finnane, *Insanity and the Insane*, p. 21.

16 They also had a regulatory function; boards of governors were entitled to issue 'begging licenses' (badges) and were responsible for the punishment of mendicants and strolling beggars not in receipt of badges, see O'Neill, 'Fever and Public Health'.

17 *Eighth Report of Prison Inspectors*, H. C. 1830 [48] xxiv, p. 80.

18 Finnane, *Insanity and the Insane*, p. 21.

19 *Third Report of Prison Inspectors*, H. C. 1825 [493] xxii, p. 8.

20 It was opened in 1788 and by 1816 could accommodate 250 patients, see *Report from the Select Committee on the Lunatic Poor in Ireland*, H. C. 1817 [430] viii (hereafter *1817 Select Committee*), pp. 35–36; M.V. Conlon, 'The Relief of the Poor in Cork', *Journal of the Cork Historical Archaeological Society* 40, 2nd series (1935), 1–13; N.M. Cummins, *Some Chapters in Cork Medical History* (Cork: Cork University Press, 1957), p. 27.

21 *Second Report of Prison Inspectors*, H. C. 1824 [294] xxii, pp. 67–69; *Sixth Report of Prison Inspectors*, H. C. 1828 [68] xii, p. 11.

22 Finnane, *Insanity and the Insane*, p. 20.

23 Finnane, *Insanity and the Insane*, pp. 18–31.

24 Williamson, 'The Beginnings of State Care of the Mentally Ill in Ireland', 281–290. Newport was first elected as MP for the Waterford constituency in 1803 and spent thirty years in Parliament. He supported Daniel O'Connell's 1820s campaign for Catholic relief, the abolition of the slave trade and the establishment of pauper lunatic asylums in Ireland. He died in Waterford in February 1843. See J. Kelly, 'Newport, Sir (Simon) John, first baronet (1756–1843)', *Oxford Dictionary of National Biography, 40* (Oxford: Oxford University Press, 2004), pp. 674–675.

25 Finnane, *Insanity and the Insane*, p. 19.

26 Finnane, *Insanity and the Insane*, p. 19; *1817 Select Committee*, pp. 10–12.

27 Scull, *The Most Solitary of Afflictions*, pp. 110–132; Bartlett, 'The Asylum and the Poor Law: the Productive Alliance', p. 48.

28 Finnane, *Insanity and the Insane*, p. 24. Richmond was Lord Lieutenant from 1807 to 1813, see T. F. Henderson, 'Lennox, Charles, fourth duke of Richmond and fourth duke of Lennox (1764–1819)', *Oxford Dictionary of National Biography, 33* (Oxford: Oxford University Press, 2004), pp. 365–366.

29 Reynolds, *Grangegorman*, pp. 20–26; Finnane, *Insanity and the Insane*, p. 24.

30 Finnane, *Insanity and the Insane*, p. 25.

31 *Report from the Committee on Madhouses in England*, H. C. 1814–15 [296] iv, p. 4; *1817 Select Committee*, p. ii.

32 Peel was Secretary of State for Ireland from July 1812 to August 1818.

33 Finnane, *Insanity and the Insane*, pp. 18–52.

34 *Ibid.*, p. 25.

35 In 1816, John Leslie Foster, a judge, re-entered Parliament as member for Yarmouth, Isle of Wight. In the same year he was made Advocate-General and two years later he was made Counsel to the Commissioners of Revenue in Ireland. He acted as a Commissioner of the Board of Education in Ireland and of the Fisheries. He was appointed a Baron of the Court of Exchequer in July 1830, see G. Goodwin, 'Foster, John Leslie (1780/81?–1842)', *Oxford Dictionary of National Biography, 20* (Oxford:

Oxford University Press, 2004), p. 516; Spring Rice, first Baron Monteagle of Brandon, entered parliament as a member for Limerick. He was made Secretary to the Treasury under Lord Althorp's administration of 1830. He was appointed Colonial Secretary after Stanley's resignation in 1834. He succeeded Lord Althorp as Chancellor of the Exchequer in April 1835, see E. Archer Wasson, 'Rice, Thomas Spring, first Baron Monteagle of Brandon (1790–1866)', *Oxford Dictionary of National Biography* (Oxford: Oxford University Press, 2004), pp. 655–657. His fifth son, William Cecil Spring Rice (1823–80) was secretary to the English Lunacy Commission from 1861 to 1865, see *Burke's Peerage and Baronetage* (London: Harrison and Sons, 1912) p. 1355.

36   Finnane, *Insanity and the Insane*, p. 28; L. D. Smith, 'Close Confinement in a Mighty Prison: Thomas Bakewell and his Campaign against Public Asylums, 1810–1830', *History of Psychiatry*, 5 (1994), 191–214; A. Digby, *Madness, Mortality and Medicine: A Study of the York Retreat* (Cambridge: Cambridge University Press, 1985), pp. 10–12; A. Digby, 'Changes in the Asylum: the Case of York, 1777–1815', *Economic History Review*, 2nd series, 36:2 (1983), 218–239.

37   *1817 Select Committee*, pp. 10–12. For accounts of moral treatment in Ireland and elsewhere, see chapter seven and J. Goldstein, *Console and Classify: The French Psychiatric Profession in the Nineteenth Century* (Cambridge: Cambridge University Press, 1987); Digby, *Madness, Morality and Medicine*.

38   Smith, 'Close Confinement in a Mighty Prison', 196.

39   *1817 Select Committee*, p. 10.

40   57 Geo. iii, c.106 (1817).

41   V. Crossman, *Local Government in Nineteenth-Century Ireland* (Belfast: Institute of Irish Studies, 1994), p. 25.

42   Ó Gráda, *Ireland: A New Economic History*, pp. 29–31. For a discussion of Irish landlordism, see W. E. Vaughan, *Landlords and Tenants in Mid-Victorian Ireland* (Oxford: Oxford University Press, 2nd edn, 2002).

43   National Library of Ireland (hereafter NLI), Larcom Papers, Ms 7776 Thomas Larcom, 22 April 1855.

44   These amendments included 1 Geo. iv c.98 (1820) which extended the powers of governors to obtain land. 1&2 Geo. iv, c.33 (1821) repealed the 1817 and 1820 acts, and legislated for the demarcation of asylum districts and clarified the manner by which grand juries could raise money. Subsequent amendments empowered the Lord Lieutenant to make alterations to asylum districts, and further clarified the process of raising and repaying money raised – 6 Geo. iv, c.54 (1825) and 7 Geo. iv, c.14 (1826). 8&9 Vic. c.107 (1845) removed the limitation on the size of individual asylums and empowered the Lord Lieutenant to order asylums extensions, or the construction of new buildings. It established a separate lunacy inspectorate.

45   NLI, Larcom Papers, Ms 7776, Commentary by Thomas Larcom, p. 1; *Report of Lunacy Inspectors*, H. C. 1906 [Cd.2771] xxxvii, appendix A, table 2, p. 3; Finnane, *Insanity and the Insane*, p. 227.

46   Finnane, 'Asylums, Families and the State', 143; A. Scull, 'A Convenient Place to Get Rid of Inconvenient People', in A. D. King (ed.) *Buildings and Society* (London: Routledge and Kegan Paul, 1980), pp. 37–60.

47   *Report of the Select Committee on the State of the Poor in Ireland, with Minutes of Evidence*, H. C. 1830 [667] vii, appendix I, pp. 658–698; *First Report of the Commissioners for Inquiring into the Condition of the Poorer Classes in Ireland*, H. C. 1835 [369] xxxii; *Third Report of the Commissioners for Inquiring into the Condition of the Poorer Classes in Ireland*, H. C. 1836 [43] xxx, supplement to appendix C, pp. 13–18, pp. 27–29.

48   *Thom's Irish Almanac and Official Directory of Ireland* (hereafter *Thom's Directory*), 1850–1855.

49   *1817 Select Committee*, p. 8.

50   Patient classification and separation was facilitated throughout the building, see *1817 Select Committee*, pp. 34–38.

51   B. Edginton, 'A Space for Moral Management. The York Retreat's Influence on Asylum Design', in L. Topp, J. E. Moran and J. Andrews (eds) *Madness, Architecture and the Built Environment. Psychiatric Spaces in Historical Context* (London: Routledge, 2007), pp. 85–104.

52   *Ninth Report of Prison Inspectors*, H. C. 1830–31 [172] iv, p. 9. Murray joined Johnston's architectural office in 1807 and became Johnston's official assistant at the Board of Public Works in 1822, see M. Reuber, 'Moral Management and the "Unseen Eye": Public Lunatic Asylums in Ireland, 1800–1845', in Malcolm and Jones (eds), *Medicine, Disease and the State in Ireland*, pp. 208–233, p. 222.

53   'William Murray', Dictionary of Irish Architects, 1720–1940 (Irish Architectural Archive, www.dia.ie, accessed 8 March 2010).

54   'Arthur Williams', Dictionary of Irish Architects, 1720–1940 (Irish Architectural Archive, www.dia.ie, accessed 8 March 2010).

55   W. Fogerty, 'On the Planning of Lunatic Asylums', *Irish Builder*, 9:172 (15 February 1867), 39.

56   Reuber, 'Moral Management and the "Unseen Eye"', pp. 208–233.

57   Edginton, 'A Space for Moral Management', pp. 85–104.

58   *Expense of Erecting Carlow district asylum*, H. C. 1833 [192] xxxiv, p. 2.

59   *Fourteenth Report of Prison Inspectors*, H. C. 1836 [118] xxxv, p. 32.

60   These included the Commissioners of National Education (1831), Inspectors General on the General State of the Prisons in Ireland, and the Board of Public Works Commissioners (1831). A separate Poor Law Commission was introduced to Ireland in 1847.

61   V. Crossman, 'Chief Secretary', in S. J. Connolly (ed.), *The Oxford Companion to Irish History* (Oxford: Oxford University Press, 1998), pp. 85–86.

62   1&2 Geo. iv, c.33 (1821).

63   This included William Harvey, physician general, George Renny (1757–1848), Director General of Army Medical Department in Ireland, Sir Philip Crampton (1777–1858), eminent surgeon, anatomist and Surgeon-General to the Forces, and Robert Percival. See E. O'Brien, 'The Royal College of Surgeons in Ireland: A Bicentennial Tribute', *Journal of the Irish Colleges of Physicians and Surgeons*, 13:1 (1984), 29–31; 'The Late Sir Phillip Crampton', *British Medical Journal* (1858), 521–522; *Dublin Gazette* (1860); NLI, Dublin, Larcom Papers, Ms 7776. Also included were John David and Peter La Touche junior, both sons of Rt. Hon. David La Touche, Dublin banker and Director

and Governor of the Bank of Ireland (1783–96), see E. M. Johnston-Liik, *History of the Irish Parliament 1692–1800*, 5 (Belfast: Ulster Historical Foundation, 2002), p. 62.

64 M. E. Daly, *The Buffer State: The Historical Roots of the Department of the Environment* (Dublin: Institute of Public Administration, 1997), p. 44.

65 *Fourth Annual Report of the Board of Public Works in Ireland*, H. C. 1836 [314] xxxvi, p. 4.

66 Daly, *The Buffer State*, p. 11.

67 *Inquiry into the State of Lunatic Asylums and other Institutions*, p. 5. Colonel John Fox Burgoyne, Brooke Taylor Ottley and John Radcliffe were appointed to fulfil the duties of the board of control. Sir John Fox Burgoyne (1782–1871), engineer and administrator, was chairman of the board of works in Ireland from 1831 to 1845. On his resignation in 1845, he became the Inspector-General of Fortifications. In 1847, he became Chairman of the Board of Temporary Relief Commissioners administering relief under the Temporary Relief Act, see R. Hawkins, 'Burgoyne, Sir John Fox (1782–1871)', in J. McGuire and J. Quinn (eds), *Dictionary of Irish Biography*, 2 (Cambridge: Cambridge University Press, 2009), pp. 19–20; NLI, Larcom Papers, Ms 7775, p. 2.

68 D. J. Mellet, 'Bureaucracy and Mental Illness: The Commissioners in Lunacy 1845–90', *Medical History*, 25 (1981), 221–250; N. Hervey, '"A Slavish bowing down": the Lunacy Commission and the Psychiatric Profession 1845–60', in W. F. Bynum, R. Porter, and M. Shepherd (eds), *The Anatomy of Madness: Essays in the History of Psychiatry, Institutions and Society*, II (London: Tavistock Press, 1985), pp. 98–131.

69 27 Geo. iii, c.39 s.12 (1787).

70 *DJMS*, 10 (1850), 419–420.

71 Francis White (1787–1859) was apprenticed to Abraham Colles and studied medicine at Steeven's Hospital. He was admitted Licentiate of the College of Surgeons in 1813. He opened a hospital on Ormond Quay for the treatment of diseases of the eye and spent some time as Secretary to the Board of Health. White was victim of a railway accident in 1856 and, consequently, he was unable to fulfil his duties for eighteen months. He retired, and subsequently died on 16 August 1859, see Kirkpatrick, *A Note on the History of the Care of the Insane in Ireland*, p. 37; *JMS*, 4 (January, 1858), 257; 276.

72 Finnane, *Insanity and the Insane*, pp. 41–42; 5&6 Vic., c.123 s.1 (1842).

73 Finnane, *Insanity and the Insane*, pp. 41–42; *DJMS* credited it to the initiative of Thomas Spring Rice, 'ever the friend of the insane in Ireland', see *DJMS*, 10 (1850), 420; 8&9 Vict. c. 107 (1845).

74 Mellet, 'Bureaucracy and Mental Illness', 221–250, 224–225.

75 Nugent was educated at Clongowes College and Dublin University. When he died his personal estate was valued at over £38,000. 'Sir John Nugent', *JMS*, 45:189 (April 1899), 431–432; Finnane, *Insanity and the Insane*, pp. 41–42.

76 8&9 Vic., c.107 s.23 (1845).

77 *Sixty-fifth Report of Lunacy Inspectors*, H. C. 1917–18 [Cd 8454] xvi, p. 8.

78 NLI, Larcom Papers, Ms 7775, p. 1.

79 *Ibid.*

80 *Report and Minutes of Evidence of the Select Committee on Poor Law Union and Lunacy Inquiry (Ireland)* H. C. 1878–79 [C. 2239] xxxi (hereafter *Poor Law Union and Lunacy Inquiry*), p. 72 and see chapter two.

81 NLI, Larcom Papers, Ms 7775, Memorandum from Francis White, 16 May 1855.

82 J. C. B. 'Eighth Report of the Inspectors of Lunatic Asylums in Ireland', *JMS*, 24:4 (January 1858), 257–276.

83 NLI, Larcom Papers, Ms 7775, Memorandum from Francis White, 16 May 1855; Finnane, *Insanity and the Insane*, p. 39.

84 NLI, Larcom Papers, Ms 7775, Letter from John Radcliffe to Thomas Larcom, 12 March 1853.

85 18&19 Vict., c.109 s.5 (1855).

86 *Poor Law Union and Lunacy Inquiry*, p.73. In March 1860, the four appointees were Sir Richard Griffith, Chairman of the Commissioners of Public Works in Ireland, John Nugent, inspector of lunatic asylums, John Graham McKerlie, Lieutenant-Colonel of Royal Engineers and later Commissioner of Public Works in Ireland and George William Hatchell, the second inspector of lunatic asylums. This was adjusted when McKerlie become the Chairman of the Board of Public Works and William Richard Le Fanu became the Commissioner of Public Works, see *Return of the Numbers, Names and Qualifications of Commissioners of Control in Lunacy in Ireland appointed 15 December 1864*, H. C. 1868–69 [339] xli. William Richard Le Fanu (1816–1894), was a civil engineer and Commissioner for Public Works (1863–90). He was involved in the expansion of the railway system in Ireland, see S. P. Jones, 'Le Fanu, William Richard (1816–94)', in J. McGuire and J. Quinn (eds), *Dictionary of Irish Biography, 5* (Cambridge: Cambridge University Press, 2009), pp. 419–420.

87 NLI, Larcom Papers, Ms 7775, p. 1.

88 *Inquiry into the State of Lunatic Asylums and other Institutions*, pp. 26–28; *First Report of the Committee appointed by the Lord Lieutenant of Ireland on Lunacy Administration (Ireland)*, H. C. 1890–91 [C. 6434] xxxvi (hereafter *Committee appointed on Lunacy Administration*), p. 5.

89 *Poor Law Union and Lunacy Inquiry*, p. c.

90 61&62 Vict., c.37 (1898).

91 57 Geo. iii, c.106 (1817).

92 The boards of directors were obliged to meet only twice a year – the second Wednesdays in February and July – when a quorum of five directors was necessary, *Report of the Lunacy Inspectors* H. C. 1845 [645] xxvi, appendix no 4, p. 58.

93 These boards were required to hold a meeting on the first Tuesday of every month when a quorum of three governors was necessary.

94 *Report of the Lunacy Inspectors*, H. C. 1845 [645] xxvi, appendix no 4, p. 58; 57 Geo. iii c.106, s.14 (1817).

95 Scull, *The Most Solitary of Afflictions*, p. 247; Finnane, *Insanity and the Insane*, p. 38.

96 57 Geo. iii, c.106 s. 84 (1817).

97 Finnane, *Insanity and the Insane*, p. 38.

98 *Inquiry into the State of Lunatic Asylums and other Institutions*, p. 8.

99 NLI, Larcom Papers, Ms 7775.

100 *Inquiry into the State of Lunatic Asylums and other Institutions*, p. 7.

101 Melling and Forsythe, *The Politics of Madness*, p. 15.

102 Six additional appointments were made to the board between November 1867 and January 1868; *Wexford Lunatic Asylum. Returns of the Names of the Governors of the Wexford Lunatic Asylum*, H. C. 1867–68 [442] lv.

103 *Thirty-fifth Report of the Lunacy Inspectors*, H. C. 1886 [C 4811] xxxiii, appendix no. 24, pp. 86–87.

104 St Dymphna's Psychiatric Hospital, Carlow (hereafter DPH), Carlow Lunatic Asylum (hereafter CLA), Minute Book, 9 June 1858, 12 January 1859.

105 DPH, CLA Minute Book, May–December 1893 and March–June 1894.

106 DPH, CLA Minute Book, 1832–1850.

107 The Bruen family owned a residence at Oak Park in county Carlow, described as 'a handsome, spacious, building, consisting of a centre and two wings, situated to the north of the town in a fine demesne embellished with stately groves of full-grown oak', see Lewis, *A Topographical Dictionary of Ireland*, I, p. 261.

108 S. O'Shea, 'Carlow Poor Law Union: the Early Years', *Carloviana*, 52 (2003), 28; E. Malcolm, 'The Reign of Terror in Carlow', *Irish Historical Studies*, 32:125 (2000), 59–74.

109 Other representatives of the landlord class included Sir Thomas Butler, baronet of Ballintemple and magistrate for county Carlow, who attended meetings intermittently in the 1830s and 1840s.

110 *Thirteenth Report of the Lunacy Inspectors*, H. C. 1864 [3369] xxiii, p. 124.

111 *District Directory and Almanac for 1888 for the counties of Carlow, Kildare and Queen's County and portions of Wicklow and Kilkenny* (Carlow, 1888), pp. 17–19; *Carlow Post* (10 December 1870).

112 *Carlow Sentinel* (17 October 1840).

113 Francis Haly (b. c1783) entered College of Maynooth in 1807. He was ordained a priest in 1812 and was consecrated Bishop of Kildare and Leighlin on 25 March 1838 and acted as bishop for seventeen years. Dr Haly was one of the Prelates assembled at the National Synod held at Thurles in 1850. He died in 1855, see M. Comerford *Collections relating to the Diocese of Kildare and Leighlin* (Dublin: J. Duffy, 1886), pp. 140–145.

114 DPH, CLA Minute Books, 1832–1922; Dr James Walshe (b.1803) was elected Bishop of Kildare and Leighlin on 28 January 1856. He was educated at St Peter's College, Wexford, and St Patrick's College, Carlow. He was ordained in 1830 and appointed successively Professor of Humanities, of Moral Philosophy and Theology in Carlow College. He served as Curate and later as Administrator of the Cathedral Parish Carlow, acting as Secretary to the Bishop Dr Francis Haly. He rejoined Carlow College as Vice-President and Professor of Greek and Sacred Scripture, and on the retirement of Dr Taylor was appointed President in 1850. He was granted a Coadjutor (Dr James Lynch) in 1869. See Comerford *Collections relating to the Diocese*, pp. 150–151.

115 E. Ó Cathaoir, 'The Poor Law in County Carlow, 1838–1923', in T. McGrath (ed.), *Carlow: History and Society. Interdisciplinary Essays on the History of an Irish County* (Dublin: Geography Publications, 2008), p. 688.

116 DPH, CLA Register of Admissions, May 1832–November 1845, February 1846–November 1887, January 1888–July 1894.

117 P. Barlett, *The Poor Law of Lunacy*, p. 94. See also C. Smith, 'Parsimony, Power and Prescriptive Legislation: the Politics of Pauper Lunacy in Northamptonshire, 1845–1876', *Bulletin of the History of Medicine*, 81:2 (2007) 359–385; Melling and Forsythe, *The Politics of Madness*, p. 24.

118 V. Crossman, *Politics, Pauperism and Power in late Nineteenth-Century Ireland* (Manchester: Manchester University Press, 2006), p. 46.

119 Crossman, *Politics, Pauperism and Power*, pp. 42–43; W. Feingold, *The Revolt of the Tenantry: The Transformation of Local Government in Ireland, 1872–1886* (Boston: Northeastern University Press, 1984).

120 Crossman, *Politics, Pauperism and Power*, p. 43.

121 *Inquiry into the State of Lunatic Asylums and other Institutions*, p. 6.

122 Finnane, *Insanity and the Insane*, pp. 60–61.

123 *Irish Times* (4 April 1890).

124 P. Maume, 'Sir Thomas Henry Grattan Esmonde', in J. McGuire and J. Quinn (eds), *Dictionary of Irish Biography*, 3 (Cambridge: Cambridge University Press, 2009), pp. 650–653.

125 J. McConnel, 'John Redmond and Irish Catholic Loyalism', *English Historical Review*, 125:512 (2010), 90–94.

126 He was the grandfather of John Redmond, see McConnel, 'John Redmond', 92.

127 His nephew, also Thomas, was a Home Rule MP, see Maume, 'Sir Thomas Henry Grattan Esmonde', p. 651.

128 Crossman, *Politics, Pauperism and Power*, p. 41.

129 Feingold, *Revolt of the Tenantry*, p. 204.

130 S. J. Connolly, *Religion and Society in Nineteenth Century Ireland* (Dundalk: Dundalgan Press, 1985), p. 56.

131 DPH, CLA Minute Book, 14 February 1900.

132 61&62 Vict., c.37 (1898); Crossman, *Local Government in Nineteenth-Century Ireland*, pp. 91–97.

133 61&62 Vict., c.37, s.9 (1898).

134 DPH, CLA Minute Book, 14 April 1899; *Thom's Directory, 1898*.

135 On Walshe's death in 1917, Anderson sent a letter of condolence to the Archbishop of Dublin, William Walshe (1841–1921), see Dublin Diocesan Archives (hereafter DDA), Walsh Papers, 1917, 379/5 Laity, 16 February 1917.

136 Governey condemned the 1916 Rising, see T. McGrath, 'Politics, Education and Religion in the Age of Revolution', in McGrath (ed.) *Carlow: History and Society*, pp. 834, 840.

137 In July 1920 staff at Enniscorthy asylum hoisted republican flags – subsequently removed – to welcome the incoming board, see W. Murphy, 'Enniscorthy's Revolution', in C. Tóbin (ed.) *Enniscorthy. A History* (Enniscorthy: Wexford County Library, 2010), p. 432 ft. 140.

138 See chapters two and five.

139 DPH, CLA Minute Book, 5 April 1832.

140 Williamson, 'The Beginnings of State Care for the Mentally Ill in Ireland,' 285.

141   A.P. Williamson, 'The Origins of the Irish Mental Hospital Service, 1800–1843' (M.Litt dissertation, Trinity College, Dublin, 1970), p. 148.

142   Chapter seven.

143   Finnane, *Insanity and the Insane* pp. 39–47.

144   *Eleventh Report of the Lunacy Inspectors*, H. C. 1862 [2975] xxiii, pp. 55–59; *Fourteenth Report of the Lunacy Inspectors*, H. C. 1865 [3556] xxi; *Twentieth Report of the Lunacy Inspectors*, H. C. 1871 [C. 440] xxvi, p. 159; *Forty-seventh Report of the Lunacy Inspectors*, H. C. 1898 [C. 8969] xliii, p. 228; *Forty-eight Report of the Lunacy Inspectors*, H. C. 1899 [C. 9479] xl, pp. 245–246; *Rules for the Regulation and Guidance of Attendants and Servants and Other Persons in the Service of Carlow District Asylum* (Naas, 1898).

145   Finnane, *Insanity and the Insane*, p. 33.

146   NLI, Larcom Papers Ms, 7775, Memorandum, 21 April 1855.

147   See Finnane, *Insanity and the Insane*, pp. 37–38 and chapter two.

148   18&19 Vict., c.109 (1855).

149   *Twenty-second Report of the Lunacy Inspectors*, H. C. 1873 [C. 852] xxx, p. 9

150   *Ibid.*; L. Cullen, *Economic History of Ireland Since 1660* (London: Batsford, 2nd edn, 1972), pp. 146–149.

151   Finnane, *Insanity and the Insane*, p. 57.

152   40&41 Vict. c.27 (1877); *Twenty-seventh Report of the Lunacy Inspectors*, H. C. 1878 [2037] xxxix, p.13.

153   Finnane, *Insanity and the Insane*, pp. 55–59.

154   *Thirty-first Report of the Lunacy Inspectors*, H. C. 1882 [C. 3356] xxxii, p. 7.

155   K. O'Neill, *Family and Farm in Pre-Famine Ireland: The Parish of Killashandra* (Madison and London: University of Wisconsin Press, 1984), p. 146.

156   *Instruction Book for the Government and Guidance of Dublin Metropolitan Police* (Dublin: Thom, 1879), p. 177.

157   *Eighth Report of the Lunacy Inspectors*, H. C. 1857 session 2 [2253] xviii, p. 12.

158   *Fifteenth Report of the Lunacy Inspectors*, H. C. 1866 [3721] xxxii, p. 17.

159   C. Coleborne, *Madness in the Family. Insanity and Institutions in the Australasian Colonial World, 1860–1914* (Houndmills: Palgrave Macmillan, 2010), p. 6.

160   Scull, *Most Solitary of Afflictions*, pp. 77–82; Jones, *Trade in Lunacy*, pp. 221–280.

161   'Recent Publications on Insanity', *DJMS*, 10 (1850), 424.

162   *Eighteenth Report of Prison Inspectors*, H. C. 1840 [240] xxvi, p. 12; *Eighth Report of the Lunacy Inspectors*, H. C.1857 session 2 [2253] xvii, p. 12.

163   *Fourteenth Report of Prison Inspectors*, H. C. 1836 [118] xxxv, p. 32; DPH, CLA, Minute Book, 5 January 1836.

164   DPH, CLA, Minute Book, 5 January 1836.

165   DPH, CLA, Minute Book, 21 December 1842.

166   *Ibid.*, 17 April 1844, 19 February 1845, 15 February 1854, 20 July 1863.

167   'Bill to Explain and Amend the Acts relating to the Lunatic Asylums in Ireland', H. C. 1856 [1856] lxxxiii; 19&20 Vict., c.99 (1856).

168   *Cork Examiner* (11 July 1862).

169   *Twentieth Report of Lunacy Inspectors*, H. C. 1871 [C. 440] xxvi, p. 163.

170   *Thirty-second Report of Lunacy Inspectors*, H. C. 1883 [C. 3675] xxx, p. 8.

171   *Thirtieth Report of Lunacy Inspectors*, H. C. 1881 [C. 2933] xlviii, p. 15.

172 SPH, ELA Letter Book, 24 October 1885.
173 *Ibid.*, 16 September 1884, 23 November 1886.
174 *Thirty-first Report of Lunacy Inspectors*, H. C. 1882 [3356] xxxii, p. 17; *Fortieth Report of Lunacy Inspectors*, H. C. 1890–91 [6503] xxxvi, appendix A, p. 50.
175 McConnel, 'John Redmond', p. 90.

2

Expansion and demand

'all towns of significance ... should possess hospitals and asylums of good quality'.[1]

During the four decades following the opening of Carlow asylum in 1832, the original asylum district, comprising four counties, was divided. The decisions to remove counties Kilkenny and Wexford were taken in 1847 and 1860 respectively, leading to the opening of additional institutions in 1852 and 1868. The original asylum in Carlow town continued to serve counties Carlow and Kildare and the building was extended. Carlow district was not unique in this regard. By the 1840s, most asylums were overcrowded or under pressure due to high admission rates. Consequently, the asylum districts throughout the country were divided as demands for the expansion of asylum services emerged from several quarters. This process of expansion was contentious and placed national and local lunacy administrations under extreme pressure. This chapter will examine the events and debates surrounding the division of Carlow asylum district and the expansion of the original asylum, a process that involved intense disputes between local boards, the lunacy inspectorate and the board of control. As will be highlighted, in response to the supervision, censure and constraints imposed by the national inspectorate, asylum governors, many of whom were magistrates, clung tighter to the vestiges of their autonomy and resisted change. The expansion of public asylums and the high rates of pauper admissions also prompted debates on the susceptibility of the Irish to mental illness, particularly as the rates of confinement in Ireland appeared to higher than elsewhere in the United Kingdom. Thomas Drapes at Enniscorthy asylum, among others, made important contributions to debates explaining these patterns, and as this chapter will elucidate, commentators linked high rates of confinement to late nineteenth-century theories of degeneration and hereditary insanity.

Pressure and expansion

Two years after the opening of Carlow asylum in May 1832, the building was full and the governors delayed or rejected new applications until resident patients were discharged or had died.[2] Indeed, only one year after the asylum was completed and nine months after the first admissions, the lunacy inspectors noted with palpable relief that 'No order for any increased accommodation has been made.'[3] The large number of applicants came from the general community, from local gaols, such as Kilkenny and Carlow, and other institutions, including the Richmond asylum in Dublin.[4] While the inspectors expected that the pressure would dissipate when other institutions were cleared, this was not the case.[5] As figure 2.1 demonstrates, though admissions into the asylum decreased,[6] pressure for places remained high; in 1844, there were seventeen patients on the waiting list.[7] Thus, while admissions declined during the remainder of the decade, the asylum frequently failed to accommodate new patients.

Responding to the pressure, the Carlow governors adopted a series of short-term strategies that required the reconfiguration of patients' cells and other living spaces. This policy compromised the original architectural design of the asylum space, which was an intrinsic part of the institution's therapeutic regime. The design of the early asylums was intended to 'privilege' 'ideas of cure, care and safe custody' and not 'reproduce prisons or workhouses'.[8] When Carlow asylum was originally opened, patient accommodation generally consisted of single cells, in addition to large dormitories intended for multiple occupancy by convalescent patients. Segregation of the sexes was also facilitated in the design of the asylum. When managing the high demand for admissions, Patrick McCaffry, the asylum's lay manager from 1834 to 1842, placed incurable patients in a single large dormitory, releasing accommodation for an additional fifty-one patients.[9] The number of single cells was steadily reduced: by 1843 there were eighty-eight, with an additional twelve large cells and three large sleeping rooms for 'idiot' and tranquil patients.[10] This process of re-configuring the use of space continued throughout the 1840s as the asylum governors accepted more patients than the building could accommodate within the original layout. In 1843, the conversion of a 'straw-house' into patient accommodation facilitated eleven admissions and by the following year the institution could house 180 patients though the original building had not been extended.[11] This piecemeal response to the problem was unsuccessful. Not only did it undermine the curative component of the asylum's architectural design, shifting the emphasis onto the custodial role of the institution, each new facility was quickly filled with patients and during a visit in 1845, the inspectors found that the asylum was overcrowded.[12]

The Famine further contributed to the problem of overcrowding. The Carlow asylum district did not experience the extreme privation evident in other parts of Ireland, particularly the western seaboard, during the Famine. Joel Mokyr has suggested that there were relatively low excess mortality rates in counties Kilkenny, Kildare, Wexford and Carlow, though counties Kildare and Kilkenny suffered more.[13] None the less, by 1847, most workhouses in counties Carlow, Kilkenny, Kildare and Wexford were overcrowded, while the numbers in receipt of outdoor relief soared.[14] The workhouses became sites of fear for a population anxious to avoid contact with diseases endemic within their walls. Fever – typhus,

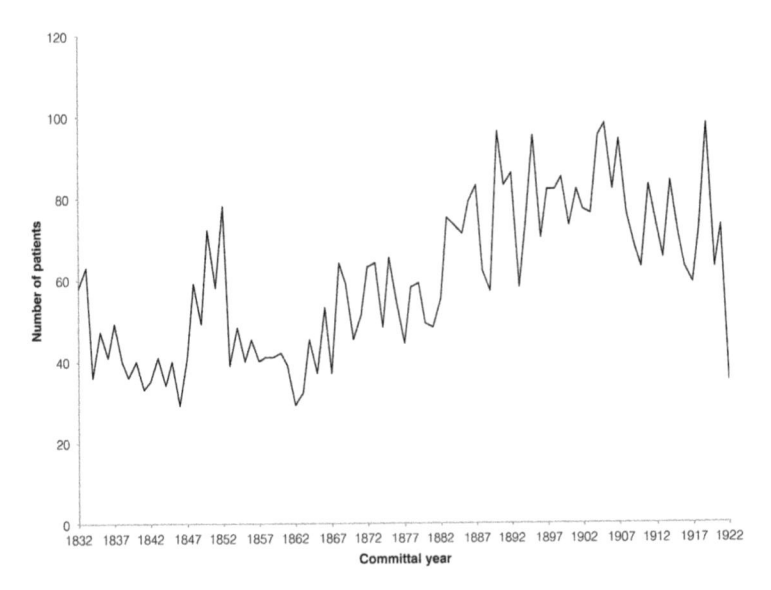

Figure 2.1   Annual admissions to Carlow Asylum, 1832 to 1922

relapsing, and dysentery – appeared in workhouses in county Kildare. The master of Naas workhouse, James Butler, died of typhus fever in August 1847.[15] Cholera broke out in Carlow workhouse between July and September 1849.[16] In spite of the presence in the region of these contagious diseases, Carlow asylum was relatively successful in limiting its spread. Though it was one of the few asylums to report an outbreak of cholera to the lunacy inspectors, there were no deaths.[17] During the latter period of the Famine-related crisis – 1847 to 1852 – admissions to Carlow asylum increased, suggesting that the asylum was incorporated into the population's survival strategies.[18] Families initiated most of these admissions, implying that most patients, though not all, were maintained at home prior to institutionalisation.[19] The relatively tardy increase in asylum admissions, in the terms of the chronology of the Famine, is related to the difficulties communities experienced in gaining access into Irish workhouses at the height of the crisis, as well as to changes in emigration patterns. By 1847, emigration had become one of the many survival mechanisms deployed by individuals and families in response to the Famine, contributing to the dramatic population decline in the four counties.[20] Some 8,157 migrants left county Carlow alone between May 1851 and 1855.[21] Workhouses and individual landlords also organised some assisted emigration schemes.[22] Family members able to migrate did so and, consequently, relatives were admitted into asylums. The number of 'dangerous lunatic' certifications climbed during this period and there was an increase in the transfer of this group of the mentally ill from local gaols (table 2.1). Approximately 33 per cent (111) of patients transferred into Carlow asylum from local gaols between 1838 and 1867 were moved between 1848 and 1852, peaking in 1850, 1851 and 1852. Gaol and workhouse officials were actively clearing institutions of inmates suitable for asylum care.

Local asylum authorities responded to the Famine crisis in various ways. The Carlow governors alleviated Famine overcrowding by discharging patients; there was an increase in the rate of release between 1847 and 1852 and there was a particular surge in patients released as 'relieved' between 1848 and 1851. There was an increase in mortality in the institution across these five years: deaths peaked in 1847 and thereafter slowly declined. Although denied by the governors, lunacy inspectors attributed this to 'epidemic dysentery'.[23] The asylum mortality rate would never return to its pre-Famine level.[24] Some asylum boards lobbied for the commencement of an asylum-building programme to provide employment for the destitute.[25]

Table 2.1   Patients transferred from gaols to Carlow Asylum, 1848 to 1868

Year	No.	%
1848	12	3.5
1849	11	3.2
1850	28	8.2
1851	24	7.1
1852	36	10.6
1853	9	2.6
1854	10	2.9
1855	13	3.8
1856	8	2.4
1857	15	4.4
1858	14	4.1
1859	15	4.4
1860	14	4.1
1861	17	5.0
1862	7	2.1
1863	5	1.5
1864	18	5.3
1865	14	4.1
1866	31	9.1
1867	16	4.7
1868	14	4.1
Year Missing	9	2.6
Total	340	100.0

Most asylum governors, including the Carlow board, were anxious to avoid policies that increased costs to ratepayers and demonstrated a reluctance to expand institutions both before and during the crisis.[26]

Surprisingly, there were relatively few references to the Famine in the lunacy inspectors' annual reports. In 1848, the inspectors acknowledged the impact the extreme conditions had upon the pauper population, arguing that 'in many cases it would seem that the insanity arising from starvation was a mere prelude to death, as the comforts and remedial treatment of our hospitals were found inoperative to restore either health or reason'.[27] It appears that only in retrospect was the Famine seen as having a potentially devastating impact on Irish minds when links were made with the high rates of admission and the psychological impact of living through Famine conditions – starvation, the loss of friends and family, and bearing witness to horrific conditions. In 1913, the inspectors speculated that the 'nervous equipment' of children who were either born during or lived through the Famine was significantly impaired rendering them more susceptible to mental disease.[28]

By the 1840s, there appeared to be an inexhaustible demand for admissions. The 1843 House of Lords Select Committee reported that the asylums, originally designed to accommodate 1,220 patients, contained 2,028 patients. It recommended an expansion in the number of institutions and the capacity of individual asylums.[29] The committee requested that the lunacy inspector, Francis White, produce estimates of the country's future accommodation needs.[30] The lunacy inspectors were committed to institutionalisation and this fuelled the growth of asylum provision in Carlow and nationally. From 1834, the Carlow governors were repeatedly requested by the lunacy inspectors to expand the asylum.[31] With the additional pressure placed upon the asylum following the introduction of the 1838 Dangerous Lunatic Act, in May 1840 the Carlow governors eventually conceded that a permanent solution was required and resolved that the building should be extended to accommodate a further fifty patients.[32] A significant obstacle to expansion was the limitation placed on the size of asylums by the original lunacy legislation.[33] Partly in response to the findings of the 1843 House of Lords Select Committee, this limitation was removed in 1845 by an amendment to the lunacy legislation, which facilitated a second major phase in asylum construction.[34] This resulted in the establishment of six new asylums providing an additional 1,722 beds.[35]

Following the introduction of the 1845 amendment, central government invited the lunacy inspectors to offer their views on the 'best mode of providing increased accommodation'. The initial proposals for the province of Leinster included enlarging Richmond asylum in Dublin and the asylums at Carlow and Maryborough. County Kildare would be removed from Carlow asylum district and attached to the Maryborough district. A new asylum would be erected in Mullingar town.[36] These suggestions were approved and the architect of the board of works, Jacob Owen, in conjunction with the inspectors, surveyed Carlow asylum with a view to enlargement.[37] The extension was expected to house fifty patients and accommodation for an additional fifty-five patients would be made available by the removal of county Kildare from the district.

The reaction to the expansion of 'asylumdom' varied; there were a series of debates at a county level regarding the potential benefits. While

Carlow asylum district was being divided, members of local grand juries – comprised in the 1850s of representatives from the landed gentry – fought to secure an asylum in their respective counties. The construction of asylums, hospitals and workhouses in provincial Irish towns brought significant financial benefits – contracts for the supply of foodstuffs, clothing, furniture and employment.[38] Medical and welfare institutions contributed to a town's civic identity;[39] their presence displayed a county's humanity and progressive nature. A separate asylum also gave magistrates, poor law guardians and local elites control over their own institution rather than obliging them to negotiate with representatives from other counties. Consequently, the location of the new 'wave' of asylums became contentious as the original proposals were contested, delaying work on the proposed new asylums until 1849.[40]

These tensions were played out during the revision of asylum provision in the Carlow district. In spite of the general agreement with the decision to separate county Kildare from the Carlow asylum district, in July 1846 a local committee representing the interests of Kilkenny city and county, with Charles Vignoles as chairman, forwarded a petition containing an assessment of asylum provision in that county, to the Lord Lieutenant.[41] The petition argued that the existing institutional facilities – the lunatic wards attached to the Kilkenny house of correction and the city gaol – were inadequate and requested that the local house of industry be converted into an asylum to serve county Kilkenny.[42] The lunatic inspectors once again reviewed the accommodation in Leinster in 1847 and, in this instance, favoured the removal of Kilkenny from the district and the construction of a separate institution in that city.[43] And so, Kilkenny rather than Kildare became the first county to be removed from the Carlow asylum district. An order in council was issued on 29 June 1847 for work to commence on a new asylum, to house 150 patients from Kilkenny city and county. It was the smallest of the asylums built during this phase: the total cost 'in land, building, furniture and fittings' amounted to £24,920.[44] The Kilkenny governors took possession of the building in 1852 and, in September, the Carlow governors were directed to remove fifty-four Kilkenny patients from Carlow asylum.[45] As a result of the decision to build Kilkenny asylum, the inspectors postponed the proposed extension to Carlow asylum.[46] The Carlow governors were compelled to wait six years for work to commence. There were significant financial repercussions in the removal of county Kilkenny. Counties

Carlow, Kildare and Wexford were obliged to repay Kilkenny county and city the money – £5,710 19s 7d and £800 18s 8d respectively – initially paid towards the construction of Carlow asylum.[47]

The cost of this second wave of asylum construction was extremely contentious. In spite of Larcom's efforts to defend it,[48] some counties protested 'about the high cost and imperfect work in some asylums'.[49] Local county officials had assumed that estimates for the cost of the new asylums would be submitted to the grand juries for approval and then communicated to the board of works.[50] This had been the policy prior to 1835. However, the estimates did not require the grand juries' approval and this caused resentment at local level.[51] The lunacy inspectors and the board of works became the targets of local criticism, while poor communication between these two bodies resulted in financial inconsistencies during the building programme.[52] As alluded to in chapter one, the controversy resulted in the establishment of a Treasury Inquiry, comprising London architect T. L. Donaldson and James Wilkes, medical officer at Stafford Lunatic Asylum. They were appointed in August 1855 to investigate the cost of the erection of the new asylums and visited every asylum built by the board of works 'with a view to determining whether any useless and unnecessary expenditure has been occurred'. They were also to advise on whether there should be remission of the original expenditure.[53] During their tour, which lasted from 31 August to 24 September, Donaldson and Wilkes inspected twelve asylums, visiting Kilkenny on 20 September. They identified a series of structural problems with the new asylums, and recommended that money be remitted in four cases – Sligo, Killarney, Cork and Mullingar. At Kilkenny asylum, they identified a serious problem with damp and recommended that the walls be rendered dry and weather tight. The plasterwork, sections of the woodwork and the airing yard required improvement. Donaldson and Wilkes recommended that the expense of repairing the defects should not be charged to the ratepayers.[54] Kilkenny asylum was later visited by the Lord Lieutenant, in the company of the lunacy inspectors, in August 1863.[55]

With the exception of Kilkenny, the asylums constructed during the 1850s were significantly larger than their predecessors. Cork catered for 500 patients, Sligo for 250, Killarney for 200 and Omagh for 300.[56] By the 1850s the orthodoxy that smaller asylums facilitated successful curative regimes no longer suited exigencies.[57] By this time in England, larger institutions, such as the Devon County Asylum at Exminster, which opened in July 1845, were explicitly designed to accommodate large numbers.[58] While most commentators agreed that larger asylums could be designed to facilitate a therapeutic environment, others, such as the Irish architect William Fogerty, cautioned that they should not become too large.[59] During the second building programme, the Irish board of works stressed that the new asylums were 'hospitals … not prisons'.[60] Donaldson and Wilkes found that several new asylums were not in keeping with this ethos, criticising the design of the internal space and the failure to adhere to the board of works' guidelines. For example, they reported there were insufficient single rooms at Belfast, Kilkenny and Sligo, while the long corridors were draughty. They also noted that the furniture was 'scanty' and constructed from the 'commonest description'.[61]

Finnane has suggested that the controversy surrounding the cost and quality of asylums constructed under the management of the board of works and the inspectors reflected a declining enthusiasm for asylums at a local level.[62] However, this should not be overstated. Counties that experienced difficulties in securing admissions into institutions they supported through taxation continued to lobby for separate asylums. Over the next decade, the construction of six new asylums – Castlebar (county Mayo), Downpatrick (county Down), Ennis (county Clare), Letterkenny (county Donegal), Monaghan (county Monaghan) and Enniscorthy (county Wexford) – was authorised and in the cases of Wexford, Clare and Donegal, county officials actively lobbied for separate institutions. Officials and grand juries responsible for the original asylums were anxious about the associated cost. For example, the Limerick asylum governors did not support the decision to divide their district and construct a separate institution in Ennis town to serve county Clare. Clare grand jury, however, voted unanimously in favour of separation.[63] Similarly, the Londonderry asylum board objected to the separation of county Donegal and the construction of a second asylum. While county Donegal officials were anxious to secure another institution, they were divided on the most suitable location. In this instance, the debate on the construction of another asylum became embroiled in ongoing clashes as to the form local government should take in Ireland and these broader political concerns informed the controversy. A division emerged between those who felt the asylum should be located in Lifford, the county town, and those who preferred the location of Letterkenny. John Nugent, the lunacy inspector, insisted that Letterkenny was the most appropriate location, describing the town in April 1860 as 'a very rising town in a fertile, populous and well-supplied district'. Nugent felt the centrality of Letterkenny was a key consideration; the towns of Lifford, Stranolar, Ballybofey, Milford, Castlefinn, Raphoe and Rathmelton were within a thirty-mile radius.[64] The choice of Letterkenny was not, however, popular among the magistrates and the landed proprietors of county Donegal. Viscount Lifford, speaking in the House of Lords, demanded that the asylum be sited in Lifford town. He suggested the decision to locate the asylum in Letterkenny reflected the Lord Lieutenant's attempt to 'set aside' the county gentry and landed proprietors in local government in Ireland.[65] The controversy raged on from April to December 1860 and occurred after the failure of the Irish Lunacy Bill, tabled by the Chief Secretary, Lord Naas in 1859. It proposed devolving control of the asylum system away from Dublin Castle to the grand jury system, which was still dominated by Protestant landed proprietors such as Lifford. Nugent opposed the bill and saw it as a threat to his position, while Catholic interests were likewise dissatisfied.[66] In county Donegal, a separate asylum was built in Letterkenny much to the dissatisfaction of Lifford.

In the Carlow district, the proposal to construct a further asylum in Wexford county – it opened in Enniscorthy in 1868 – had significant support from that town's local elites. In spite of the opening of Kilkenny asylum, by the 1860s Carlow asylum was again in a state of crisis while Kilkenny asylum was nearly full by 1856.[67] As a result, there were difficulties securing new admissions and this seemed to be particularly problematic for county Wexford. Group transfers of patients certified as 'dangerous lunatics' from county Wexford into the asylum generated a series of acrimonious communications between the Carlow governors, the lunacy administration and Wexford gaol.[68] In May and June 1846 the pressure of applicants from Wexford was particularly acute.[69] Responding in August 1847, Nugent suggested that the construction of a separate asylum in Wexford would resolve the problem and also eliminate the need to expand Carlow asylum.

At the time Nugent's proposal was not adopted, but it was prescient. A decade later, Wexford grand jury lobbied the government for a separate institution.[70] The proposal was not popular among the grand juries of counties Carlow and Kildare. In October 1856, the governors sent a deputation to the lunacy inspectors arguing that it was more economical to enlarge Carlow asylum.[71] They estimated it would cost between £10,000

and £20,000 and counties Carlow and Kildare would contribute proportionately.[72] The governors pointed out that a new asylum required the
duplication of staff, that the cost of maintaining Carlow asylum would fall
on two counties, and that county Wexford would have to be reimbursed
for the funds they contributed to the construction of the first asylum.[73]
The proposal to open an asylum in Wexford was also one of the recommendations in the 1857–58 *Report of the Commission of Inquiry into the
State of Lunatic Asylums*.[74] Although county Wexford did not meet the
lunacy inspectors' guideline that a county should have a population of
approximately 200,000 to warrant a separate asylum,[75] the inspectors and
central government decided that a separate asylum was required there.[76]
The order in council, authorising its construction in or near Enniscorthy,
was issued on 4 February 1860.[77]

    In spite of the controversy surrounding the cost of asylums built in
the 1850s, and the inspectors' anxiety to justify the continued expansion
of the asylum system, the architectural plans for the exterior of Wexford
asylum were quite ornate.[78] The architects, James Farrell and James
Bell, were both county surveyors while the contractor, Patrick Kerr, was
experienced in asylum building.[79] He had been clerk of works on Belfast
lunatic asylum from 1850 to 1854. The elevated position of Enniscorthy
asylum outside the town, its dramatic water towers – two of 112 ft, two
of 100 ft and one of 90 ft – and 'the decoration composed of contrastive
colours, mainly in the brick and stone' ensured that the building became a
regional landmark. As an editorial in the *Irish Builder* commented, 'there
is no timidity observable here; a little would have been salutary'. The
interior plans were less dramatic but still quite expansive: there were two
separate T-shaped wings for male and female patients at the end of which
were separate infirmaries. The central block, 124 ft long, contained the
physicians' residence and offices, the boardroom, the chapel, the dining-
hall, housekeeper's room and other shared or 'common' spaces. There
were also separate buildings for the kitchen, laundry and other support
services.[80]

    Work on the new asylum proceeded slowly, partly due to the size
and elaborate structure of the building. Its opening was eagerly awaited in
the region, but there were some false starts. In 1867, the lunacy inspectors prematurely announced that the asylum was complete, but only in
April 1868 were Wexford patients in Carlow asylum finally transferred
and, even then, the building was incomplete.[81] Dr Thomas W. Shiell, the

Resident Medical Superintendent at Enniscorthy asylum from 1868 to 1874, agreed to 'open a portion of the house' following repeated requests from Carlow asylum.[82] While waiting, Carlow governors requested that all new dangerous lunatic certifications from county Wexford gaols be sent directly to Enniscorthy asylum. Until the Lord Lieutenant's order declared the house to be ready, this was illegal.[83] Attempting to expedite the situation, the Carlow governors threatened to rent an auxiliary asylum to house surplus patients, the cost of which would be forwarded to the Lord Lieutenant. The Lord Lieutenant approved the proposal but the Carlow board hastily retreated, insisting it could not locate a suitable building to rent and the proposal silently disappeared.[84] Wexford patients were removed from Carlow in small groups and by July the transfer process was complete.[85]

The opening of the new asylum in Enniscorthy town was generally welcomed. The poor law guardians at Enniscorthy workhouse were keen to make use of the new facility and in March they contacted Shiell with a view to transferring some workhouse inmates.[86] The guardians were particularly anxious to remove two certified dangerous lunatics who had been accepted into the workhouse when the authorities at the gaol had refused to admit them under the 1867 amendment to the 1838 Dangerous Lunatic Act.[87] Enniscorthy guardians agreed to accommodate the patients but were concerned about the potential for violent behaviour, insisting that the asylum was the most appropriate locus of care for 'dangerous' insanity. The poor law guardians hastily transferred the two dangerous lunatics to the asylum in May 1868.[88] The new asylum also provided employment opportunities in the town. John Doyle, the Enniscorthy workhouse porter, and James Farrell, a wardsman at the workhouse 'idiot' ward, were both employed in the new institution, while most of the medical staff were local doctors.[89] The visiting physician was the Enniscorthy dispensary medical officer, Dr Thomas G. Cranfield.[90] Dr Joseph Edmundson succeeded Shiell in 1874, and, following Cranfield's death in 1872, Drapes was appointed visiting physician in March 1872.[91] In 1884 he was appointed Resident Medical Superintendent at Enniscorthy asylum, and Dr Nicholas Furlong assumed the post of visiting physician.

The completion of Enniscorthy asylum and the second programme of asylum building engendered a new sense of optimism, locally and nationally, in the curative functions of the asylums.[92] The lunacy inspectors were convinced that the problems of overcrowding at Carlow asylum had finally been resolved through the provision of 300 extra beds in Enniscorthy.[93] Initially, the population of Carlow asylum was reduced by over one-third. However, new patients quickly filled the available accommodation. The opening of Enniscorthy asylum coincided with the passage of the 1867 amendment to the 1838 Dangerous Lunatic Act and this resulted in a determined campaign on behalf of the lunacy inspectors and gaol officials to transfer dangerous lunatics, committed under the 1838 act, into asylums. Between 1867 and 1868 there was a rise in dangerous lunatics transfers to Carlow asylum as the local gaols were cleared.

After 1868, the board's reluctance to expand Carlow asylum became more determined and this sparked a dispute with county Kildare's grand jury. A threat to divide the district again emerged when the county Kildare authorities experienced difficulties in securing admissions during the first half of 1870.[94] County Kildare ratepayers became aggrieved that they were contributing taxes for the upkeep of an asylum they could not use and, consequently, the Kildare grand jury established a committee to consider the 'desirability of separation'.[95] The Carlow governors were strongly opposed to the proposal, fearing that Carlow asylum would be too large for the needs of one county and too great a burden on Carlow taxpayers. They made repeated representations to the Lord Lieutenant, requesting that county Kildare remain in Carlow asylum district and promised in return to facilitate the county's needs.[96] The governors sought the support of the ratepayers of both counties, enlisting the press in the campaign. The *Carlow Sentinel* ominously warned Kildare ratepayers that the cost of erecting a separate asylum would be £40,000. This estimate was clearly based on the cost of Enniscorthy asylum.[97] The cost of an extension to Carlow asylum was estimated to be £4,000.[98] A month later the paper published a report on the state of the institution, commissioned by the Carlow governors and compiled by two Carlow asylum doctors, the medical superintendent, Dr Michael Howlett and the visiting physician, Dr Thomas O'Meara. The report was essentially a justification of the governors' opposition to the division of the district and stressed the virtues of Carlow asylum. These were listed as its convenient location for the population of both counties and the staff's success in withstanding the spread of various epidemic diseases. The article outlined in full the structural additions completed by various managers to extend the available accommodation.[99] The report was published in the *Irish Builder* and in the *Leinster Express*, a Kildare-based newspaper. Both articles were accompanied by critical editorial commentary. The editor of the *Irish Builder* was scathing of the failure to provide new lavatories to replace the converted bathrooms, which rendered the governors 'guilty of most culpable negligence' particularly in light of the high levels of diarrhoea.[100] The *Leinster Express* echoed many of these comments and defended the actions of the Kildare grand jury, insisting that they would remove their proposal for separation when in receipt of assurances from the Carlow governors that the existing building would be augmented.[101] Such assurances had been issued the previous July, but building work had not started. The county Kildare grand jury was clearly using the threat of separation as a means of overcoming the Carlow governors' reluctance to expand the asylum. In spite of the manoeuvring, the lunacy inspectors were not in favour of separating county Kildare from the Carlow district, agreeing that the cost of erecting a new asylum and the annual expense of a separate staff would be excessive.[102]

As the debates on dividing Carlow asylum district indicate, the failure to anticipate the level of demand for asylum accommodation prompted a fundamental reassessment of the configuration of Irish asylum provision. This in turn prompted a myriad of responses at a local level. While individual county officials were concerned about the burden asylums placed on ratepayers, those without a separate institution became increasingly frustrated. From their viewpoint, they endured the financial hardships of maintaining an asylum with few of the benefits as time and again applications for admission were rejected. In some counties, the logical conclusion was to lobby for a separate institution. Individual towns and county officials perceived asylums not only as important economic and welfare providers but also as symbols of progress and modernity. These debates were not just local squabbles. They intersected with broader questions about the most effective form of local government for Ireland. As suggested in chapter one, the governance of the Irish asylum system was heavily centralised and this was resented at local level. Therefore, decisions concerning the funding of new asylums and the selection of sites became embroiled in attempts to devolve power to a local level. As discussed in the next section, this struggle to wrest more power to a local level was heightened further when counties, particularly those responsible for the first generation of asylums now in poor physical condition, were obliged to fund extensive renovation and expansion programmes.

Renovation: Local and national politics

By the 1870s Carlow asylum was in urgent need of renovation. Though the governors were obliged to delay works until the construction of Wexford asylum was completed, in June 1869 the board of control criticised them for not initiating structural alterations earlier.[103] The governors refuted the accusation that the asylum was in a 'dilapidated state', but very few improvements had been made since it was first opened in 1832.[104] The 1857–58 Inquiry into the State of Lunatic Asylums found that sanitary conditions were poor and patients were obliged to wash in open courts.[105] Although the construction of two asylums provided an additional 450 beds in the original asylum district, the pressure on accommodation continued and the institution admitted more patients than it could accommodate. Efforts to resolve these problems within the asylum included the completion of a series of renovations and extensions that were carried out between 1870 and the turn of the twentieth century after which the asylum could house 500 patients.

This process was not without its difficulties. Drawing on the controversies surrounding the renovation of the original Carlow asylum, the next section of this chapter will examine the acrimonious disputes that arose between the Carlow governors, the board of control and the lunacy inspectors concerning the cost of works and, perhaps more fundamentally, the authorisation of the work. These disputes occurred in a period that witnessed 'the disintegration' of the lunacy inspectorate.[106] Nugent and George Hatchell, who had dominated the inspectorate for decades, were now quite elderly.[107] Throughout his time on the inspectorate, Nugent had proved to be a particularly difficult personality; there were complaints from both asylum governors and from central government about his failure to fulfil his duties and he was regarded as extremely interfering and domineering. Hatchell, who was a less controversial figure, was often too ill to carry out his duties during this crucial period of expansion.[108] Thus during an important period, the lunacy inspectorate was increasingly enfeebled.

Following the removal of Wexford patients, the lunacy inspectors attempted to initiate a building programme at Carlow asylum by bringing urgent items in need of renovation to the attention of the governors.[109] Initially the board did not hesitate to instigate plans for improvements, forwarding the proposed alterations to the board of control architect in February 1869, and requesting plans and estimates.[110] By then, the architectural design of older asylums was generally regarded as outdated. William Fogerty identified the main defects as 'the limited size of the airing grounds or yards,' and the failure to provide 'separate infirmaries, day or dining-rooms and chapels.'[111] Also by the 1860s, the size and the internal layout of Irish asylums had changed considerably. Both Kilkenny and Enniscorthy asylums possessed large common rooms for patient recreation and there was a reluctance to depend exclusively on single cell accommodation. In 1860, Joseph Lalor, Resident Medical Superintendent of Kilkenny and, later, Richmond asylums, argued that large institutions such as the Colney Hatch asylum outside London could be improved as therapeutic spaces through systematic internal reorganisation rather than through ad hoc arrangements.[112] Lalor advocated dispensing with single cell accommodation and introducing larger dining halls and other communal spaces such as recreational halls and large dormitories. This would eliminate the difficulties of supervising patients in spaces divided into smaller cells and rooms.[113] Although by the 1880s Lalor had a tense relationship with Nugent, he was an influential voice in the Irish asylum system. Larcom included a copy of his article among his papers on the Irish asylum system, while the Treasury commissioners, Wilkes and Donaldson, had been favourably impressed by his methods. Lalor had been the Resident Medical Superintendent at Kilkenny asylum during their inspection in 1855, where they witnessed the recreation hall being used as a communal dining space. Previously, patients had eaten meals in separate cells. Reflecting Lalor's views, Wilkes and Donaldson opined that the collection of tranquil patients in one area would facilitate supervision and have 'moral effects on the patients themselves'.[114] The move towards increased provision of communal patient dormitories and day rooms had both a therapeutic and an economic rationale. The communal wards that replaced single cell accommodation were strictly divided by sex and there were ward divisions between chronic or tranquil patients and convalescents.

The proposals drawn up by the Carlow governors incorporated changing theories on asylum design. The board proposed three main areas for development – enlarging the dayrooms and associated dormitories, a new dining hall with additions to the kitchens and laundry rooms, and improvements to the sewerage system including the renovation of bathrooms and privies. The board of control architect, George Wilkinson, who was appointed in August 1860, produced the plans. Wilkinson is better known as the architect responsible for the design of Irish workhouses in the 1840s, which were based on two basic models, both incorporating communal spaces such as large dining halls, dormitories and separate infirmaries. During his time at the board of works, he designed asylums at Castlebar and Letterkenny.[115] The Carlow governors approved Wilkinson's plans and by March they resolved to borrow £900 to pay for the alterations to the dining hall, kitchen and laundry, plus an additional £500 to complete other repair works, including the replacement of a section of the original lead roof.[116] It was expected that these minor works would be finished by 1870.[117] The governors successfully applied to central government for an advance of £2,500 to complete the cost of the smaller alterations and the more substantial works to be carried out on the dormitories.[118]

The completion of the more substantial work was, however, delayed. By June 1870, overcrowding in the male side of the asylum was acute. There was accommodation available in the female ward for thirty-one patients but the inspectors were not willing to allow male and female patients to share wards.[119] This, and the demands from Kildare grand jury for a separate asylum, resulted in a reappraisal of the alterations proposed for Carlow asylum. In February 1871, the lunacy inspectors informed the asylum governors of an ambitious plan to extend Carlow asylum that incorporated 'two wings capable of accommodating 150 additional patients.'[120] Additional land was to be purchased to allow for a separate Gothic structure, containing two chapels, for Protestant and Catholic worship. It was estimated that the extension and the two chapels, would cost under £15,000.[121] The work received the Lord Lieutenant's sanction in 1871, although it was February 1872 when the board was notified that an order in council had been made issuing a loan of £13,000. Priority was given to the extension of the male side of the house, intended for completion by September 1872.[122] It is not clear when exactly the extension and the chapel were completed.[123] The 1874 lunacy inspectors' report included these works in an itemised list of completed work. In addition to the extension, land was purchased to extend the farm and improvements were made to the hospital. The overall cost of the work was £20,000, exceeding the original estimate considerably.[124]

In spite of the very significant expansion to the asylum, the problem of overcrowding re-emerged in the 1880s. Harvest failures caused considerable economic hardships in the period 1879 to 1883. While the worst affected regions were in the west of Ireland, other regions suffered.[125] As figure 2.1 demonstrates, admissions into Carlow asylum in this period increased and by December 1884, the asylum was once again under pressure. O'Meara, who had been appointed the Resident Medical Superintendent in 1880, converted an old dayroom into a temporary sleeping apartment and in February 1885 a room used to store timber was converted to house patients.[126] O'Meara also requested additional staff be employed to assist, particularly as the building work was causing further disruption in an already overcrowded institution. Nugent and Hatchell suggested that O'Meara place his requests before the Carlow governors, which he did in December 1889.[127] No immediate action was taken; some improvements and additions were agreed to but without any real sense of urgency. Faced with an uncooperative local board, Nugent and Hatchell did not have any appetite to compel the governors to act. In any case, by 1889 the inspectorate had all but collapsed. Hatchell retired in February 1889 while Nugent left later that year. The weakness of the inspectorate ensured that asylum governors could ignore deteriorating conditions and, as a consequence, the male side of the house, where overcrowding was again acute, became seriously dilapidated. Dayroom accommodation was insufficient, as the available space had been converted into dormitories. This left little room for daily amusements, particularly for women who worked indoors at sewing and other domestic pursuits. Patients suffering from epilepsy were confined in the few remaining single rooms, and the use of restraint, generally disapproved of, became more widespread.

With the departure of Nugent and Hatchell, a new inspectorate comprising George Plunkett O'Farrell and E. Maziere Courtenay was appointed. Although they remained 'essentially narrow' and committed to the expansion of the asylum system, O'Farrell and Courtenay brought new energy to the inspectorate and were less complacent about poor conditions in asylums.[128] Carlow asylum encountered the inspectors' new approach almost immediately in a damning account of conditions in 1890:

> Unprovided with a sufficient water supply, with its drainage system defective and obsolete, overcrowded, with insufficient accommodation and appliances for cooking and washing, with flagged stone in some parts, with wards meagrely furnished and devoid of all those comforts universally seen in modern public asylums, this institution must be looked upon as inferior to all other public asylums in Ireland, and calls for the serious consideration of all responsible for its management.[129]

The governors responded with anger, reminding the inspectors that they had 'procured plans' and had applied for a loan to complete works nearly two years previously during the declining days of Nugent's and Hatchell's inspectorate. In reality, Nugent's and Hatchell's indifference had suited the Carlow governors, who were fundamentally opposed to expansion and had adopted a policy of obstructionism. In October 1891, they refused to approve a set of plans and estimates to renovate the asylum characterising them as too expensive.[130] Throughout 1891 there was a stream of acrimonious exchanges between the Carlow governors and the board of control concerning planned renovations as the governors sought to reduce costs. While this was ongoing, O'Meara made repeated representations to the governors expressing concern over the rates of admissions and the overcrowded conditions.[131] He also adopted a policy of discharging patients to the local workhouses.[132] In spite of the crisis, the governors resisted attempts to initiate what they regarded as unnecessary alterations. There was a strong class bias in their arguments, as they attempted to protect the interests of the ratepayers against the increasing financial encroachments of the pauper classes. Though the board of control had the power to compel local boards of governors to comply with requests for expansion, the argument between the governors and the board of control continued throughout the early months of 1892. At the lunacy inspectors' suggestion, the governors appointed a committee to negotiate with the board of control and this produced a series of comprehensive 'modifications,' that halved the expense.[133] In July 1892 a compromise was reached and the inspectors reported that the board of control would carry out work on a new laundry and the laying of a new sewerage system.[134] Once this work had been started, plans for extending the accommodation were agreed upon and work commenced on the construction and remodelling of a laundry, kitchen and stores, a new male block, and the erection of padded rooms. The poor washing and sanitary facilities were to be improved with the construction of sanitary blocks.[135] By November 1894, the inspectors were pleased with progress on the dayroom and the enlargement of the kitchen.[136] The asylum was also re-decorated, to be 'bright, cheerful, well-warmed and well-ventilated'.[137] At this point it was decided to build a separate building for Protestant worship.[138] The sanitary conditions in the asylum had improved due to the work completed on the drainage system and the water supply.

Notwithstanding these improvements, the restructuring of asylum administration under the 1898 Local Government Act inhibited further progress on the renovations. As discussed in chapter one, under the 1898 act, local asylum governance was transferred into the hands of a joint asylum committee dominated by elected county councillors. The county councils were responsible for voting the money necessary for building work and, as elected representatives, councillors were even more reluctant to increase the tax burden that the asylum placed on their constituents. After 1898, the Carlow management committee, together with Sligo and Leitrim, refused or delayed authorisation of loans for renovations. While much of the renovation work on the female side of Carlow asylum was complete by 1898, due to this delay, eight months elapsed before the completed accommodation was equipped. The dayrooms on the male side remained unoccupied because there was no furniture.[139] In August 1899, E.T. Quilton, the Carlow county surveyor, requested a loan from the asylum management committee to cover escalating costs of ongoing works, but it was slow to materialise.[140] Eventually, in March 1900, the joint committee agreed to seek a loan of a further £3,500.[141] However, the Local Government Board did not sanction the loan until November 1900 and by the time of the inspectors' visit in December 1900 the male dayroom remained unoccupied.[142] Finally, during an inspection in 1905, the inspectors reported that most of the work had been completed.[143] The renovations had only limited impact on the problem of overcrowding, which was more acute on the male side. Consequently, structural alterations to the building continued: the female dayroom and the dining hall were both enlarged. The committee continued to make improvements to the house, focusing on the sanitary conditions both inside and outside the asylum, but the demand for further accommodation did not relent.

The increase in insanity?

The expansion in the number and size of asylums and high rates of pauper lunatic confinement was a national and international phenomenon. As Scull and others have demonstrated for England, Wales and Scotland, welfare provision for the insane was systematically expanded in the nineteenth century. In England and Wales the asylum population doubled between 1844 and 1860, while the general population grew by 20 per cent.[144] In Ireland, the expansion of the asylum population presented a more intractable and perplexing problem as it occurred in the context of a persistent decline in the population after the Famine. According to census returns, the number of 'lunatics and idiots' in Irish asylums almost trebled between 1871 and 1911, while the population declined by just under 20 per cent and there were additional numbers of 'lunatics and idiots' maintained in the country's workhouses.[145] Dublin Castle was primarily concerned with the financial burden the Irish asylum system placed on the exchequer.[146] However, the increase also prompted extensive debate among alienists, including the lunacy inspectorate and asylum doctors, on the prevalence and causes of mental illness in Britain and Ireland. The commentary centred on whether the increase in the number of certified patients in asylums represented a real or apparent increase and considered whether the Irish were particularly susceptible to mental illness and institutionalisation.

Theories of degeneration and hereditary insanity occupied a central place in the debate.[147] Between 1850 and 1900 these theories were extremely influential in European intellectual culture and, according to Pick, degeneracy was a 'European Disorder.'[148] In the late 1850s, theories of heredity were used to explain the accumulation of acquired pathological characteristics such as alcoholism and tuberculosis in individual patients. Bénédict-Augustin Morel (1809–73) developed the concept further, arguing that the accumulation of pathological characteristics in families across generations was part of a degenerative process, the 'key element' of which was heredity. Heredity did not produce a predisposition to a particular disease but a 'flawed condition of the nervous system – nervous disathesis – that could produce a variety of neurological and psychical disturbances'. These had the potential to spread beyond the individual.[149] While there was some resistance to Morel, the conviction that in some families hereditary influences transferred 'an organic condition that tended to make the nervous system respond to stimuli pathologically' thereby producing 'nervous disorders and diseases such as hysteria, alcoholism, scrofula, tuberculosis and rickets' gained adherents from the 1860s to the 1880s in France.[150] By the 1880s, the idea of the 'neuropathic family' was generally accepted and 'few doctors believed mental and nervous diseases could be acquired'.[151] In Britain, Henry Maudsley's elucidation of theories of degeneration and hereditary insanity, which became more explicitly bleak and pessimistic towards the end of the century, were particularly influential.[152] Maudsley was joint editor of the *Journal of Mental Science* from 1862 to 1878 and was president of the Medico-Psychological Association, which had a number of Irish members.[153] Under the influence of these late-Victorian medical theories, there was an acceptance of the existence of incurable and chronic insanity, which contrasted sharply with Thomas Spring Rice's optimistic characterisation of mental illness as a predominantly transitory and curable condition during the 1817 Select Committee hearings.[154]

The commentary on the increase in the size of the Irish asylum population was embedded in these intellectual theories and was also influenced by a similar debate on the growth of the English asylum population.[155] Pointing to the evidence in the annual reports of the commissioners in lunacy and the significant extension in asylum accommodation since the 1870s in England and Wales, Dr Frederick MacCabe, Resident Medical Superintendent at Waterford asylum, and W. J. Corbet, Chief Clerk at the Irish lunacy office, argued that the increase in admissions reflected the emergence of new cases of insanity. While acknowledging that there was a relatively low death rate in asylums and a disappointing rate of recovery, Corbet and MacCabe insisted that these factors alone could not account for the size of the English patient population. Dr Rooke Ley, Resident Medical Superintendent at Prestwich asylum, evoking theories of degeneration and hereditary insanity, argued that there was an increased incidence of specific forms of mental disease, such as general paralysis, and that the premature removal of patients from asylums allowed them to reproduce thereby contributing to the degeneration of the population.[156] Ley argued that there was a predisposition to insanity in the population rather than in an individual.

The English commissioners in lunacy discounted these arguments claiming that previous methods of gathering statistics had been inadequate, which meant cases went unrecorded and that there had been a failure to certify patients during the early stages of disease. They argued that contemporary improvements in patient treatment, greater accuracy in medical identification of illnesses and the development of a more nuanced understanding of the deleterious effects of a 'mechanical civilisation' on the mind, resulted in an increase in institutionalisation rather than the emergence of new cases.[157] Daniel Hack Tuke, Charles Lockhart Robertson[158] and Noel A. Humphreys argued along similar lines. Tuke had succeeded Maudsley as the editor of the *Journal of Mental Science*, holding the post for seventeen years before his death in 1895.[159] He published several articles in the *Journal* in which he disaggregated the statistics gleaned from the reports of the English commissioners in lunacy and the Irish lunacy inspectors, as did Lockhart Robertson and Noel Humphreys.[160] Their overarching thesis was that the increase in certified patients in asylums represented the accumulation of chronic cases and transfers from workhouses encouraged by the 1867 Metropolitan Poor Act in England. Combined, this produced the impression that the size of the asylum population had increased to an alarming degree since the 1870s. Transfers from the workhouses were regarded as particularly prob-lematic as they included a large proportion of chronic cases previously left without specialist care in workhouse 'idiot' wards. This cohort was a statistical anomaly as these patients were recorded as new certifications in the commissioners' reports and not identified as workhouse transfers. Tuke, Lockhart Robertson and Humphreys also echoed the findings of the commissioners noting there was a greater awareness of insanity as a disorder, an acceptance of asylums as appropriate sites of treatment and an expansion of definitions of insanity.[161] They concluded there was little evidence to suggest that there were an increase in new cases of insanity in England since 1878.[162]

Like his French colleagues, by the 1880s Tuke argued that 'new' cases of insanity emerged amongst 'neuropathic' families among whom nervous disorders represented the cumulative effects of hereditary influences over several generations. He therefore lamented the lack of evidence pointing to a decline in insanity in spite of the increase in scientific understanding and the expansion of asylum services. Tuke argued that the apparent increase in general paralysis amongst male and female patients, particu-larly the young, demonstrated that mental health hygiene had failed to actively combat the spread of mental diseases. He advocated that men and women be vigilant in the promotion of mental hygiene to protect new generations from disease. Lockhart Robinson also argued that the population should guard against the corrosive influence of race degenera-tion. Focusing on the impact of migration on the rural English population, Lockhart Robinson contended that not only was migration 'depriving' the insane of their 'protectors', the social and economic conditions that produced emigration contributed to the occurrence of insanity, particu-larly amongst a population deprived through 'emigration of the best and boldest of the peasantry'.[163] As Scull has noted, in promoting guidance on choice of marriage partners, Lockhart Robinson and Tuke were more optimistic than Maudsley.[164]

Tuke also reported on the rise in the Irish asylum population, exploring not only whether mental illness was on the increase, but also considering whether it was increasing at a disproportionate rate to England, Wales and Scotland. According to Dr Thomas More Madden, despite population decline in Ireland, there was one lunatic to every 214 inhabitants compared with one to every 414 in England and Wales.[165] Consequently, the discussion on Ireland focused on factors that were regarded as peculiar to the Irish asylum system and population. From the late 1850s, the Irish lunacy inspectors were faced with a degree of disquiet over disappointing recovery rates, the escalating cost of asylums and the apparently endless demands for expansion. Several editorials in the *Irish Times*, drawing in part on the inspectors' reports, were devoted to the topic.[166] The inspectors sought explanations in the different usage of certification procedures in Ireland, particularly the dangerous lunatic legislation. As demonstrated in chapters three and four, the inspectors insisted that magistrates and families used the legislation inappropriately, certifying people unsuitable for asylums and thereby contributing to the growth of the Irish asylum population. In other respects, the inspectors' analysis was similar to explanations advanced in the English lunacy commission reports. They argued that patients' improved life expectancy, public acceptance of asylums as appropriate sites of care, the expansion in definitions of mental illness, the identification of new cases and the redistribution of patients between asylums and workhouses accounted for the increase in patients.[167] By the 1870s Nugent and Hatchell concluded that lunacy in Ireland was 'not so progressive' as feared; rather there was an apparent increase caused by the accumulation of the chronically insane in the asylums. They argued that the actual proportion of the insane in the population would decrease were this category to die.[168]

Over a decade later, the continued growth in the size of the Irish asylum population was difficult to dismiss and the lunacy inspectors conceded that 'relative to a decreasing population' insanity was on the increase throughout Ireland.[169] In their first report, published in 1890, O'Farrell and Courtenay acknowledged that while changing definitions of insanity, inaccuracies in statistics and other trends affected the figures, these were 'not sufficient' to explain the extent of the increase.[170] More Madden agreed and, in a paper presented to the Academy of

Medicine in 1884, he insisted that insanity had increased among 'all classes'. However, when the Chief Secretary, John Morley, canvassed the opinions of Irish asylum doctors late in 1893, they concluded that the increase was 'due to accumulation and it is so far, an apparent and not a real increase'.[171]

Tuke and Drapes presented papers on the subject at a meeting of the Medico-Psychological Association in 1894.[172] Drapes was one of the relatively few Irish asylum doctors to publish on the causes of mental illness in Ireland and during World War I he was editor of the *Journal of Mental Science*.[173] Following the methodology adopted by Tuke in his study of admissions to English asylums, Drapes argued that the increase in Ireland was not as rapid as the stark statistics implied. Comparing figures for England and Ireland, Drapes focused primarily on the differences in the timing of asylum expansion, the lower discharge and death rates, the allegedly greater number of readmissions into Irish asylums, and the distorting effect caused by the representation of workhouse transfers in the asylum statistics. Drapes conceded that there was a higher proportion of the insane – 'certified and uncertified' – in Ireland than in England, and that the rate of increase was 'more rapid in Ireland.'[174] However, he argued that the picture was not as alarming as the statistics implied. The 'far higher proportion of readmissions in Ireland along with a great increase in admissions from workhouses' caused this increase, not the identification of new cases of insanity. While there was evidence for a 'real' but declining increase in insanity, Drapes argued that this was a result of the negative effects of hereditary insanity in the Irish population. He also acknowledged that the chronically insane would always form part of the asylum population. His arguments were echoed in the inspectors' reports in the first decades of the twentieth century.[175]

When explaining the high rates of institutionalisation of the Irish, commentators identified trends in Irish society that marked the country apart from the remainder of the United Kingdom. The high levels of emigration, political agitation surrounding the land war, campaigns for greater political autonomy and the excitable nature of the 'Celt' were identified as contributing factors.[176] Echoing Lockhart Robinson's reflections on the influence that emigration had on English rates of admissions, the Irish inspectors argued that emigration contributed in several ways. The departure of emigrants produced a vacuum in families' support mechanisms while some returned Irish migrants suffered from mental illness.[177] Emigration was believed to be detrimental to the quality of the Irish population, as the 'stronger' and more ambitious left while the remaining population was mentally inferior. The quality of the population was further undermined by 'intermarriage' among families with pathologies and nervous disorders ensuring that hereditary insanity was passed on.[178]

Towards the end of the century, these arguments were increasingly contested. Drapes claimed that the influence of emigration was 'over-estimated' and while he argued that the weaker portion of the population remained, emigrants were not always the 'stronger' members of Irish society; the return of emigrants with mental disorders was evidence of diseased nervous systems.[179] Tuke dismissed the arguments on emigration as 'absurdly illogical' and contended that the influence of emigration was limited to the increased stress placed upon family members remaining in Ireland. The relationship between emigration and asylum admissions was indirect.[180] Drawing from a comparative analysis of the ten asylum districts that exhibited the highest and lowest rates of emigration during the previous two decades, Tuke argued that though the districts with high emigration rates demonstrated a larger increase in the asylum population this was due to the factors that led to emigration such as poverty and economic stress.[181] In their responses to John Morley's 1893 request to identify the number of asylum certifications that were a result of the emigration of a family's wage earner, asylum doctors working in districts with high rates of emigration, such as Ballinasloe, Castlebar, Killarney and Maryborough, commented extensively on its influence.[182] While they acknowledged that the departure of wage earners was a factor, most doctors reported a relatively high incidence of certification among returned emigrants.[183] Two asylum doctors, Dr. W. H. Garner at Clonmel asylum and MacCabe at Waterford asylum, explicitly connected emigration with the degeneration of the race. Garner characterised emigration as 'drain[ing] the country of its bone and sinew', while MacCabe lamented that it caused the 'removal of the fittest' members of Irish society.[184]

Although Finnane has suggested that by 1900 Irish psychiatrists such as Dr Norman Connolly and Dr William Dawson were sceptical of the concept of an 'insane predisposition',[185] throughout the previous decades lunacy inspectors, asylum doctors and alienists reported hereditary factors as contributing to the rise in Irish insanity. From the 1850s, White and Nugent repeatedly asserted that 'hereditary predisposition' was one of the main 'feeders' of patients into Irish asylums and subsequent inspectors shared this conviction.[186] In 1907 O'Farrell and Courtney argued that an 'unstable nervous system' was the predisposing cause of insanity and that this was a product of a 'hereditary taint'.[187] Asylum doctors generally agreed. Drapes regarded hereditary disposition as the 'most powerful predisposing cause', but was unsure whether it was on the increase.[188] He estimated that it accounted for 20 per cent of admissions but noted that there was significant divergence between different asylums, which he attributed to faults in the collection of statistics. Drapes insisted that the increase was due to the number of transfers from the workhouses.[189] Hereditary predisposition featured prominently in the asylum doctors' evidence in 1893, and it was often linked to the failure to prevent injudicious marriages. The 'neuropathic' family, 'identified' by Dr Charles Féré, was sought in Ireland. For example, Dr A. S. Merrick, at Belfast asylum, traced 186 patients whose parents were asylum inmates, and argued that by releasing patients and allowing them to marry, the asylum was in fact assisting in the spread of mental disease.[190]

In eliciting the views of asylum doctors, the lunacy inspectors were relatively prescriptive in the directions issued to them, requiring doctors to focus on 'new attacks' of the disease, and to specifically comment on the relationship with hereditary insanity, alcohol and diet. In response, asylum doctors identified the familiar pathologies associated with theories of degeneration, particularly alcoholism. The extent and significance of alcoholism as an aetiology of insanity was contested throughout the nineteenth century. Social attitudes towards the consumption of alcohol and its illicit distillation by the Irish had been a matter of concern throughout the nineteenth century and earlier.[191] The government tightened the regulation of 'licensed drinkshops' and regulated the sale of drink at fairs, patterns and other outdoor festivals.[192] A series of restrictions were placed on the supply of drink for out-door consumption and increasingly the pub became more popular as a clearly defined site of predominantly male alcohol consumption after 1850.[193] While drink consumption at outdoor events did not disappear, by the middle of the century 'drink laws were significantly harsher in Ireland than in England'.[194] Alcohol became the subject of campaigns advocating moderation and abstinence. The temperance societies that emerged between 1829 and 1835 were successful in parts of Ulster, in contrast to Father Mathew's crusade, which had diminished by 1840. Temperance did not re-emerge as a national concern until the 1870s and even then had only limited impact on the lunatic asylums in Ireland, where it was reflected in staff's request for tea to be supplied in place of beer at Christmas dinner at Carlow asylum.[195]

There were changing medical attitudes towards alcohol that increasingly linked excessive consumption with insanity. In 1804, in a treatise primarily concerned with the typical English 'nervous patient,' Thomas Trotter argued that '[t]he habit of drunkenness is a disease of the mind.'[196] Subsequent commentators were less assured of the relationship. In 1878, the Irish lunacy inspectors commented on the increase in the number of patients exhibiting 'actual delusions', whose aetiology was identified as the abuse of alcohol. However, these cases did not result in 'genuine lunacy' rather they terminated 'for the most part in epilepsy or in disease of the brain.'[197] Nugent and Hatchell also connected alcoholism with the production of children who were born 'imbecile, idiotic, mutes or malformed'.[198] Alcoholism was a symptom of degeneracy rather than 'genuine lunacy' and was regarded as an 'exciting cause' amongst a population with a hereditary predisposition towards insanity.[199]

Nugent and Hatchell, however, shared the medical optimism in the curability of alcoholism that Stephen Snelders, Frans J. Meijman and Toine Pieters identified in medical discourses in the Netherlands. There, doctors argued that the 'manifestation of the problem [alcoholism] … was dependent on environment and circumstances' and consequently the treatment needed to be specific to patients' requirements. This required the removal of patients to a more appropriate curative environment solely devoted to their care.[200] Nugent and Hatchell supported the introduction of the Habitual Drunkards Act in 1879, which allowed 'local authorities' to issue a license to any person wishing to establish a 'retreat' for the cure of 'drunkards'.[201] Their support was coloured by an expectation that it would reduce the number of alcoholics admitted into asylums. However, the 1879 act was not as successful as the inspectors hoped and ten years after its introduction no retreat had opened in Ireland.[202]

By 1912, the inspectors' interpretation of the deleterious impact of alcohol on the mind was shifting. Courtney and O'Farrell argued that factors previously identified as 'moral' and 'physical' causes of insanity, including religion, disappointment, 'toxic agents' – alcohol and tea – 'are now looked upon as little more than the stumbling blocks, at which the unstable brain breaks down'.[203] Asylum doctors had previously identified the increased use of 'nervous stimulants' including tea, alcohol, ether and tobacco, as aggravating factors and regarded the changes in the Irish diet – the shift away from potatoes and porridge to bread and tea – as particularly deleterious. Bread was believed to be less nourishing while tea, particularly a strong concoction, was regarded as an exciting stimulant. While alcohol consumption was cited in the 1893 submission to the Chief Secretary, asylum doctors did not always identify it as a direct cause of insanity. R. V. Fletcher, Resident Medical Superintendent at Ballinasloe asylum, stated that few asylum admissions were directly caused by alcohol while Merrick claimed it was the direct cause of 11.5 per cent of admissions.[204] In the annual report published in 1912, Courtney and O'Farrell attempted to establish a statistical connection between high rates of certification, social behaviour including alcohol consumption, poverty and emigration. Their results confirmed the 1893 evidence from asylum doctors, which did not identify any significant correlation between the size of the asylum population and rates of drunkenness.[205] These changing social and medical attitudes towards alcohol were similar to the shifts Pick identified in Europe, whereby the influence of alcoholism was believed to be more evident in the effects it produced on an enfeebled portion of the population.[206]

Commentators linked the extreme poverty of the Irish population to high levels of mental illness. During the 1870s and 1880s – a period that witnessed an increase in certifications – there were several agricultural depressions that created hardship throughout Ireland, particularly in regions in the west.[207] Tuke argued that 'the poverty of the land' – meaning the poor quality of the land and living conditions – was 'well calculated to produce mental weakness and insanity',[208] while the asylum doctors cited poverty and the inferior diet as contributing factors. Courtney's and O'Farrell's comparative, county-by-county survey of rates of asylum certifications suggested that among the ten counties exhibiting the highest rates of certifications – Waterford, Kilkenny, Westmeath, Monaghan, Clare, Carlow, Meath, Tipperary, Limerick and Wexford – there was particularly high levels of pauperism. Poverty was regarded as one of the most common environmental causes of mental illness.[209]

The sheer size of the Irish asylum population also led to some speculation among medical circles as to whether the Irish as a race were more susceptible to insanity. Walsh has suggested that theories of race were influential in asylum practice in Ballinasloe asylum, linking it specifically to asylum doctors' examination of patients' physical characteristics.[210]

As historians of colonial psychiatry have argued, racial differences frequently featured in medical constructions of susceptibility to mental illness and colonial discourses were particularly pertinent where there were non-white populations.[211] Walsh is correct in noting that the inspectors commented on race, and some asylum doctors, including Drapes, explicitly used theories of racial susceptibility to mental illness. Among late nineteenth-century intellectuals, such as Francis Galton and John Beddoes, there was a rising interest in anthropology and in racial hierarchies that prompted an assessment of the nature of the Irish 'Celtic' race. L. P. Curtis has suggested that nineteenth-century anthropological interest in the Irish and ethnic differences between the Celt and the Anglo-Saxons resulted in the identification of the Irish as simianised in British literature and newspapers.[212] However, late nineteenth-century Irish scientists were less committed to the characterisation of the 'Celt' within the category of the ape and the less evolved. Peter Bowler has argued that race theorists did not 'attempt to link the Irish with an early stage in human evolution' as this would undermine the imperial project to assert the superiority of white races.[213] Instead, the 'more ancient race in Ireland' was defined as the Iberians not the Celts and though some argued that the Celtic brain was slightly smaller, differences in behaviour was due to the 'Celtic blood' and an excitable nature.[214]

In a similar vein, Drapes suggested that the 'passionate, versatile and vivacious Celtic' temperament while 'charming' ensured that the Irish were more susceptible to insanity. The Irish were an emotional race and created a large 'amount of mental excitement.' The stresses of civilisation on the nervous system of such a constitution were detrimental. While acknowledging that there were relatively few urbanised regions in Ireland, and that most of the asylum population originated in rural districts, Drapes argued that the speed with which new innovations in transport and communication had revolutionised rural life combined with the growth of new ambitions among the 'plodding' peasantry had a deleterious impact on the Irish peasantry's mental state.[215]

Drapes went on to argue that the inherently excitable temperament was not sufficiently robust to withstand the disruptive influence of Irish social and political life. When Drapes was writing in 1894, the country had gone through two decades of turbulent and disruptive events. From the 1870s onwards, political agitation over land ownership and tenants' rights had resulted in evictions, boycotts and a high level of political activity across rural communities. By 1884 this political energy was being subsumed into the movement for Home Rule. Enniscorthy town itself had a history of political unrest. Drapes maintained that these conditions were 'the ingredients for producing a large amount of mental excitement':

> Disappointed often, but still not despairing, betrayed as he has often been, he still clings with a wonderful tenacity to a picture of an ideal Ireland … Both hopes, fears and anxieties, the stirring up of emotions, some evil some generous, engendered by this almost chronic condition of political unrest can hardly fail to have a more or less injurious effect on a not-over stable kind of brain.[216]

The lunacy inspectors and Tuke also identified these disruptive elements, particularly the fear of eviction and associated poverty, as detrimental to Irish minds already destabilised through hereditary influences and disorders.[217]

Conclusion

The increase in the size of the Irish asylum population during the nineteenth century produced several contradictions and tensions for the medical and administrative management of the mentally ill. The problem of overcrowding was eventually alleviated when a balance between supply and demand of asylum beds was reached in the twentieth century. Prior to this, local authorities actively sought the construction of institutions in counties not only to secure the practical advantages that an asylum brought to a county town, but also because the lunatic asylums had become emblems of civic pride. As one Kildare councillor commented 'all towns of significance … should possess hospitals and asylums of good quality'.[218] Once institutional development was achieved and individual institutions were pressured to expand, local concerns quickly morphed, and politicians and magistrates baulked at the associated tax burden. The events following the introduction of the 1898 act indicates that the devolution of certain financial power to a local level allowed asylum boards to obstruct building work quite effectively. The construction of new asylums was also part of broader debates on the form and efficiency of local government in Ireland. In the struggle to retain local autonomy, the asylum system, in addition to the poor law unions, became an arena in which the infringe-ments of central government were resisted.

The expansion of the Irish asylum system, fuelled by the seemingly inexhaustible pressure for asylum admissions, produced some worrying statistics. By the late nineteenth century, Ireland boasted the highest per capita rate of certification in the United Kingdom, leading some to conclude that there was a greater propensity towards mental illness among the Irish. In explaining this phenomenon, commentators disagreed on the most important 'aggravating' or 'exciting' causes as emigration, political and social agitation, fear of eviction, extreme poverty and shifting dietary habits were identified as aggravating factors.[219] While debates on racial difference also featured, by the late nineteenth century commentators on Ireland, in line with the European intellectual climate, deployed theories of degeneration and hereditary influences to account for the size of the Irish asylum population.

Notes

1   *Leinster Leader* (24 March 1900).
2   *Fourteenth Report of Prison Inspectors*, H. C. 1836 [118] xxxv, p. 32.
3   *Returns Relating to District Asylums in Ireland*, H. C. 1833 [695] xxxiv, p. 21.
4   DPH, CLA Minute Book, 3 May 1832, 6 September 1832.
5   *Sixth Report of Prison Inspectors*, H. C. 1828 [68] xii, p. 11; *Seventh Report of Prison Inspectors*, H. C. 1829 [10] xiii, p. 13.
6   *Ninth Report of Prison Inspectors*, H. C. 1830–31 [172] iv, p. 9.
7   *Report of Lunacy Inspectors*, H. C. 1845 [645] xxvi, p. 21.
8   Edginton, 'A Space for Moral Management', p. 94; Reuber, 'Moral Management and the "Unseen Eye"', pp. 221–223.
9   *Sixteenth Report of Prison Inspectors*, H. C. 1837–38 [186] xxix, p. 36.
10 *Report of Lunacy Inspectors*, H. C. 1844 [567] xxx, p. 25.
11 *Ibid.*; *Report of Lunacy Inspectors*, H. C. 1845 [645] xxvi, pp. 19–21.
12 *Report of Lunacy Inspectors*, H. C. 1845 [645] xxvi, pp. 19–21.
13 J. Moykr, *Why Ireland Starved? A Quantitative and Analytical History of the Irish Economy, 1800–1850* (London: George Allen and Unwin, 1983), pp. 264–268.
14 Ó Cathaoir, 'The Poor Law in County Carlow, 1838–1923', pp. 691–700; K. Kiely, 'Poverty and Famine in county Kildare, 1820–1850', in W. Nolan and T. McGrath (eds), *Kildare: History and Society. Interdisciplinary Essays on the History of an Irish County* (Dublin: Geography Publications, 2006), pp. 507–514.
15 Kiely, 'Poverty and Famine', p. 510.
16 Ó Cathaoir, 'The Poor Law in County Carlow', p. 702.

17 *Fifth Report of Lunacy Inspectors*, H. C. 1851 [138] xxiv, p. 8.
18 O. Walsh, '"A Lightness of Mind": Gender and Insanity in Nineteenth-Century Ireland', in M. Kelleher and J. H. Murphy (eds), *Gender Perspectives in Nineteenth-Century Ireland* (Dublin: Four Courts Press, 1997), p. 163; C. Ó Gráda, *Black '47 and Beyond: the Great Irish Famine in History, Economy and Memory* (New Jersey: Princeton University Press, 1999), pp. 178–182.
19 The exact family relationship was not always provided.
20 D. Fitzpatrick, *Irish Emigration 1801–1921* (Dublin: Dundalgan Press, 1984), pp. 9–13.
21 Ó Cathaoir, 'The Poor Law in County Carlow', p. 706.
22 *Ibid.*, p. 703.
23 *Ninth Report of Lunacy Inspectors*, H. C. 1849 [1054] xxiii, p. 3.
24 Chapter seven.
25 Finnane, *Insanity and the Insane*, p. 36.
26 *Report of Lunacy Inspectors*, H. C. 1845 [645] xxvi, pp. 19–21.
27 *Report of Lunacy Inspectors*, H. C. 1849 [1054] xxiii, p. 6.
28 *Sixty-third Report of Lunacy Inspectors*, H. C. 1914 [Cd. 7527] xli, p. xvi.
29 Finnane, *Insanity and the Insane*, p. 34.
30 *Ibid.* and chapter one, fn 71.
31 *Sixteenth Report of Prison Inspectors*, H. C. 1837–8 [186] xxix, p. 36.
32 DPH, CLA Minute Book, 20 May 1840.
33 57 Geo. iii c.106 (1817).
34 Finnane, *Insanity and the Insane*, p. 32.
35 *Ibid.*, p. 37 and appendix table A.
36 *Report of Lunacy Inspectors*, H. C. 1846 [736] xxii, pp. 6–7.
37 *Third Report of Lunacy Inspectors*, H. C. 1847 [820] xvii, p. 31.
38 Walsh, 'Lunatic and Criminal Alliances in Nineteenth-Century Ireland', pp. 132–152.
39 H. Marland, *Medicine and Society in Wakefield and Huddersfield, 1780–1870* (Cambridge: Cambridge University Press, 1989), p. 124.
40 Finnane, *Insanity and the Insane*, pp. 36–37.
41 Vignoles was the Dean of Ossory and a founding member of the Kilkenny Archaeological Society, see F. Carson Williams, 'Vignoles, Charles Augustus', in J. McGuire and J. Quinn (eds), *The Dictionary Irish Biography*, 9 (Cambridge: Cambridge University Press, 2009), pp. 665–666.
42 National Archives of Ireland (hereafter NAI), Chief Secretary's Office Registered Papers (hereafter CSORP), G12292, Letter from Charles Vignoles to the Lord Lieutenant, 22 July 1846.
43 *Third Report of Lunacy Inspectors*, H. C. 1847 [820] xvii, p. 12, p. 30.
44 *Eighth Report of Lunacy Inspectors*, H. C. 1857 session 2 [2253] xvii, p. 7.
45 DPH, CLA Minute Book, 20 October 1852; *Eighth Report of Lunacy Inspectors*, H. C. 1857 session 2 [2253] xvii, p. 6.
46 *Fourth Report of Lunacy Inspectors*, H. C. 1849 [1054] xxiii, p. 5.
47 *Report of the Commissioners Appointed to Ascertain the Equitable Amount to be Repaid by Counties in Ireland Transferred to other Lunatic Asylum Districts*, H. C. 1857 [277] xvii, p. 4.
48 NLI, Larcom Papers, Ms 7775, p. 3.

49 Finnane, *Insanity and the Insane*, p. 37.
50 See the example of Cork asylum, NLI, Larcom Papers, Ms 7775.
51 NLI, Larcom Papers, Ms 7775, p. 3.
52 Chapter one; Finnane, *Insanity and the Insane*, p. 37.
53 NLI, Larcom Papers, Ms 7775, Letter from James Wilkes to Thomas Larcom, 13 August 1855.
54 NLI, Larcom Papers, Ms 7775: *Copy of Treasury Minute, dated 10 August 1855, Appointing a Commission for Inquiring into the Erection of District Lunatic Asylums in Ireland; of the Report of the said Commissioners, dated 14 December 1855; and of further Treasury Minute, dated 18 December 1855*, H. C. 1856 [9] liii.
55 *Express* (29 August 1863).
56 Finnane, *Insanity and the Insane*, p. 32; Reuber, 'Moral Management and the "Unseen Eye"', p. 229.
57 Reuber, 'Moral Management and the "Unseen Eye"', p. 226.
58 A. Scull, C. MacKenzie and N. Hervey, *Masters of Bedlam. The Transformation of the Mad-Doctoring Trade* (New Jersey: Princeton University Press, 1996), pp. 191–192.
59 Fogerty, 'On the Planning of Lunatic Asylums'.
60 *Copy of Treasury Minute, dated 10 August 1855*, H. C. 1856 [367] liii, p. 5.
61 *Ibid.*, pp. 6–8.
62 Finnane, *Insanity and the Insane*, p. 37.
63 NLI, Larcom Papers Ms 7776, Newspaper cuttings, *Clare Journal* (1 December 1859).
64 NLI, Larcom Papers Ms 7776, Memorandum to John Nugent, 30 April 1860.
65 NLI, Larcom Papers Ms 7776, Newspaper cuttings, *Express* (12 May 1860).
66 Finnane, *Insanity and the Insane* p. 39.
67 *Eighth Report of Lunacy Inspectors*, H. C. 1857 session 2 [2253] xvii, p. 64.
68 DPH, CLA Minute Book, 16 June 1841.
69 *Ibid.*, 18 August 1847.
70 *Eighth Report of Lunacy Inspectors*, H. C. 1857 session 2 [2253] xvii, p. 6.
71 NAI, OLA/1, Minute Book of the Office of the Lunatic Asylums (Ireland), 16 October 1856.
72 DPH, CLA Minute Book, 15 October 1856, 19 November 1856.
73 *Ibid.*, 19 November 1856.
74 *Inquiry into the State of Lunatic Asylums and other Institutions*, p. 23.
75 NLI, Larcom Papers, Ms 7776, Newspaper cuttings, *Express* (25 October 1861).
76 *Eighth Report of Lunacy Inspectors*, H. C. 1857 session 2 [2253] xvii, p. 6.
77 *Tenth Report of Lunacy Inspectors*, H. C. 1861 [2901] xxvii, p. 4.
78 *Eleventh Report of Lunacy Inspectors*, H. C. 1862 [2975] xxiii, p. 7, p. 26.
79 'James Farrell' and 'James Bell', Dictionary of Irish Architects, 1720–1940 (Irish Architectural Archive, www.dia.ie).
80 'Lunatic Asylum, Enniscorthy', *Irish Builder*, 8:146 (15 January 1866), 20.
81 *Seventeenth Report of Lunacy Inspectors*, H. C. 1867–68 [4053] xxxi, p. 10.
82 SPH, ELA Letter Book, letter from Thomas W. Shiell to the Lunacy Inspectors, 2 April 1868.
83 SPH, ELA Letter Book, letter from Thomas W. Shiell to Joseph Gladwin, governor Wexford gaol, 22 February 1868.

84   DPH, CLA Minute Book, 17 February 1868.
85   *Seventeenth Report of Lunacy Inspectors*, H. C. 1867–68 [4053] xxxi, p. 10; *Eighteenth Report of Lunacy Inspectors*, H. C. 1868–69 [418] xxvii, p. 16.
86   Wexford County Archives Service (hereafter WCA), WX/BG 87/1/1/41, Enniscorthy Board of Guardians Minute Book, 25 January 1868, 7 March 1868.
87   *Ibid.*, 11 April 1868.
88   *Ibid.*, 23 May 1868.
89   *Ibid.*, 30 May 1868.
90   *Wexford Lunatic Asylum. Returns of the Names of the Governors of the Wexford Lunatic Asylum, Specifying by Whom Appointed*, H. C. 1867–68 [442] lv.
91   WCA, WX/BG 87/1/3/1, Enniscorthy Dispensary Minute Book, 6 August 1878; SPH, Proceedings of the Governors and Directors of the Wexford District Lunatic Asylum, Enniscorthy, Minute Book, 21 March 1872.
92   NLI, Larcom Papers, Ms 7776, Thomas Larcom 'New Lunatic Asylums', p. 1.
93   *Eighteenth Report of Lunacy Inspectors*, H. C. 1868–69 [418] xxvii, p. 16.
94   *Ibid.*
95   DPH, CLA Minute Book, 26 July 1870.
96   *Ibid.*, 26 July 1870, 17 October 1871.
97   *Carlow Sentinel* (3 September 1870); 'Lunatic Asylum, Enniscorthy', *Irish Builder*, 8:146 (January, 1866), 20.
98   *Carlow Sentinel* (3 September 1870).
99   *Ibid.*
100 'Carlow District Lunatic Asylum', *Irish Builder*, 12:266 (October, 1870).
101 *Leinster Express* (8 October 1870).
102 DPH, CLA Minute Book, 20 February 1871.
103 *Ibid.*, 14 June 1869.
104 *Carlow Sentinel* (23 July 1870).
105 *Inquiry into the State of Lunatic Asylums and other Institutions*, p. 13.
106 Finnane, *Insanity and the Insane*, p. 65.
107 *Ibid.*
108 *Ibid.*, pp. 63–67.
109 *Eighteenth Report of Lunacy Inspectors*, H. C.1868–69 [418] xxvii, p. 16.
110 DPH, CLA Minute Book, 8 February 1869.
111 Fogerty, 'On the Planning of Lunatic Asylums', 39.
112 'J. Lalor', *JMS*, 32:139 (October, 1886), 462–463.
113 J. Lalor, 'Observations on the Size and Construction of Lunatic Asylums', *JMS*, 7: 35 (October 1860), 104–111.
114 *Copy of Treasury Minute, dated 10 August 1855*, H. C. 1856 [9] liii.
115 'George Wilkinson', Dictionary of Irish Architects, 1720–1940 (Irish Architectural Archive, www.dia.ie).
116 DPH, CLA Minute Book, 15 March 1869.
117 *Nineteenth Report of Lunacy Inspectors*, H. C. 1870 [C. 202] xxxiv, p. 12.
118 DPH, CLA Minute Book, 28 June 1869.
119 *Ibid.*, 13 June 1870; *Carlow Sentinel* (23 July 1870); *Nineteenth Report of Lunacy Inspectors*, H. C. 1870 [C. 202] xxxiv, p. 12.

120 DPH, CLA Minute Book, 19 February 1872, 20 February 1871.

121 'Carlow District Lunatic Asylum', *Irish Builder*, 13:278 (July, 1871), p. 188.

122 DPH, CLA Minute Book, 19 February 1872.

123 Minute Books for the period 1873–1879 have not survived.

124 *Twenty-fourth Report of Lunacy Inspectors*, H. C. 1875 [C. 1293] xxxiii, p. 31.

125 Crossman, *Politics, Pauperism and Power*, pp. 106–143; Ó Cathaoir, 'The Poor Law in County Carlow'.

126 DPH, CLA Minute Book, 12 December 1884, 13 February 1885. Dr Thomas O'Meara (d. 1903) M.B. T.C.D. LRCSI (1872). He served as assistant house-surgeon to the Borough Hospital at Birkenhead in England prior to his appointment as Resident Medical Superintendent at Carlow Asylum in 1880 where he remained until 1903, see *Medical Press and Circular* (10 November, 1880), (24 November 1880).

127 DPH, CLA Minute Book, 13 December 1889.

128 Finnane, *Insanity and the Insane*, pp. 68–70.

129 *Fortieth Report of Lunacy Inspectors*, H. C. 1890–91 [C. 6503] xxxvi, p. 119.

130 DPH, CLA Minute Book, 9 October 1891.

131 For examples, see *Ibid.*, 10 April 1891, 8 May 1891, 12 June 1891 and 11 September 1891.

132 *Forty-second Report of Lunacy Inspectors*, H. C. 1893–4 [C. 7125] xlvi, p. 97.

133 *Forty-first Report of Lunacy Inspectors*, H. C. 1892 [C. 6803] xl, p. 9.

134 DPH, CLA Minute Book, 8 July 1892.

135 *Forty-third Report of Lunacy Inspectors*, H. C. 1894 [C. 7466] xliii, p. 15.

136 *Forty-fourth Report of Lunacy Inspectors*, H. C. 1895 [C. 7804] liv, pp. 97–98.

137 *Forty-eighth Report of Lunacy Inspectors*, H. C. 1899 [C. 9479] xl, p. 131.

138 *Forty-seventh Report of Lunacy Inspectors*, H. C. 1898 [C. 8969] xliii, p. 21.

139 *Ibid.*, p. 117; *Forty-ninth Report of Lunacy Inspectors* H. C. 1900 [Cd. 312] xxxvii, p. 119.

140 DPH, CLA Minute Book, 9 August 1899.

141 *Ibid.*, 14 March 1900, 11 April 1900.

142 *Annual Report for the Local Government Board for Ireland 1901*, H. C. 1902 [Cd. 1259] xxxvii, p. 105; *Fiftieth Report of Lunacy Inspectors*, H. C. 1901 [Cd. 760] xxviii, p. 93.

143 *Fifty-fifth Report of Lunacy Inspectors*, H. C. 1906 [Cd. 3164] xxxix, p. xxix.

144 Scull, *The Most Solitary of Afflictions*. pp. 335–336.

145 Vaughan and Fitzpatrick (eds), *Population Historical Statistics*, p. 3; *Sixty-second Nineteenth Report of Lunacy Inspectors*, H. C. 1913 [Cd 6935], xxxiv, p. x; Finnane, *Insanity and the Insane*, p. 53.

146 Finnane, *Insanity and the Insane*, p. 53.

147 L. J. Ray, 'Models of Madness in Victorian Asylum Practice', *Archives of European Sociology*, 22 (1981), 229–264.

148 D. Pick, *Faces of Degeneracy. A European Disorder, c.1848–c.1918* (Cambridge: Cambridge University Press, 1989).

149 I. R. Dowbiggan, *Inheriting Madness: Professionalisation and Psychiatric Knowledge in Nineteenth-Century France* (California and Oxford: University of California Press, 1991), pp. 117–119.

150 Dowbiggan, *Inheriting Madness*, pp. 120–121.

151 *Ibid.*, p. 123.
152 Scull, MacKenzie and Hervey (eds), *Masters of Bedlam*, pp. 226–267; Ray, 'Models of Madness'.
153 D. Healy, 'Irish Psychiatry. Part 2: Use of the Medico-Psychological Association by its Irish Members – Plus ça Change!', in H. Freeman and G. H. Berrios (eds), *150 Years of British Psychiatry* (London: The Athlone Press, 1996), pp. 314–320.
154 Ray, 'Models of Madness', 234, 246 and see chapter one.
155 D. H. Tuke, 'Alleged Increase of Insanity', JMS, 40:169 (April, 1894), 219–231; C. Lockhart Robertson, 'Further Notes on The Alleged Increase in Insanity', JMS, 16:76 (1871), 473–497; N. A. Humphreys, 'The Alleged Increase of Insanity', *Journal of the Royal Statistical Society*, 70: 2 (1907), 203–241.
156 'The Increase of Lunacy', *North British Review Art* (March, 1869); F. MacCabe, 'On the Alleged Increase in Lunacy,' JMS, 15:71 (October, 1869), 363–366; W. J. Corbet, 'The Increase of Insanity', *Fortnightly Review*, 61:362 (1897), 321–442; Tuke, 'Alleged Increase of Insanity'.
157 Ray, 'Models of Madness', 232.
158 President of the Medico-Psychological Association, Medical Superintendent of the Sussex Lunatic Asylum, Hayward's Heath and Lord Chancellor's Visitor in Lunacy, see Scull, MacKenzie and Hervey, *Masters of Bedlam*, p. 261.
159 A. Digby, 'Tuke, Daniel Hack (1827–1895)', *Oxford Dictionary of National Biography*, 55 (Oxford: Oxford University Press, 2004), pp. 535–537.
160 D. H. Tuke, 'Alleged Increase in Insanity', JMS, 32:139 (October, 1886), 360–376'; D. H. Tuke, 'Alleged Increase in Insanity', JMS, 40:169 (April, 1894), 219–331; D. H. Tuke, 'Increase in Insanity in Ireland', JMS, 40:171 (October 1894), 549–361; C. Lockhart Robinson, 'The Alleged Increase in Insanity', JMS, 15:69 (April, 1869), 1–23; Lockhart Robinson, 'Further Notes on The Alleged Increase in Insanity'; Humphreys, 'The Alleged Increase of Insanity'.
161 Tuke, 'Alleged Increase in Insanity', JMS (October 1886); Tuke, 'Alleged Increase in Insanity', JMS (April, 1894); Lockhart Robinson, 'The Alleged Increase in Insanity'; Lockhart Robinson, 'Further Notes on The Alleged Increase in Insanity'; Humphreys, 'The Alleged Increase of Insanity'.
162 Tuke, 'Alleged Increase in Insanity', JMS, 32:139 (October, 1886), 363.
163 Lockhart Robinson, 'Further Notes on The Alleged Increase in Insanity', 494–496.
164 Scull, *Masters of Bedlam*, p. 261.
165 T.M. Madden, 'On the Increase of Insanity, with Suggestions for the Reform of Lunacy Laws and Practice,' DJMS, 78 (July–December, 1884), 303–314, 304–305.
166 *Irish Times* (23 September 1859); *Irish Times* (22 October 1861); *Irish Times* (22 July 1864); *Freeman's Journal* (20 July 1864).
167 Scull, *The Most Solitary of Afflictions*, pp. 338–340; *Tenth Report of Lunacy Inspectors*, H. C. 1861 [2901] xxvii, p. 14, *Thirteenth Report of Lunacy Inspectors*, H. C. 1864 [3369] xxiii, pp. 9–10; *Twenty-second Report of Lunacy Inspectors*, H. C. 1873 [C. 852] xxx, pp. 5–6, *Twenty-fourth Report of Lunacy Inspectors*, H. C. 1875 [C. 1293] xxxiii, p. 6.
168 *Twenty-third Report of Lunacy Inspectors*, H. C. 1874 [C. 1004] xxvii, p. 7.
169 *Thirty-sixth Report of Lunacy Inspectors*, H. C. 1887 [C. 5121] xxxix, p. 6.
170 *Forty-second Report of Lunacy Inspectors*, H. C. 1893–94 [C. 7125] clvi, p. 3.

171 *Forty-third Report of Lunacy Inspectors*, H. C. 1894 [7466] xliii, p. 4.

172 T. Drapes, 'On the Alleged Increase of Insanity in Ireland', *JMS*, 40:171 (October, 1894), 519–548; D. H. Tuke, 'Increase of Insanity in Ireland', *JMS*, 40:171 (October, 1894), 549–561.

173 Drapes, 'On the Alleged Increase of Insanity in Ireland'; T. Drapes, 'Psychology in Ireland', *DJMS*, 87: 7 (1889), 109–116. Educated at Trinity College Dublin, Drapes achieved his medical degree and his license in midwifery from the Rotunda Hospital in 1871, see *Irish Times* (31 July 1871); (7 October 1919); (16 October 1919).

174 Drapes, 'On the Alleged Increase of Insanity', 529.

175 *Sixty-second Report of Lunacy Inspectors*, H. C. 1913 [Cd 6935], xxxiv, pp. xiv–xvi.

176 A broader analysis of causes deployed in Irish asylum practise is discussed in chapter seven.

177 *Tenth Report of Lunacy Inspectors*, H. C. 1861 [2901] xxvii, p.14; *Thirteenth Report of Lunacy Inspectors*, H. C. 1864 [3369] xxiii, p. 6; *Thirty-second Report of Lunacy Inspectors*, H. C. 1883 [C. 3675] xxx, p. 7, p. 12; *Twenty-fourth Report of Lunacy Inspectors*, H. C. 1875 [1293] xxxiii, p. 5.

178 *Forty-first Report of Lunacy Inspectors*, H. C. 1892 [C. 6803] xl, pp. 2–3.

179 Drapes, 'On the Alleged Increase of Insanity', 536.

180 Tuke, 'Increase of Insanity in Ireland', 551.

181 *Ibid.*, 552–553.

182 *Alleged Increasing Prevalence of Insanity in Ireland. Special Report from the Inspectors of Lunatics to the Chief Secretary*, H. C. 1894 [C. 7331] xliii, p. 4.

183 *Ibid.*, p. 6, p. 8, p. 9.

184 *Ibid.*, p. 6, p. 12, pp. 15–16.

185 M. Finnane, 'Irish Psychiatry. Part 1: The Formation of a Profession', in H. Freeman and G. E. Berrios (eds), *150 Years of British Psychiatry* (London: Tavistock, 1996), p. 311.

186 *Eighth Report of Lunacy Inspectors*, H. C. 1857 session 2 [2253] xvii, p. 13; *Twenty-third Report of Lunacy Inspectors*, H. C. 1874 [C. 1004] xxvii, p. 8; *Twenty-seventh Report of Lunacy Inspectors*, H. C. 1878 [C. 2037] xxxix, p. 9.

187 *Fifty-seventh Report of Lunacy Inspectors*, H. C. 1908 [4302] xxxiii, p.xxvi.

188 Drapes, 'On the Alleged Increase', 534.

189 *Alleged Increasing Prevalence of Insanity in Ireland*, p. 7.

190 *Ibid.*, p. 5.

191 E. Malcolm, 'Ireland Sober, Ireland Free' Drink and Temperance in Nineteenth Century Ireland* (Dublin: Gill and Macmillan, 1986); K. H. Connell, *Irish Peasant Society* (Oxford: Clarendon Press, 1968), pp. 1–50.

192 E. Malcolm, 'The Rise of the Pub: A Study in the Disciplining of Popular Culture', in J. S. Donnelly Jr. and K. A. Miller (eds), *Irish Popular Culture* (Dublin: Irish Academic Press, 1998), pp. 50–77.

193 D. McCabe, 'Open Court: Law and the Expansion of Magisterial Jurisdiction at Petty Sessions in Nineteenth-Century Ireland', in N. M. Dawson (ed.), *Reflections on Law and History* (Dublin: Four Courts Press, 2006), pp. 144–145; Malcolm, 'The Rise of the Pub', p. 71.

194 McCabe, 'Open Court', p. 145.

195   For example, see DPH, CLA Minute Book, December 1850.

196   W. F. Bynum, 'The Nervous Patient in Eighteenth- and Nineteenth-Century Britain: the Psychiatric Origins of British Neurology', in W. F. Bynum, R. Porter and M. Shepherd (eds), *Anatomy of Madness: Essays in the History of Psychiatry*, I (London: Tavistock, 1988), pp. 89–102; R. Hunter and I. MacAlpine, *Three Hundred Years of Psychiatry 1535–1860* (London: Oxford University Press, 1963), p. 589.

197   *Twenty-third Report of Lunacy Inspectors*, H. C. 1874 [C. 1004] xxvii, p. 7.

198   *Ibid.*

199   *Twenty-seventh Report of Lunacy Inspectors*, H. C. 1878 [C. 2037] xxxix, p. 9.

200   S. Snelders, F. J. Meijman and T. Pieters, 'Heredity and Alcoholism in the Medical Sphere: the Netherlands, 1850–1900', *Medical History*, 51 (2007), 219–236.

201   42&43 Vict. c.19 (1879).

202   *Ninth Report of the Inspectors of Retreats under the Inebriates Acts, 1879 and 1888*, H. C. 1889 [C. 5841] xviii; G. Bretherton, 'Irish Inebriate Reformatories, 1899–1902: an Experimentation in Coercion', in I. O'Donnell and F. McAuley (eds), *Criminal Justice History. Themes and Controversies from Pre-Independence Ireland* (Dublin: Four Courts Press, 2003), pp. 214–232.

203   *Fifty-seventh Report of Lunacy Inspectors*, H. C. 1908 [4302] xxxiii, pp. xxvi–xxvii. *Sixty-first Report of Lunacy Inspectors*, H. C. 1912–13 [C. 6386] xxxix, p. xix.

204   *Alleged Increasing Prevalence of Insanity in Ireland*, p. 5.

205   *Ibid.*

206   *Twenty-seventh Report of Lunacy Inspectors*, H. C. 1878 [C. 2037] xxxix, p. 9; Pick, *Faces of Degeneracy*, pp. 201–202.

207   Crossman, *Politics, Pauperism and Power*, pp. 106–143.

208   Tuke, 'Increase of Insanity in Ireland', 553.

209   *Sixty-first Report of Lunacy Inspectors*, H. C. 1912 [Cd 6386], xxxix, p. xiv–xxi.

210   O. Walsh, '"The Designs of Providence": Race, Religion and Irish Insanity', in Melling and Forsythe (eds), *Insanity, Institutions and Society*, pp. 235–236.

211   S. Mahone and M. Vaughan (eds), *Psychiatry and Empire* (Houndmills: Palgrave Macmillan, 2007), p. 3.

212   L. P. Curtis, *Apes and Angels. The Irishman in Victorian Caricature* (Washington and London: Smithsonian Institution Press, 1997); Pick, *Faces of Degeneracy*, p. 177.

213   P. Bowler, 'Race Theory and the Irish', in S. Ó Síocháin (ed.), *Social Thought on Ireland in the Nineteenth Century* (Dublin: University College Dublin, 2009), p. 142.

214   Bowler, 'Race Theory', pp. 140–141.

215   Drapes, 'On the Alleged Increase of Insanity', 531–532.

216   *Ibid.*, 532.

217   *Forty-third Report of Lunacy Inspectors*, H. C 1894 [C. 7466] xliii, pp. 4–5; Tuke, 'Increase of Insanity in Ireland', 553.

218   *Leinster Leader* (24 March 1900).

219   Tuke, 'Increase of Insanity in Ireland', 555.

3

Routes into the asylums

In Ireland, most patients were institutionalised using one of three certification procedures. Asylum governors were entitled to certify patients
– referred to as 'ordinary' certification – while asylum physicians authorised
'urgent' admissions. Most patients were certified however as 'dangerous
lunatics'. Certification 'divided the sane from the insane' and represented
'the crucible in which medical approaches to insanity were mixed with lay
ideas of insanity.'[1] A thorough understanding of certification procedures
and forms facilitates an analysis of the importance of medical evidence
and authority in the confinement of the mentally ill in this period when
medicine was established as a profession. Asylum staff transcribed lay
and medical evidence, recorded in original certification documents, into
asylum casebooks. This ensured that the certification documents shaped
clinical histories and influenced patients' experiences in the asylum. It
is therefore not only important to understand the legal framework that
governed certification procedures, but also how certification forms were
constructed and how families, legal, medical and administrative officials
interacted with both the procedures and the documentation.

By the early twentieth century over 70 per cent of male and 60
per cent of female patients in Irish asylums were certified as 'dangerous
lunatics' and, consequently, that legislation has preoccupied scholars.[2]
There is general agreement that the legislation facilitated committal
and established an overt link between lunacy and criminality.[3] Finnane
has exposed the limitations of the legislation and explored attempts to
eliminate abuses of the act, while Pauline Prior has focused on the official
debate that surrounded its use.[4] Walsh has looked at the legislation in the

context of Connaught asylum district in county Galway, and, like Prior, has situated the extensive use of the legislation within the context of state concern for national security, land agitation and political disaffection.[5]

The main aim of this, and the succeeding chapter, is to reconsider these interpretations by assessing the evolution of the different certification procedures in Ireland, and the negotiations that surrounded the use of each procedure. The regulation of 'ordinary' certifications has received limited scholarly attention and we know relatively little about the procedures and how they evolved. As will be demonstrated, over the course of the nineteenth century the evolution and regulation of certification procedures and forms encompassed attempts to enhance the importance of medical evidence and to harmonise differing procedures. It also reflected changes in medical preoccupations and understandings of mental illness.[6] Medical participation in dangerous lunatic certifications was enhanced over time though magistrates and family members mediated these admissions. The lunacy inspectors introduced a series of changes to the regulations governing 'ordinary' certifications that endeavoured to establish asylum resident medical superintendents as 'gatekeepers'. Finnane argues that this was successful and by the end of the century, resident medical superintendents exercised a monopoly over 'ordinary' certifications.[7]

Drawing heavily from local asylum records, this chapter suggests that the process was not as successful as previously argued. The statistics cited here are gleaned from Carlow asylum admission registers, 1832 to 1922. By focusing on Carlow asylum, the older of the two institutions, a thorough assessment of shifts and continuities in the use of differing admission procedures throughout the nineteenth century is possible. For the purpose of analysis the period was divided into two phases: 1832 to 1867 and 1868 to 1922. This methodology allowed for an analysis of the use of 'ordinary' certification procedures before the 1867 amendment to the 1838 Dangerous Lunatic Act came to dominate certification procedures.

Regulating certification procedures

The principle of legal certification of pauper lunatics was introduced to Ireland in the eighteenth century under vagrancy and prison legislation. Though the legislation was primarily concerned with containing vagrancy and criminality, section twelve of the 1787 Prisoners (Ireland)

Act specified that two magistrates could certify and confine idiots and the insane in separate wards in prisons.[8] The medical and legal certification of private patients was established in 1842 under the Private Asylums (Ireland) Act, which required two doctors to separately examine individuals before signing a certification form.[9] In contrast to the English lunacy legislation, the Irish 1817 Lunacy Act, and the subsequent 1821 amendment, did not include details of certification procedures.[10] Due to the absence of specific legislation and the delay in devising the privy council rules, most district asylums modified the admission regulations in operation at the influential Armagh asylum.[11] The Armagh rules ensured that certification was at the discretion of lay asylum governors and managers. The rules advised governors and managers to establish 'a principle of selection' and admit 'those cases which come strictly under the denomination of lunatics.' As a result, idiots and epileptics were to be excluded.[12] To document the procedure, the Armagh governors devised certification forms and in these the criteria that determined the certification of pauper admissions to Irish asylums were established. Relatives and friends were required to swear to the poverty of the person and to an inability to pay for accommodation in private lunatic asylums.[13] Two relatives had to agree to remove the patient when he/she recovered or ceased to pose any danger. Additional testimony provided by a magistrate, parish minister or church-warden confirmed that the individual was both dangerous and poor.[14] Finally, a medical certificate of insanity accompanied the application providing the medical 'legitimisation' of pauper committals. This medical certificate asserted that the individual was curable, however, it did not include descriptions of the behaviour that led to a diagnosis of mental illness. The doctor confirmed he had examined the patient, and that the individual was dangerous and suitable for confinement in an asylum.[15] Thus, similar to the regulations in England, pauper certifications required only one medical signature while private asylum certifications required two.[16] On the completion of the documentation, the forms were placed before the asylum governors and manager for approval; the final authority to certify patients lay with them.

Over the subsequent decade, changes were introduced to the certification forms and procedures. By 1842, at Clonmel asylum 'ordinary' certification forms contained fourteen questions concerning patients' social, moral and medical history.[17] Reflecting changing medical preoccupations, the forms were explicitly concerned with tracking hereditary insanity. When finally issued in 1843, the certification procedure laid down in the privy council rules were very similar to the Armagh rules and reiterated the asylum governors' authority over the procedure. The rules also permitted the asylum physician to admit urgent cases, but he was obliged to seek retrospective approval from the governors.[18] The rules specified that asylum managers provide applicants with printed admission forms that contained a series of questions, which were subsequently transferred into casebooks, and formed the foundation of clinical histories. As Nancy Tomes has observed, the asylum physician seldom examined individuals prior to admission.[19] In Ireland a local doctor provided the medical testimony. The admission form was returned to the asylum manager who then submitted it to the physician, and he used it as the basis of his diagnosis. He then advised the governors whether the individual was suitable for admission.[20] The privy council rules ensured that the physician's influence over certifications increased but it did not supersede the governors.[21] Towards the end of the nineteenth century, certifying doctors were required to personally assess individuals. Guidelines issued to dispensary doctors specified that the medical officer 'should complete a personal inquiry' and that a 'physician and surgeon who has personally examined the lunatic' should complete medical certificates.[22] Also in 1862, a revision to the privy council rules required asylum medical superintendents to examine individuals on the submission of certification documents.[23] This not only confirmed the importance of medical evidence in the certification of 'ordinary' lunatics, it enhanced the asylum medical superintendent's influence over 'ordinary' certifications. However, the governors' approval was still required.

In spite of the availability of these methods of certification, over the course of the nineteenth century the most frequently used certification procedure was the *Act for the more effectual provision for the prevention of offences by insane persons in Ireland*, otherwise known as the Dangerous Lunatic Act, passed in June 1838 and later amended in 1867.[24] The introduction of the legislation in 1838 was relatively uncontroversial. According to Francis White, the act was introduced following the murder in July 1833 of Nathaniel Sneyd, bank director with the House of Sneyd, French and Barton, by John Mason. The murder, and subsequent inquest, received considerable coverage in English and Irish newspapers. It transpired that Mason's family had attempted to place him under restraint before the attack on Sneyd, however the police had refused to do so.[25]

In 1843, White claimed that Mason was 'well-known to be going about deranged' and maintained that the government and the Chief Secretary were so concerned 'to remedy a recurrence of such an Evil' that they passed the Dangerous Lunatic Act.[26] Despite the notoriety of the case there was no parliamentary debate on the legislation.

The passage of the 1838 legislation resulted in the construction of a new legal category of insane, known as 'dangerous lunatics'. The terms under which an individual could be certified were open to broad interpretation. The stated aim of the act was to 'protect' society from individuals who displayed a propensity to commit an indictable crime while denoting a 'derangement of mind' and who were perceived to represent a threat to the community.[27] The act also allowed for the confinement in district lunatic asylums of prisoners who had become mentally ill. Certification under the legislation required the signature of two magistrates. As it was a legal procedure, the merits of the case were heard before petty sessions court hearings. Although it was not mandatory, magistrates were permitted to seek medical advice during the procedure. Witnesses, who were usually relatives, provided testimony during hearings and from 1845 onwards it was given on oath.[28] Until 1867, 'dangerous lunatics' were initially confined in county gaols and bridewells and subsequently transferred to asylums though they were not charged with an offence.[29] The equivalent 1800 English Act also permitted the confinement of individuals in gaols, however this was amended in 1838 and, consequently, they were sent directly to county asylums.[30]

Journeying to the asylum

The workings of the dangerous lunatic certification procedure drew in a series of protagonists including the individual's relatives, the police, and legal and medical officers. Scholars have identified the central role the family played in the identification of insanity, and as demonstrated in greater depth in chapter four, families were central to the certification procedure throughout the four counties. Having determined that a relative was potentially dangerous and required institutionalisation, contact was made with a member of the Irish constabulary, and legal proceedings were initiated.[31] As Finnane has suggested 'the police were an indispensable part of the practical business of confining lunatics'.[32] A police force was introduced to Ireland in 1822, reconstituted in 1836 as the Irish Constabulary and designated as the Royal Irish Constabulary in 1867.[33] As a point of contact, the constabulary were readily accessible within Irish communities and there were high levels of policing in Ireland.[34] Vaughan has suggested that by 1870 there were twice as many police in Ireland as in England and Wales, though this varied according to settlement patterns.[35] The counties in Carlow asylum district had a population of 543,000 in 1831. Prior to 1846, there were 1,212 representatives of the constabulary and this subsequently expanded. County Carlow alone contained one county inspector, five sub-inspectors, six head constables and constables and 151 sub-constables. Kildare contained one county inspector, six sub-inspectors, eight head constables and constables, and 250 sub-constables. Between Kilkenny county and city there was one county inspector, ten sub-inspectors, fourteen head constables and constables, and 450 sub-constables. Finally, county Wexford, in addition to a county inspector, had eight sub-inspectors, twenty head constables and constables, and 280 sub-constables.[36] There was also a military station at the Curragh camp in county Kildare. The size of the police presence in the four counties fluctuated during the century and there were variations in the dispersal in each county. Nevertheless, accessing the constabulary forces in Ireland and in the Carlow district was relatively easy.

The policeman was 'someone with whom Irish people would expect to have regular contact'[37] and while police duties were mainly devoted to the 'prevention and detection of crime',[38] the force acquired a number of civil duties.[39] Recruits were advised to 'know the members of their communities very well' and 'acquire a thorough knowledge of his district'.[40] The evolving civil nature of the role allowed the constabulary to move with ease from the public into the private sphere thus facilitating the invocation of the dangerous lunatic legislation. Police manuals and instruction books contained procedural advice on the apprehension of putative lunatics and on the interpretation of the dangerous lunatic acts.[41] They were entitled to apprehend people found wandering in the streets and not under 'proper control'.[42] Also specific advice was provided in cases when alcohol was suspected to be the cause of aberrant behaviour.[43] When satisfied that someone was mentally ill and dangerous, constables were required to record the individual's personal and family details. Police manuals contained sample certification forms.[44] The police then placed individuals under safe custody until cases came before the petty session court. While the police were important to the process, they usually acted at the behest of a family. Amongst patients certified in counties Wexford, Kilkenny, Kildare and Carlow, the constabulary sought the institution-alisation of lunatics in only fifteen cases between 1843 and 1868. This contrasted with the use of similar legislation in Australia, where in New South Wales, the police force, largely modelled on the Irish one, was responsible for the identification of mental illness and for the 'arrest of large numbers of people in public spheres'.[45]

Following arrest, individuals usually appeared before two magis-trates at the local petty session hearing where the magistrates signed the certification warrants. This process was sometimes subverted as an alter-native practice had developed whereby individuals were brought before each magistrate at their private homes.[46] In response in 1874, a circular reminded magistrates of the requirement to bring cases before the petty session hearings.[47] Under the 1838 act, magistrates were advised that it was lawful to seek the assistance of a medical officer contracted to local gaols, workhouses or dispensaries when examining individuals.[48] They were not obliged to do so and Finnane has argued that 'medical opinion was dispensable'.[49] However, in 1847, Francis White and John Nugent recommended that both 'a medical certificate and sworn informations [sic] should accompany the committal of every so called dangerous lunatic or idiot'.[50] Thus, magistrates were urged to mimic certification procedures in England and Wales, where committing justices were required to include a medical certificate signed by one 'medical man'.[51] The certifying magis-trates in counties Kildare, Kilkenny, Wexford and Carlow followed the inspectors' directives and amongst 'dangerous lunatics' certified between 1843 and 1868, 96.5 per cent included a medical certificate. This was relatively commonplace by 1849 and dangerous lunatic certifications had become an established part of doctors' duties under medical juris-prudence. Medical officers completed their examinations of the mentally ill prior to the petty session hearings though occasionally an adjudicating magistrate would defer a hearing to allow a doctor to personally examine an individual.[52] In other instances, family members sought the advice of local dispensary doctors before contacting the police.[53]

The original dangerous lunatic certification forms contained only two questions that could be described as medical in nature. However, in 1848 the inspectors introduced new forms that required the signature of the certifying medical officer. It contained columns for the insertion of

social and medical information, including the cause of mental derangement, the presence of hereditary insanity and 'other particulars connected
with the previous history of the lunatic'. There were similarities between
the new form and medical certificates required for ordinary certifications,
pointing to an attempt to standardise the documents. The gaol governor
was obliged to ensure that the completed form, together with all other
relevant documents, accompanied people when transferred from the gaol
to the asylum.[54]

The insistence that individuals brought before petty session hearings
were medically assessed also suggests that there was a reluctance among
magistrates to base judgments solely on lay accounts. Magistrates, in
conjunction with the inspectors, were undoubtedly aware of debates in the
English press concerning doctors' role in the confinement of the mentally
ill and the heightened fear of wrongful confinement. In the late 1820s
and early 1830s there were two highly publicised scandals involving the
successful London alienist George Man Burrows during which it emerged
that Burrows had based his medical assessment on relatives' evidence and
had not personally examined the individuals. Following the revelations,
the public suspected that medical witnesses were actively colluding with
families to secure wrongful certification.[55] Other notorious cases emerged
in the 1850s and the 1870s, receiving widespread publicity.[56] The details
of Lawrence Ruck's and W. F. Windham's wrongful confinements were
reported in popular Irish newspapers, including the Freeman's Journal
and the Irish Times.[57] Mindful of the controversy surrounding allegations
of wrongful committal, magistrates increasingly sought medical advice
during the certification of dangerous lunatics. Yet these controversies
would have alerted them to the potential limits of that advice.

Once magistrates had signed the certification forms, dangerous lunatics were confined in local gaols or bridewells and awaited transfer to an
asylum; the practice ended in 1867 when the legislation was amended.
This created an overt link between asylums and prisons, and was widely
criticised. The prison inspectors, Majors Woodward and Palmer, regularly
criticised the dangerous lunatic legislation, specifically condemning the
practice of accommodating the insane in gaols. They feared the certified
would become long-term inmates of gaols and would be disruptive to
prison discipline. They also argued that the paucity of specialised medical
care in gaols inhibited recovery rates.[58] Most medical treatises emphasised that the key to recovery was early treatment.[59] Nonetheless, the

inspectors' primary concern was that the mentally ill were 'destructive to the discipline of the County Gaols' and they regarded the asylums 'as an adjunct to the smooth running of the gaols'.[60]

White and Nugent generally concurred that the practice was 'subversive to prison discipline', particularly in institutions which operated a separate classification system.[61] They were less critical of the effects penal incarceration had on dangerous lunatics, noting that some recovered while in gaols. These recoveries were accredited to interacting with sane prisoners and attendants during a curative phase of illness, and to the elimination of the exciting causes of insanity, particularly alcohol and an intemperate lifestyle.[62] In addition, the improved diet and shelter provided 'a temporary refuge' for people who were otherwise neglected and maltreated.[63] Thus the Irish inspectors were echoing the English lunacy commissioners' assertion that institutionalisation was preferable to domestic care. Nonetheless, the inspectors argued that most suffered while in gaols, confined 'in narrow cells, and cheerless passages, without a single break to the monotony of their existence'. The lack of classification ensured that volatile individuals were shackled to maintain order, a practice denounced in the age of moral treatment.[64] Spring Rice supported the inspectors' criticisms in his evidence to the 1843 House of Lords Select Committee.[65]

Relatives of those confined as dangerous lunatics were also uneasy; in 1853, Edward F., a thirty-three year-old labourer, was committed as a dangerous lunatic to Wexford gaol after an assault on a relative and an attempt to hang himself. While he was confined his mother sent a memorial to the Lord Lieutenant requesting that his transfer to the asylum be expedited.[66] Similarly, in 1867 the father of James C., who was confined in Athy gaol in county Kildare, petitioned for his transfer to Carlow asylum or Waterford asylum.[67] Families therefore tried to prevent relatives spending periods in gaol, a preference commented on by at least one Dublin magistrate.[68] In these memorials, relatives also argued that removal to the asylum would assist the recovery process.

Accommodating dangerous lunatics in gaols was characterised as a considerable burden on the system. The prison inspectors claimed that 'each Prison of the Kingdom has charge of from five to ten Lunatics, and even more'.[69] White and Nugent also argued that large numbers accumulated in gaols. However, there was considerable variation in the numbers. In the Carlow asylum district there was an average of two or three dangerous lunatic certifications annually between 1838 and 1843.

As a result, there were nine dangerous lunatics scattered across five gaols in the towns of Carlow, Wexford, Naas, Athy and Kilkenny. According to the *Freeman's Journal*, by May 1862 there were 282 dangerous lunatics confined in forty gaols throughout Ireland. Two hundred and nine were in ten gaols situated in counties without asylums. In counties with an asylum, most local gaols did not accommodate any 'dangerous lunatic' inmates. Among the seven gaols that did, there was an average of five inmates in each gaol.[70] There was therefore significant variation in the accumulation of dangerous lunatics in gaols and this was related to the distribution of asylums.

Transferring 'dangerous lunatic' inmates from gaols to local asylums was a protracted, bureaucratic process, particularly during the years immediately after the introduction of the 1838 act. Both the prison and lunacy inspectors were highly critical of delays.[71] Transferring an inmate required an additional medical certificate that confirmed the prisoner was dangerous and mentally ill, in addition to a warrant issued by the Lord Lieutenant.[72] The gaol physician and a second physician signed the second medical certification, rubberstamping the original findings. Physicians often used formulaic phrases that emphasised the potential for recovery and confirmed that the person was dangerous.[73] Transfers were delayed further when asylums were overcrowded and asylum governors were pressurised to admit dangerous lunatic inmates. According to asylum regulations, the admission of dangerous lunatics took precedence over 'ordinary committals', regardless of the urgency of the latter cases. Thus the Carlow governors were obliged to defer ordinary admissions and this created considerable tension between gaol and asylum administrators when Carlow officials attempted to delay transfers.[74] In 1839, the governors negotiated an agreement with the prison inspectors that required gaol officials to notify the asylum manager before transferring patients.[75] However, the difficulties continued. In June 1841, the Carlow board informed the governors of Wexford gaol that 'it was utterly impossible' to admit five dangerous lunatics until the institution was enlarged and harmless patients transferred elsewhere. The asylum was overcrowded and there was an extensive waiting list.[76]

The length of time dangerous lunatic inmates were confined in gaols was also related to the date of the initial certification. In the Carlow district, the first dangerous lunatic certifications took place in 1843, however, transfers to the asylum started in 1848 thereby confirming

Walsh's characterisation of the process as 'appallingly slow'.[77] The substantial increase in the number of certifications between 1847 and 1851 – the number doubled – resulted in the systematisation and regularisation of the process.[78] As table 2.1 (see chapter two) highlighted, after the Famine the transfer of inmates from local gaols to the asylum settled into a relatively efficient system. Most transfers occurred within a few months of the original certification at the petty session hearing. Finnane found that by 1857 'less than 20 per cent of dangerous lunatics in gaols had been there for longer than twelve months.'[79] In the Carlow district, the improvement occurred earlier and was partly prompted by the Famine crisis.

The dangers and problems associated with accommodating dangerous lunatic inmates in gaols were brought into sharp relief by several highly publicised cases in the 1860s. In January 1861 a twenty-one-year-old woman, Elizabeth Fitzgerald, died in Grangegorman penitentiary. An inquest sought to establish the circumstances surrounding Elizabeth's death and to ascertain whether the Adelaide hospital in Dublin was responsible as alleged by the widower, Christopher. During the inquiry it emerged that a week after the birth of her first child Elizabeth had become delirious and was removed to the Adelaide. Her condition deteriorated and her husband was advised that the 'only hope of curing her' was to admit her to Richmond asylum. He certified Elizabeth as a dangerous lunatic and she was removed from the Adelaide to Grangegorman penitentiary to await transfer to the asylum. She arrived at the prison on Tuesday between twelve and one o'clock, but was found dead on Thursday morning. During the inquest, Dr John K. Barton, surgeon to the Adelaide, admitted that he did not believe that transferring Elizabeth to the prison was 'good for her' rather that 'it was for the benefit of the other patients in the hospital that she be removed'. The inquest jury found that Elizabeth had 'died of puerperal mania but that her death was accelerated by her removal from the Adelaide Hospital' into a prison.[80] Elizabeth was not the only certified dangerous lunatic to die while in gaol. Julia Doyle had been an inmate of south Dublin union workhouse when she was certified as a dangerous lunatic. She was moved to Grangegorman prison until she could be transferred to Richmond asylum. However in May 1862 she died in prison.[81] Similarly, Charles Read, who had been returned to Kilmainham gaol following his certification as a dangerous lunatic, died. His return to prison was cited as the cause of his death during the inquest.[82] These cases received considerable media attention and there were other, less publicised, instances. In July 1863, Patrick Gormill, a certified, dangerous lunatic, died in Armagh gaol.[83] Nicholas Lawless, who had been committed to the lunatic ward in Harold's Cross prison in Dublin as a dangerous lunatic, also died. He was scalded while being bathed.[84] Newspaper reports on the cases were frequently accompanied by editorial commentaries that demanded the reform of the legislation, specifically seeking an end to the practice of committing the mentally ill to gaols.[85]

These cases formed part of the context informing the decision to amend the dangerous lunatic legislation. From early on, the 1838 act was heavily criticised, initially by the prison inspectors, and after 1845, by the lunacy inspectorate. The inspectors argued that the act was abused by relatives of the insane[86] and by the magistrates,[87] and was responsible for overcrowding in Irish asylums.[88] White, Nugent and, later, Hatchell were particularly critical of families, insisting that they used it to relieve themselves of inconvenient relatives.[89] This criticism featured regularly in the inspectors' reports and claims were made that the legislation was used to commit relatives who had previously been 'refused admission by the Local Board' and were subsequently 'forced on the institution'.[90] The inspectors argued that 'the question of land' and disputes over property inheritance motivated some dangerous lunatics certifications.[91] While asylum governors supported these accusations, as Finnane has shown, certifying magistrates did not always concur.[92] In an attempt to monitor dangerous lunatic certifications, the inspectors established a 'General Registry of Criminal and Dangerous Lunatics' and from November 1847 gaol governors were requested to forward details of all dangerous lunatic certifications.[93] They requested that asylum medical superintendents provide detailed returns on the suitability of asylum care for dangerous lunatic patients.[94]

The lunacy inspectors also lamented that as a result of the legislation asylum 'Governors and Medical Officers' had limited influence over 'the selection of cases' for admission.[95] This informed their commentary on the use of the legislation. As discussed in chapter seven, the inspectors tried to bolster the position of the asylum medical superintendent within the asylum as well as during certifications. However, during petty session hearings dispensary doctors provided medical advice, and prior to 1867 this evidence was introduced at the discretion of magistrates. This challenged the value of medical expertise and the status of the emerging nineteenth-century alienist. In addition, the inspectors had greater regulatory powers over patients certified by asylum governors and physicians. The inspectors, asylum governors and physicians could only challenge dangerous lunatic certifications on precise, legal and bureaucratic grounds. However, neither the inspectors nor asylum administrators could prevent dangerous lunatic certifications, as the judiciary and the office of the Lord Lieutenant governed and regulated the procedure.

The legislation was also heavily criticised during two parliamentary committees on the Irish asylum – the 1843 House of Lords Select Committee and the 1857–58 Commission of Inquiry into the State of Lunatic Asylums. In spite of their criticisms, proposals to amend the legislation repeatedly failed.[96] For example, in 1857 Lord Naas introduced a bill that integrated certification procedures in Ireland with the poor law system, but the bill was defeated.[97] Finally, he was successful in July 1867, when he introduced a bill that amended the 1838 act.[98] The 1867 act contained several important innovations; it ended the practice of confining dangerous lunatics in gaols after certification, instead they were to be sent directly to local lunatic asylums where asylum officials were obliged to admit them, irrespective of the level of overcrowding in the asylum.[99] In addition, the amendment required magistrates to call the nearest available dispensary medical officer to examine patients and sign certification forms. From 1875, dispensary doctors and other medical officers were paid a fee for the service, which by the 1890s was one pound.[100] As Finnane has noted, the 1867 amendment excluded doctors in private practice; however, it also ensured that asylum medical superintendents could not sign dangerous lunatic certification forms. Nonetheless magistrates sometimes called upon local asylum doctors to provide evidence during petty session hearings and perform examinations. In 1870, O'Meara, from Carlow asylum was called upon to provide evidence in the case of Edward F., however, the magistrates were still obliged to request that Dr Shrewbridge J. Connor, the local dispensary medical officer, sign the medical certification.[101]

A new, more detailed certification form was circulated following the 1867 amendment. The form was intended to compel certifying magistrates to adhere 'more strictly' to the provisions of the legislation and to bring the dangerous lunatic certification form in line with 'ordinary' certification forms.[102] The inspectors and asylum governors had previously complained of problems with older forms, which were sometimes left incomplete. Incomplete or incorrect documentation was brought to the attention of the Chief Secretary's office and due to the continued failure to complete the correct forms, an 1875 amendment to the legislation specified that corrected defective forms could be submitted within fourteen days.[103] This did not eliminate the problem. Until the 1880s, Enniscorthy asylum continued to report defective forms to the lunacy inspectors.[104] Patients sometimes arrived at the asylum without case histories and certification warrants thereby inhibiting asylum authorities' ability to supply 'the facts that might serve to guide the Medical Officers in the course of treatment'.[105] The 1867 amendment re-enforced the requirement that completed certification documentation accompany patients to the asylum.[106]

The new certification forms facilitated the inclusion of more detailed lay and medical testimony and reflected changes in medical theories of insanity. There were similarities with the 'ordinary' certification forms introduced in 1842. Medical officers providing testimony responded to questions on the species of insanity, aetiology, symptomatology, the patient's physical condition, whether there were signs of epilepsy or idiocy, and, finally, they provided an assessment of the potential danger posed to society. Relatives and friends provided additional evidence on the person's social standing and habits. Relatives were also required to provide information on the duration of the illness and the presence of hereditary insanity. The section completed by the medical officer was the briefer of the two testimonies. Certifying magistrates were responsible for ensuring that medical certificates and other testimonies were fully completed and signed and therefore continued to exert significant authority over certifications.

The inspectors were initially well disposed towards the amendment, describing it as 'salutary reform' that 'had for a long time pressed itself on the attention of the Executive.'[107] Carlow asylum governors, however, were more critical and forwarded their objections to the government in October 1867.[108] A year later, the lunacy inspectors agreed, insisting that they had supported the amendment because it ended the practice of committing lunatics to gaols.[109] They now argued that the amendment removed 'one evil by the substitution of another'[110] as it reduced further the control asylum governors and lunacy inspectors had over the admission of a large cohort of patients.[111] Once again, the inspectors began to call for changes to the legislation, making comparisons with certification procedures in England and Scotland where the number of dangerous lunatic admissions was significantly lower.[112] In spite of repeated requests for the amendment of Irish lunacy legislation, the Dangerous Lunatic Act remained in place until 1945.

Patterns in certification

Figure 3.1 shows the proportion of admissions into Carlow asylum under each certification procedure between 1832 and 1921. During the decade following the asylum's opening, the governors authorised most admissions, however, after 1842, the impact of the dangerous lunatic legislation became apparent. Between 1838 and 1868 one fifth of admissions to Carlow asylum were under the dangerous lunatic legislation and it was used extensively throughout the four counties. Most admissions continued to be certified by the governors or the physician though, as figure 3.1 demonstrates, the proportion of these steadily declined in the late nineteenth century. According to the Carlow asylum registers, there was, however, a rise in 'ordinary' certifications at the start of the twentieth century, when the asylum was enlarged. This also coincides with the period when the asylum boards were reconstituted as management committees under the 1898 Local Government Act (figure 3.1). As discussed in chapter one, by 1900, the active members on these committees were elected county councillors and local clergymen and, initially, they appeared to be more willing to admit patients. The public were fully aware of the changes to the committee's composition as the monthly meetings and committee members' names were recorded in local newspapers, including the *Carlow Sentinel* after 1898. The increase in these certifications was brief and, after 1908, the number of 'ordinary' certifications declined.

Finnane has suggested that by the 1870s asylum governors' authority over admissions was diminished due to the facility that allowed medical superintendents to certify patients as 'urgent' cases arguing that this 'proved to be a loop-hole in the system of control over admissions'. [113] The inspectors' annual statistics support his argument, indicating that from 1869 most 'ordinary' certifications in Carlow were described as 'urgent by the Resident Medical Superintendent'. 'Urgent' certifications still required the governors' retrospective authorisation. In contrast, Carlow asylum admission registers indicate that only 7 per cent of admissions were explicitly recorded as 'urgent' certifications. According to this source, between 1868 and 1922, the asylum physician certified 11 per cent (180) of Carlow

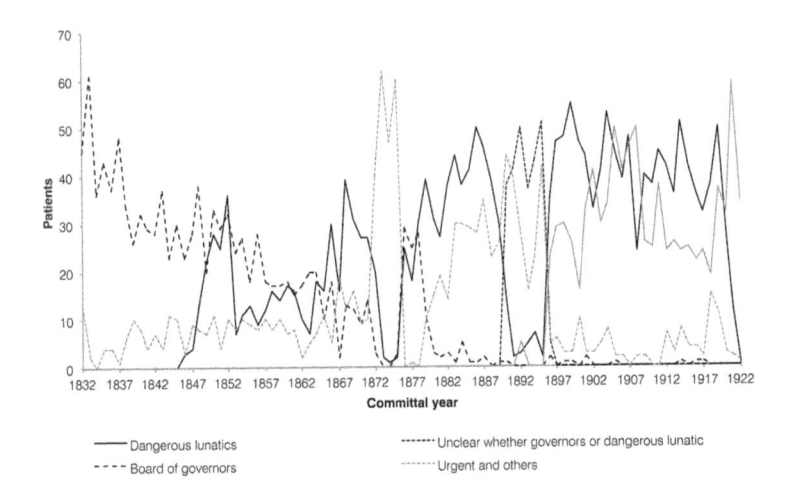

Figure 3.1   Forms of certification into Carlow Asylum, 1832 to 1922

patients and 9.6 per cent (205) of Kildare patients. The inconsistencies between the two sets of records are striking. For example, in 1871 the inspectors' published statistics indicate that the medical superintendent certified 74 per cent of non-dangerous lunatic admissions. For the same year, Carlow asylum register recorded that 26 per cent of admissions were 'urgent' while the remainder were certified 'on the authority of the board of governors'.[114]

In the 1880s, the inspectors' published statistics were consistent with the asylum registers. During this period, O'Meara was medical superintendent at Carlow asylum and he was responsible for submitting the admission returns to the inspectors. Following the 1862 amendment to the privy council rules, asylum resident medical superintendents were required to submit admission statistics to the Office of the Lunatic Asylums. After O'Meara's departure there was a return to previous recording practises, though 'ordinary' certifications were now given the nomenclature 'houseform'. After 1904, the asylum registers no longer differentiated between the two forms of non-judicial certifications while the inspectors' reports returned all such certifications as 'urgent'. Therefore, the presentation of admission statistics in the annual reports depended on the resident medical superintendent's reporting of them to the inspectors. This complicates a linear narrative of asylum medical superintendents' ever increasing control over 'ordinary' certification as tracked by Finnane in the inspectors' statistics. It is unclear whether the apparent rise in 'urgent' admissions in the inspectors' annual statistics reflects an increase in the authority of the asylum medical staff or anomalies in gathering statistics.

As figure 3.1 shows, the number of dangerous lunatic admissions into Carlow asylum rose significantly throughout the century and between 1868 and 1922, 44.5 per cent (3857) of certifications were dangerous lunatics.[115] Numerous factors encouraged the increasing use of the legislation. As suggested above, relatives disliked the requirement that under the 1838 act, dangerous lunatics were first confined to gaols and tried to avoid the stigma of criminalisation. Distance from the asylum was also a factor. Distance has been conceptualised in various ways; it can denote 'social distance' and 'the different ways in which information about services filtered into an area which Clifford Geertz termed as "local knowledge."'[116] In this chapter, distance is analysed in terms of physical proximity to the asylum, and the relationship between it and use of the dangerous lunatic legislation. Other definitions of 'distance' are explored in greater depth in the next chapter.

The architects of the Irish asylum system were mindful that distance would impact on the population's ability to access the asylum and, according to Jarvis' classic analysis, the 'probability of admission decreases' in relationship to a population's distance from the asylum.[117] Sections of the Carlow asylum district were at a considerable distance from the asylum. Therefore, when securing 'ordinary' admissions, relatives and friends were obliged to travel significant distances to the asylum to consult the manager, governors and asylum medical staff. While the privy council rules did allow 'ordinary' certification forms to be submitted by post to the asylum, relatives were still obliged to bring the person to the asylum. This required travelling significant distances, the cost of which was sometimes beyond the resources of the poor.[118] By the mid-nineteenth century, railways[119] – the Southern and Western Railway and the Irish South-Eastern Railway – canals, coaches and cars operated in the district. In 1854, the average cost of a third class ticket on the Irish South-Eastern Railway line was approximately one penny per mile, which was relatively expensive when compared to other railway lines. By 1899 a third-class fare from Kildare to Carlow towns was two shillings.[120] The Grand Canal and the Barrow navigation served parts of Kildare and Carlow counties and were an expensive form of transport.[121] The cheapest form of transport was the Bianconi coaches and car hire, however managing a fractious relative on these coaches would have been difficult. The dangerous lunatic legislation eliminated many of these difficulties. Not only was the local petty session hearing rather than the district asylum the gateway, but, as the inspectors observed, families secured free transport of relatives to the asylum.[122] The police brought the person to the asylum on the railway or coach and expenses were paid.

Physical distance from the asylum therefore affected the use of different certification procedures and, from early on, dangerous lunatic certifications were more common in counties at a greater distance from the asylum.[123] Between 1832 and 1868, most county Carlow admissions – 79.4 per cent – were 'ordinary' certifications. This was significantly higher than the number from the other three counties during the same period. Ordinary certifications comprised 64.8 per cent (295) of admissions from county Kildare, 56.2 per cent (291) from county Wexford and 63.9 per cent (106) from county Kilkenny. The number of dangerous lunatic admissions from these counties was higher than the proportion from county Carlow. Between 1832 and 1868, 33 per cent of admissions from county Wexford were certified as dangerous lunatics while 30 per cent and 22.6 per cent of admissions from counties Kilkenny and Kildare were dangerous lunatics. It was 20 per cent among county Carlow admissions.

Following the 1867 amendment, the relationship between distance and the use of the dangerous lunatic legislation was diluted. Between 1868 and 1922 the number of ordinary admissions declined in each county. These represented only 31.2 per cent (511) of county Carlow admissions and 24.3 per cent (520) of county Kildare admissions. During this period the asylum was frequently overcrowded and securing an ordinary admission was difficult. However, as discussed above, under the privy council rules dangerous lunatic admissions took precedence over ordinary certifications and this rule was reiterated in the 1867 amendment. Consequently, after 1867, dangerous lunatic admissions became more common. This was evident in both counties Carlow and Kildare. Between 1869 and 1922, 47.1 per cent (1008) of county Kildare admissions and 41.4 per cent (679) of county Carlow admissions were dangerous lunatics.[124] County Kildare was at a greater distance from the asylum suggesting that distance still mattered. In addition, the presence of petty session hearings in these county towns and the visibility of dangerous lunatic certifications during hearings had an impact. As discussed in chapter four, the public nature of these certifications ensured that knowledge about certification procedures was communicated to observers.

Conclusion

Changes to the frameworks regulating ordinary and dangerous lunatic certification procedures and the concomitant development of medical certificates indicate that from the late 1840s medical evidence was provided during most certification procedures. Among ordinary admissions, signed medical certificates were required from the 1830s. Finnane and Walsh have argued correctly that medical evidence was not mandatory for dangerous lunatic certifications before 1867, however, by the 1840s it was provided frequently. This suggests that enhanced medical involvement in dangerous lunatic certification had occurred well in advance of the 1867 amendment to the 1838 Dangerous Lunatic Act. The period also saw the introduction of regulations to enforce greater conformity between ordinary and dangerous lunatic certification procedures in terms of medical evidence, while the changes introduced to the certification forms from the 1840s – the increase in medical questions and the notable focus on hereditary insanity – reflected contemporary understandings of aetiologies of mental illness. Nonetheless, as discussed in chapter four, these changes to certification forms did not silence lay articulations of aetiologies of mental illness.

While revisions to dangerous lunatic certification procedures attempted to enhance medical authority, dispensary and poor law doctors, not asylum superintendents, certified patients and they acted at the behest of lay magistrates. Asylum superintendents seldom completed examinations prior to admission and they were therefore marginalised during dangerous lunatic certifications. Whoever provided the medical evidence, the authority to certify a dangerous lunatic remained with legal rather than medical experts. This informed the lunacy inspectors' hostility towards the legislation. Changes introduced in 1862 to 'ordinary' certifications indicate that the inspectors desired to establish asylum superintendents as 'gatekeepers'. The 1862 revision to the privy council rules allowed asylum superintendents to accept or reject ordinary applications though dispensary and poor law doctors continued to sign certification forms. Asylum superintendents also authorised admissions as 'urgent' and by the late nineteenth century this appeared to give them even greater control over ordinary admissions.[125] However, statistics in the local asylum admission registers seem to indicate that asylum governors continued to exert considerable influence over ordinary certifications, while 'urgent' admissions may have been less frequent than the official sources indicate. These findings suggest that medical superintendents' authority over the majority of asylum admissions continued to be contested in spite of regulatory reforms that endeavoured to consolidate their position.

Notes

1 Wright, 'The Certification of Insanity', 269.

2 Finnane, *Insanity and the Insane*, p. 100.

3 Finnane, *Insanity and the Insane*, pp. 88–128; Prior, 'Dangerous Lunacy', 534; Walsh, '"The Designs of Providence"', p. 225; Walsh, 'Lunatic and Criminal Alliances', pp. 132–152; Prior, 'Mad, Not Bad', 501–516.

4 Prior, 'Dangerous Lunacy', 525–541

5 Walsh, 'Gender and Insanity in Nineteenth-Century Ireland', p. 85.

6 D. Wright, 'Delusions of Gender?: Lay Identification and Clinical Diagnosis of Insanity in Victorian England', in Andrews and Digby (eds), *Sex and Seclusion, Class and Custody*, p. 160.

7 Finnane, *Insanity and the Insane*, pp. 18–52.

8 27 Geo. iii, c.39 s. viii (1787).

9 5&6 Vict. c.123 (1842).

10 For England, see Wright, 'The Certification of Insanity', 272–276.

11 Williamson, 'The Origins of the Irish Mental Hospital Services', p. 142.

12 *Copies of all Correspondence and Communications between the Home Office and the Irish Government during the year 1827, on the Subject of Public Lunatic Asylums*, H. C. 1828 [234] xxii, pp. 22–23.

13 *Ibid.*

14 *Ibid.*

15 *Ibid.*

16 Melling and Forsythe, *The Politics of Madness*, p. 13; Wright, 'The Certification of Insanity', 272–277.

17 NAI, CSORP, 1842/G14406, Form of Admission for Clonmel District Lunatic Asylum, County Tipperary.

18 *Report of Lunacy Inspectors*, H. C. 1845 [645] xxvi, p. 58.

19 N. Tomes, *A Generous Confidence. Thomas Story Kirkbride and the Art of Asylum-Keeping, 1840–1883* (Cambridge: Cambridge University Press, 1984), p. 120.

20 *Report of Lunacy Inspectors*, H. C. 1847 [820] xvii, p. 95.

21 See chapter seven and *Report of Lunacy Inspectors*, H. C.1844 [567] xxx, pp. 45–46. See Wright, 'The Certification of Insanity', p. 273.

22 T. A. Mooney, *Compendium of the Irish Poor Law* (Dublin: Thom, 1887), pp. 481–482.

23 *Report of Lunacy Inspectors*, 1865 [3556] xxi, p. 126.

24 1&2 Vict. c.27 (1838); 30&31 Vict c.118 (1867).

25 *The Times* (3 August 1833); *Dublin Times* (30 July 1833); *Dublin Times* (31 July 1833); *Dublin Times* (1 August 1833).

26 *Report from the Select Committee of the House of Lords appointed to Consider the State of the Lunatic Poor in Ireland*, H. C. 1843 [625] x, p. 12.

27 1&2 Vict., c.27 (1838); P. Prior, 'Women, Mental Disorder and Crime in Nineteenth-Century Ireland', in A. Byrne and M. Leonard (eds), *Women and Irish Society: A Sociology Reader* (Belfast: Beyond the Pale Publications, 1997), p. 225.

28 8 & 9 Vict., c.107, s.10 (1845).

29 *Judicial Statistics for Ireland 1863*, H. C.1864 [3418] lvii.

30 1& 2 Vict., c.14 (1838); J. Saunders, 'Institutionalised Offenders'.

31 For a later example see Malcolm, 'Ireland's Crowded Madhouses', pp. 315–333.

32 Finnane, *Insanity and the Insane*, p. 107.

33 E. L. Malcolm and W. J. Lowe, 'The Domestication of the Royal Irish Constabulary', *Irish Economic and Social History*, 19 (1992), 27–48, 27.

34 B. Griffin, 'Prevention and Detection of Crime in Nineteenth-Century Ireland', in N. W. Dawson (ed.), *Reflections on Law and History. Irish Legal History Society Discourses and Other Papers, 2000–2005* (Dublin: Four Court Press, 2006), pp. 99–125; Lowe and Malcolm, 'The Domestication of the Royal Irish Constabulary'; E. Malcolm, *The Irish Policeman 1822–1922: A Life* (Dublin: Four Courts Press, 2008).

35 W. Vaughan, 'Ireland c.1870', in W. E. Vaughan (ed.), *A New History of Ireland V: Ireland Under the Union* (Oxford: Clarendon Press, 1989), pp. 193–217, p. 762.

36 D. J. O'Sullivan, *The Irish Constabularies 1822–1922. A Century of Policing in Ireland*, (Dingle: Brandon, 1999), pp. 88–89.

37 Lowe and Malcolm, 'The Domestication of the Royal Irish Constabulary', 29.

38 Griffin, 'Prevention and Detection of Crime', p. 99.

39 Lowe and Malcolm, 'The Domestication of the Royal Irish Constabulary', 29; Vaughan, 'Ireland c.1870', p. 766.

40 Lowe and Malcolm, 'The Domestication of the Royal Irish Constabulary', p. 29; Griffin, 'Prevention and Detection of Crime', pp. 106–107.

41 A. Reid, *The Irish Constable's Guide* (Dublin: Thom, 1880); *Instruction Book for the Government and Guidance of Dublin Metropolitan Police* (Dublin: Thom, 1879).

42 This applied equally to paupers and non-paupers, see *ibid.*, p.177.

43 *Ibid.*, p.177.

44 *Ibid.*, pp. 364–365.

45 E. Malcolm, '"What Would People Say if I became a Policeman?": the Irish Policeman Abroad', O. Walsh (ed.), *Ireland abroad: Politics and Professions in the Nineteenth Century* (Dublin: Four Courts Press, 2003), pp. 95–107; Coleborne, 'Passage to the Asylum', pp. 129–148; S. Garton, 'Policing the Dangerous Lunatic: Lunacy Incarceration in New South Wales, 1843–1914', in M. Finnane (ed.), *Policing in Australia: Historical Perspectives* (Kensington: New South Wales University Press, 1987) pp. 75–87.

46 NAI, Carlow District Court Circulars to Petty Sessions, 2001/132/49, T. H. Burke, Dublin Castle 'Circular to magistrates', 10 March 1874.

47 See chapter four.
48 1&2 Vict. c. 27 s. 2 (1838); *Carlow Sentinel* (17 November 1860).
49 Finnane, *Insanity and the Insane*, p. 91, p. 93.
50 *Report of Lunacy Inspectors*, H. C. 1849 [1054] xxiii, p. 19.
51 Wright, 'The Certification of Insanity', 272.
52 *Carlow Sentinel* (17 November 1860); NAI, CSO CRF Wexford 1866.
53 *Leinster Leader* (3 June 1905).
54 *Fourth Report of Lunacy Inspectors*, H. C. 1849 [1054] xxiii, pp. 21–22.
55 A. Suzuki, *Madness at Home. The Psychiatrist, the Patient and the Family in England, 1820–1860* (California: University of California Press, 2006), pp. 50–64.
56 P. McCandless, 'Liberty and Lunacy: the Victorians and Wrongful Confinement', in A. Scull (ed.), *Madhouses, Mad-doctors and Madmen. The Social History of Psychiatry in the Victorian Era* (Philadelphia: University of Pennsylvania Press, 1981), pp. 339–362.
57 *Freeman's Journal* (August 1858); *Irish Times* (December 1861).
58 *Twentieth Report of Prison Inspectors*, H. C. 1842 [377] xxii, p. 8.
59 *Nineteenth Report of Prison Inspectors*, H. C. 1841 [299] xi, p. 8.
60 *Ibid.*; Walsh, 'Lunatic and Criminal Alliances', p. 136.
61 *Sixth Report of Lunacy Inspectors*, H. C. 1852–3 [1653] xli, p. 12.
62 *Eighth Report of Lunacy Inspectors*, H. C. 1857 session 2 [2253] xvii, p. 17; *Eleventh Report of Lunacy Inspectors*, H. C. 1862 [2975] xxiii, p. 25.
63 *Eleventh Report of Lunacy Inspectors*, H. C. 1862 [2975] xxiii, p. 25.
64 *Ibid.*, p. 26.
65 *Nation* (29 April 1843).
66 NAI, CSO CRF, Wexford 1853.
67 NAI, CSO CRF, Kildare 1867.
68 Finanne, *Insanity and the Insane*, p. 94.
69 *Twentieth Report of Prison Inspectors*, H. C. 1842 [377] xxii, p. 8.
70 NLI, Larcom Papers, Ms 7776, Newspaper cuttings, *Freeman's Journal* (20 May 1862).
71 *Twentieth Report of Prison Inspectors*, H. C.1842 [377] xxii, p. 8.
72 1 Vict. c. 27, s.1 (1838).
73 For example, see NAI, CSO CRF, Wexford 1848.
74 DPH, CLA Minute Book, 20 May 1840, 19 March 1845.
75 *Ibid.*,19 June 1839.
76 *Ibid.*,16 June 1841.
77 Walsh, 'Lunatic and Criminal Alliances', p. 135.
78 By 1852, the number returned to its 1847 level, and slowly decreased again.
79 Finnane, *Insanity and the Insane*, p. 93.
80 NLI, Larcom Paper, Ms 7776, Newspaper cuttings, *Irish Times* (6 January 1862).
81 *Ibid.*, Newspaper cuttings, *Express* (12 May 1862).
82 *Irish Times* (8 February 1864).
83 *Irish Times* (10 July 1863).
84 *Ibid.*, (29 March 1864); (8 July 1862).
85 See *Irish Times* (29 March 1864); (8 July 1862); (13 May 1862).
86 *Thirteenth Report of Lunacy Inspectors, 1863*, H. C. 1864 [3369] xxiii, p. 52; *Twenty-second Report of Lunacy Inspectors*, H. C. 1873 [C. 852] xxx, p. 6.

87 *Twenty-second Report of Lunacy Inspectors*, H. C. 1873 [C.852] xxx, p .9; *Eighteenth Report of Lunacy Inspectors*, H. C. 1868–69 [4181] xxvii, p. 5.

88 *Nineteenth Report of Prison Inspectors*, H. C. 1841 [299] xi, p. 8.

89 *Eighth Report of Lunacy Inspectors*, H. C. 1857 session 2 [2253] xvii, pp. 15–17.

90 *Twenty-second Report of Lunacy Inspectors*, H. C. 1873 [852] xxx, p. 6; *Eighth Report of Lunacy Inspectors*, H. C. 1857 session 2 [2253] xvii, p. 15.

91 *Thirteenth Report of Lunacy Inspectors*, H. C. 1864 [3369] xxiii, p. 52.

92 Finnane, *Insanity and the Insane*, p. 94.

93 Finnane, *Insanity and the Insane*, p. 93.

94 SPH, ELA Letter Book, Dr T. Shiell to the Lunacy Inspectors, 1 January 1868; 26 August 1869.

95 *Eighteenth Report of Lunacy Inspectors*, H. C. 1868–69 [4181] xxvii, p. 5.

96 Finnane, *Insanity and the Insane*, pp. 95–97.

97 *Ibid.*, p. 63.

98 *Ibid.*, pp. 96–97.

99 30&31 Vict c.118 (1867).

100 30&31 Vict. c.118 s.10 (1867); 38&39 Vict. c.67 s.14 (1875); *Anglo-Celt* (25 March 1893), p. 4; Finnane, *Insanity and the Insane*, p. 109.

101 *Carlow Sentinel* (4 June 1870); *Thom's Directory, 1866*.

102 NAI, Carlow District Court Circulars to Petty Sessions, 2001/132/49, T. H. Burke, Dublin Castle, Circular to Magistrates, 21 August 1869.

103 38&39 Vict., c.67 s. 5 (1875).

104 SPH, ELA Letter Book, Thomas Shiell to Register in Lunacy, Four Courts, Dublin, 27 November 1871; Robert Henderson, Clerk, to Master, Wexford Union Workhouse, 12 November 1871; Joseph Edmundson to Inspector of Lunatic Asylums, 17 November 1877; Joseph Edmundson to Inspector of Lunatic Asylum, 20 February 1882, 24 February 1882, 8 March 1882, 3 May 1882; Thomas Drapes to Inspector of Lunatic Asylum, 17 July 1886.

105 *Seventeenth Report of Lunacy Inspectors*, H. C. 1867–68 [4053] xxxi, p .6; Finnane, *Insanity and the Insane*, p. 98; DPH, CLA Minute Book, 18 May 1842, 15 June 1842.

106 *Sixteenth Report of Lunacy Inspectors*, H. C. 1867 [3894] xviii, p. 7.

107 *Seventeenth Report of Lunacy Inspectors*, H. C. 1867–68 [4053] xxxi, p. 31.

108 DPH, CLA Minute Book, 21 October 1867.

109 *Eighteenth Report of Lunacy Inspectors*, H. C. 1868–69 [4181] xxvii, p. 5.

110 *Ibid.*

111 *Thirty-second Report of Lunacy Inspectors*, H. C. 1883 [3675] xxx, p. 7.

112 *Ibid.*, pp. 7–8.

113 Finnane, *Insanity and the Insane*, p. 91.

114 *Twenty-first Report of Lunacy Inspectors*, H. C. 1872 [C. 647] xxvii, p. 72.

115 By the end of the century, constabulary rather than private prosecutions 'took up the bulk of [petty] session business', see McCabe, 'Open court', p. 159.

116 Melling and Turner, 'The Road to the Asylum', 298–332.

117 J. M. Hunter and G. W. Shannon, 'Jarvis Revisited: Distance Decay in Service Area of mid-19th Century Asylums', *Professional Geographer*, 37:3 (1985), 296.

118 *Report of Lunacy Inspectors*, H. C.1845 [645] xxvi, p. 58; NAI, Carlow District Court, Circulars to Petty Sessions 2001/132/49, T. H. Burke, Dublin Castle, Circular to Magistrates, 21 August 1869.

119 *Thom's Directory, 1848*, p. 159; *Thom's Directory, 1854*, p. 300.

120 *Irish Times* (29 September 1899).

121 *Thom's Directory, 1862*, p. 711; C. A. Power, 'The Origins and Development of Bagnelstown, c.1680–1920', in T. McGrath (ed.), *Carlow: History and Society*, pp. 435–436.

122 Prior, 'Dangerous Lunacy', p. 531.

123 Only 2.6 per cent of patients' county of origin was unrecorded and 17.4 per cent (twenty-five) of these were dangerous lunatic patients.

124 Between 1887 and 1892, the data recorded in the admission registers was not reliable.

125 Wright, 'The Certification of the Insane', 288.

4

Insanity on display:
Magistrates, doctors and families, 1840–70

In May 1849, Mathew W. appeared before a Carlow petty session hearing charged with seriously assaulting his stepdaughter, Eliza B. Eliza was attacked while trying to protect her mother from Mathew. Evidence of Mathew's 'dangerous character' was provided by several witnesses and during the hearing it emerged that he had been previously confined in an asylum. William Duckett, the presiding magistrate and a governor at Carlow asylum, informed the court that Eliza had called upon him six weeks earlier requesting that Mathew be put under restraint, 'as she feared for her life'. Mathew's hearing concluded when magistrates signed 'the usual forms' for his admission to Carlow asylum as a dangerous lunatic.[1] All this was reported in the local newspaper, the *Carlow Sentinel*

The reporting of Mathew W.'s certification in the *Carlow Sentinel* was mundane and the case was not particularly sensational, notorious or even unusual.[2] He was one of 340 dangerous lunatic certifications heard at petty session courts held in counties Carlow, Wexford, Kildare and Kilkenny between 1843 and 1868.[3] Much of the discussion in this chapter will focus on the lay and medical evidence presented by witnesses during these hearings and recorded in certification warrants. During the procedures the defendants usually remained silent in contrast to Joel Eigen's criminal lunatic defendants who 'moved to center stage'.[4] James Moran has argued that while the details contained in certification documents are not 'symptoms' of mental illness in the medical sense, they are important sources.[5] Here, they will be used to explore magistrates', doctors' and families' negotiations with the asylum. Responding to Finnane's assertion that the asylum's place in the 'popular mentality' remained fragile in late Victorian period,[6] this chapter will argue that the public nature of dangerous lunatic certifications assisted in the dissemination of medical and lay knowledge regarding legal certification procedures, and of the demarcation between 'sane' and 'insane' behaviour. In the nineteenth century, petty session hearings were popular social events and this popularity contributed to establishing a 'place' for the asylum within the consciousness of families and friends, magistrates and dispensary doctors. In spite of this it will be argued that families continued to display an ambiguous relationship with, and attitude toward, lunatic asylums.[7] While the asylum gained some legitimacy in popular discourse, this did not result in a complete replacement of domiciliary care as families continued to maintain relatives at home, a decision that could have significant economic and emotional consequences.[8]

Drawing on certification warrants, this chapter will assess how lay and medical indications of mental illness were constructed during certification and whether lay narratives shaped medical evidence.[9] Additionally, the certification documents are drawn upon to consider politics within the family.[10] David Wright, Michael MacDonald and others have argued that families were important for the identification of mental illness and the decision to commit relatives to asylums.[11] Hilary Marland has demonstrated how 'disorder' in bourgeois households and families were part of psychiatric aetiologies in cases of puerperal insanity.[12] Read closely, certification warrants provide insights into the events behind decisions to certify a family member as a 'dangerous lunatic', the role the public assigned to the asylum, and familial emotional relationships and bonds.[13]

The petty session hearings

In the nineteenth century, petty sessions court hearings were a site for 'on-going negotiation between popular belief and official regulation'.[14] Between 1823 and 1825, a network of regular petty session hearings was established in Ireland and their character and jurisdiction evolved significantly throughout the century. Most petty session summary jurisdiction dealt with the 'settlement or adjudication of specific minor injuries and offences', including cases brought under the Dangerous Lunatic Act.[15] For minor cases such as assault, larceny, trespass and employment law, magistrates were responsible for summary adjudication. In the case of more serious crimes, magistrates' duties were confined to initial investigations.

Petty session hearings were less formal than crown courts, and magistrates were empowered to adjudicate on cases 'at any time or place', though this was not encouraged.[16] From the 1820s, the cost of renting rooms to hold petty session hearings was presented at grand juries ensuring that for much of the nineteenth century, petty sessions hearings took place in 'rooms in market houses, hotels or other civic or public buildings'.[17] Dedicated courthouses were erected later in the century. Over the course of the century, a routine surrounding the hearings developed, though they continued to be relatively informal events. Petty session personnel included a clerk – salaried after 1858 – whose main task was to complete and issue summons, signed by magistrates, at a fee of six pence. The complainant paid this fee implying that bringing relatives before the hearings required financial resources. The litigant usually took out the summons.

Among cases brought under the dangerous lunatic legislation, the allegation of mental illness was made before the trial. This differed from criminal cases when the question of the defendant's mental state arose during the trial.[18] Magistrates were often reluctant to change original criminal indictments even when evidence of mental illness was presented. At Mountrath petty sessions the magistrates rejected the deposing constable's suggestion that a defendant on drunk and disorderly charges should be committed as a lunatic, insisting that they could only commit an individual charged with an indictable crime.[19] In another case, though evidence was brought to court demonstrating that the defendant was both dangerous and of 'a weak intellect', the original charge was pursued and the individual was sentenced to two years' imprisonment.[20]

During hearings, litigants informed defendants of the complaints made against them, and defendant were asked whether there was cause not to convict. When defendants failed to show cause, presiding magistrates made a conviction or an order. When complaints were denied, magistrates heard the prosecutor and his witnesses while defendants and complainants were entitled to cross-examine the 'opposing party'.[21] Magistrates could adjourn the proceedings to summons additional witnesses in specific cases, and in the case of dangerous lunatic certifications, these were usually medical witnesses. Defendants were also entitled to make statements to the court and from 1836 the provision of counsel for both sides was permitted. While petty session hearings were relatively informal, evidence presented during hearings was heard according to statutory rules – from 1845 testimony provided at dangerous lunatic hearings was made under oath. At the end of the process, 'magistrates consulted and determined the matter'.[22]

Petty session hearings became an intrinsic part of local communities' social calendar. They were extremely well attended, sometimes raucous, affairs and were more inclusive than quarter sessions or assizes.[23] Nationally, the number of petty sessions expanded during the century, increasing from 536 in the mid-1830s to 610 in the early 1880s. They were 'weekly, fortnightly and monthly' events and were most abundant in the province of Leinster.[24] By 1850, petty session hearings were held in seven different places in county Carlow, eighteen in county Kilkenny, thirteen in county Kildare and eleven throughout county Wexford.[25] The general public attended these events as litigants, defendants and interested observers. By 1870, 'most of the male adult population appeared before the petty sessions once a decade' mainly on drunk and disorderly charges.[26] Historians and contemporaries have argued that the large number of petty session cases indicates that nineteenth-century Ireland was a very litigious society. In the 1840s, one commentator remarked that 'litigation among the peasantry has superseded quarrelling and fighting at fairs'.[27] Thus the large number of dangerous lunatic certifications was part of a general trend among the Irish peasantry and the middle classes to seek legal redress over a wide range of issues.[28]

The 'dangerous lunatic' cases studied here distinguished themselves from the Irish 'sane' prison population and English criminal lunatics in terms of gender and type of offence. In the first half of the nineteenth century, there was an excess of men over women among general convictions of summary offences. Amongst the 340 dangerous lunatics certified in Carlow asylum district between 1843 and 1868, there were an equal number of men and women (51 per cent were men).[29] Later in the century, this pattern changed significantly and most dangerous lunatics certified to Irish asylums were men.[30] In pre-Famine Ireland, most petty session business comprised of common assaults, trespass and damage to property. As Desmond McCabe has shown there were more cases of assault than crimes against property.[31] In England, Eigen found that by the 1840s 'the proportion of property to personal crimes had almost reached parity' amongst criminal lunatic cases. However, most dangerous lunatic certifications were brought before magistrates as a result of a 'personal' offence – usually an assault on relatives, neighbours or institutional officials. Summary trials for assault were introduced to petty sessions in 1829, and when a conviction was secured, the

penalty was a fine of up to '£2, with costs, or up to two months imprisonment in default of payment'.[32] This penalty was more lenient than an
unspecified period of confinement in an asylum. It was unlikely dangerous
lunatic certifications were used as a means of avoiding a more draconian
gaol sentence even though there was, as noted previously, considerable
resistance to the confinement of dangerous lunatics in gaols among families.
Personal offences also encapsulated self-harm and attempted suicide, and
this featured frequently in dangerous lunatic certifications. Offences against
property – often involving fire – featured but less often.

Magistrates were central to the business of dangerous lunatic certifications. Their role extended beyond the adjudication of cases, as they
sometimes acted as a source of advice before cases appeared in court.
Implicit in the newspaper report on the certification of Mathew W. was
the suggestion that William Duckett advised Eliza B. to approach the
courts rather than the asylum to certify Mathew. Similarly, in March 1839
the *Freeman's Journal* reported on Theophilus Burrows' attempt to have
his sister certified. He had originally tried to commit her as an 'ordinary'
lunatic but the application was refused as there was no vacancy in the
asylum. He subsequently approached the local magistrates for advice on
the procedures under the Dangerous Lunatic Act. The magistrates themselves were uncertain and concluded that Alicia could not be certified
under the legislation as she was not dangerous.[33] Throughout these negotiations Burrows received advice from Dr Kelly, a medical practitioner
involved in the case. This, and other cases, indicates that sometimes
magistrates refused to certify under the legislation.[34] For example, in April
1873 a Dublin magistrate refused to certify Alice K. following an attempted
suicide, while, in 1892, an unnamed doctor refused to certify Timothy S.
when his brother and sister made an application for his certification.[35]

Staff working in hospitals and workhouses also advised families
to certify relatives as dangerous lunatics. During the inquest into the
death of Elizabeth Fitzgerald in Grangegorman penitentiary in January
1861, discussed in chapter three, her husband Christopher stated that
he had been advised by the Adelaide hospital staff – the matron and the
surgeon, Dr John Baron – that the best method of securing admission into
Richmond asylum was to swear an affidavit that Elizabeth was a dangerous
lunatic. In this case no attempt was made to communicate directly with the
asylum.[36] In the case of Julia Doyle – she died in Grangegorman prison in
May 1862, following her removal from the south Dublin union workhouse

under a dangerous lunatic warrant – the board of guardians was advised to use the legislation.[37] Members of the clergy may also have acted as advisors to families and guided relatives towards the constabulary and the petty sessions hearings, though direct evidence of clerical interventions in asylum certifications is relatively tentative. However they were educated and respected members of nineteenth-century communities, and some served as asylum governors. Two Church of Ireland and two Roman Catholic clergymen were cited as petitioners on four warrants between 1843 and 1868. In 1923, Fr James Brody, a parish priest, had arranged for the 'mentally afflicted' men of a family to be certified to Carlow asylum when they became violent, but at the final moment the family had not 'let them go'.[38] The clergy also attempted to influence decisions surrounding patients' discharge. In March 1906 Father Cullen of Wexford College contacted Thomas Drapes at Enniscorthy asylum, concerned about the proposed release of a woman previously residing in his parish. He advised Drapes that the neighbours 'have been in constant dread that she would do some mischief to them'. On this occasion she was not released and appears to have died in the asylum.[39]

It is unclear how widespread these practices were, but, the lunacy inspectors were convinced that magistrates were regularly involved in this type of behaviour and criticised them for excessive use of the legislation. They argued that magistrates were either not fully aware of the terms of the act or used it for their own convenience thereby 'disembarrassing their respective localities of characters whose troublesome proclivities afforded some colour and pretext of insanity'. As a result the elderly, and 'parties when they become troublesome at home, from old age, bad temper, physical infirmities' were certified.[40] The lunacy inspectors argued that the asylums were being diverted from their true function – the treatment and cure of the mentally ill – and were becoming 'domiciles of incurable lunatics' as inappropriate cases were certified under the legislation.[41] The Carlow governors complained of one patient, a 70-year-old Scot, committed to the asylum as a dangerous lunatic who was clearly too weak to present any significant danger. He was emaciated and so delicate that he could not move without assistance.[42] This was relatively unusual at Carlow asylum, however, in a bid to curb these practices, the inspectors issued a series of circulars to magistrates reminding them of the terms of the act.

Over the course of the century, through their attendance at petty session hearings, magistrates gained some familiarity with 'symptoms' of mental illness. As shown in chapter three, during the thirty years following the introduction of the legislation, magistrates relied on dispensary doctors' evidence. By the end of the century, however, they were more self-confident in assessing defendants' mental states. For example, during an inquiry into the case of James Dowling, an 'imbecilic' inmate of Naas workhouse 'lunatic' wards, who murdered four fellow inmates with a spade and an iron bar in 1905, the presiding judge, Mr A. W. Samuels, challenged the decision of Dr Louis Crinion, medical officer of Blessington dispensary district, not to confine Dowling to an asylum. Samuels opined that 'everybody, who knows anything knows' that 'imbeciles are easily excitable and many have excesses of insanity'.[43] His criticism of Crinion points to a belief that as an experienced magistrate he possessed sufficient experience to differentiate between the forms of mental illness that required asylum institutionalisation and those that were 'harmless' and could be dealt with in workhouses. Samuels was challenging a relatively low status dispensary doctor and it is unclear whether he would have criticised the asylum superintendent in a similar manner. His statement, however, suggests that by the later period magistrates believed they possessed a good understanding of the symptoms of mental illness.[44]

There were ample opportunities for magistrates to acquire this knowledge, notably through participating in the activities of local medical and educational institutions such as asylums and mechanics' institutions, and through personal networks. As highlighted in chapter one, a number of Carlow and Enniscorthy asylum governors were local magistrates and regularly attended board meetings. During these meetings physicians provided advice and information on patients' physical and mental condition. Magistrates therefore encountered contemporary medical theories of insanity regularly. The Carlow asylum manager and later medical superintendent, Dr Matthew Esmonde White, was himself a magistrate from 1840 to 1866 and attended petty session hearings.[45] Similarly, Dr Thomas Cranfield, the visiting physician to Enniscorthy asylum from 1868 until 1872 and a local dispensary doctor, served as a magistrate and, in this role, certified dangerous lunatics. These encounters ensured magistrates were well informed and suggests that the lunacy inspectors' claim that '[t]he board of governors exercised little or no control in regard to the selection of cases' was inaccurate as several acted as certifying magistrates.[46]

Several magistrates and asylum governors were patrons of Carlow's Mechanics' Institute; there was also an institute in Kilkenny city.[47] In 1860, the honorary secretary of the Carlow institute was also the clerk for Carlow petty sessions while White was a trustee and was involved in its foundation in 1832.[48] The Carlow institute hosted lectures on mental development and health, and maintained scientific and medical libraries.[49] Although historians have questioned whether Mechanics' Institutes enjoyed much success in educating artisans, there is agreement that they assisted in the dissemination of ideas among members.[50] Mechanics' Institutes and reading rooms were 'appropriate forums for the development and promotion of civil society'[51] and they were spaces in which those invested in 'progressive' reform movements of the period could exchange ideas and knowledge. Peter Burke has suggested that personal networks were also important in the dissemination of knowledge. Two particularly active Carlow governors and magistrates, Samuel and Thomas Haughton, were related to Samuel Haughton, the polymath, scientist, and editor of the *Dublin Medical Press*, while Henry Bruen III, who was the chairman of the Carlow asylum board and a magistrate, was Vice-President of the Statistical and Social Inquiry Society of Ireland from 1874 to 1892 – he eventually became a life-member.[52] Through these personal connections magistrates became familiar with medical discourses on the indications of mental illness.

By the second half of the nineteenth century, the certification of dangerous lunatics had become routine business for many petty session hearings; people appeared alongside neighbours fined for lighting offences, cruelty to children and other offences.[53] While it was less common in some courts – Rathangan held a special session to hear the case of Brigid D. in September 1872 – rural communities became very familiar with the certification procedures.[54] This differed from most certifications in England and Wales which were less public and were 'completed in the home of the family or the surgery of the medical officer' and in workhouses.[55] There were some exceptions, such as criminal lunatics, infanticide and lunacy commission cases. The public nature of the certifications assisted in the dissemination of medical and legal frameworks in which communities could situate certain behavioural patterns. As Burke has noted, it is difficult to differentiate between knowledge and information, between 'knowing how' and 'knowing that'.[56] The petty sessions hearings in Ireland functioned as a form of oral transmission of knowledge and information ensuring families and friends became familiar with medical evidence and behaviour that was believed to constitute mental illness. Attendees at petty sessions courts heard detailed descriptions of 'aberrant' behaviour.

In addition, local and national newspapers reported on dangerous lunatic certifications as part of the coverage of local petty session hearings, ensuring that the publicity surrounding cases went beyond the attendees of the hearings.[57] The regional press was not only important in the promotion of political movements in nineteenth-century Ireland, it also acted as an important conduit of legal and medical information. Newspapers contained advertisements for medical treatments, articles debating the alleged increase of insanity and reprinted lunacy inspectors' reports.[58] Newspapers in the four counties of the Carlow asylum district – the *Carlow Sentinel*, the *Kilkenny Journal*, the *Kilkenny Moderator*, the *Wexford Independent*, the *Kildare Express* and the *Leinster Leader* – regularly reported on the petty session hearings held across the counties. Throughout the nineteenth century these reports contained the families' and doctors' testimony. In some instances newspaper coverage was relatively brief. For example, in August 1844, *The Nation* succinctly recorded that 76 cases were due for trial before the county judge, including seven 'dangerous lunatics'. In other cases the newspaper recorded the person's name and the decision to certify them.[59] Quite often, the full colour of the petty session hearing was printed. In June 1870, Edward F. appeared before Carlow petty sessions charged with 'wantonly and maliciously injuring' 350 ash trees on the estate of William Duckett in Carlow. As Duckett was a local magistrate, the case was reported in full in the *Carlow Sentinel*. Edward F. admitted the charge, but said he was 'not right in the head' at the time. O'Meara from Carlow asylum questioned him at length on his mental state and an employee of the estate provided further evidence stating that Edward F. 'spoke in a rather nonsensical way'. His wife deposed that he was often in an unsound state of mind and when 'so attacked she was in bodily fear of him'. The hearing concluded that Edward F. was a dangerous lunatic and the magistrates signed 'the usual forms' for his committal.[60] The evidence reported in the newspaper contained all the prerequisite detail necessary for committal: 'nonsensical language', a loss of control over his will evidenced by his attack on the plants, and danger.

Newspaper coverage of certifications continued into the twentieth century, though the extent of detail was dependent on other newsworthy events. The tone of the coverage was punctuated by occasional 'lunacy' scares. Following the tragedy at Naas workhouse in May 1905, there was a substantial increase in the coverage of cases.[61] After May 1905, Naas and Baltinglass guardians expressed concern about the mentally ill being accommodated in workhouses arguing that those deemed to be 'dangerous' were more suitable for asylums.[62] There were allusions to the 'Lunacy Danger' and debate on the urgent need to transfer lunatics from workhouses to asylums.[63] More sensational reportage also emerged, representing a break with the tone of previous coverage. These more sensational cases were afforded greater 'symbolic construction by editors'.[64] For example, on 17 June 1905 the *Leinster Leader* contained the dramatic headline 'Dangerous! Raving Lunatic Amuck In Naas' when it covered the certification of Lizzie K. Lizzie had broken some windows of the local Catholic curate's residence.[65] Cases that once had merited a short sombre account were subsequently described in more sensational terms.[66] After 1898, the minutes of the Carlow governors' monthly meetings were published in detail reinforcing the presence of the asylum in the public mind.

In the nineteenth century, the local population's ability to access provincial and national newspapers varied. The tradition of farmers, schoolteachers and priests reading newspapers aloud provided access for the illiterate, or those unable to afford newspapers and the paintings of Howard Helmick, Henry MacManus and Charles Lamb encapsulate this nineteenth-century passion for listening.[67] Among middle-income social groups, nineteenth-century reading rooms and libraries provided access to newspapers. The reading-room of Carlow Mechanics' Institute subscribed to local Carlow papers, in addition to the *Times* and the *Illustrated London News*, while the Kilkenny circulating library subscribed to local newspapers after 1847. Middle-income families also bought newspapers through subscription.[68] The number and accessibility of provincial newspapers spread after the 1850s. As Marie Louise Legg and others have shown changes in Irish society, the decline in the price of newspapers, the concomitant improvement in communication systems – including the arrival of the railway – and the rise in literacy levels contributed to an increase in the number and distribution of Irish newspapers and their consumption by the reading public.[69] The railway had reached the towns of Bagnelstown, Carlow, Kilkenny and Kildare by 1855, and the canals formed an important source of trade and communication. In the Carlow asylum district, levels of literacy in English were high. From 1841, significant proportions of the populations of Leinster and Ulster over the age of five were able to read and write.[70]

The public dissemination of events surrounding dangerous lunatic certifications outlined above demonstrates 'the different ways in which information about services such as a lunatic asylum filtered into an area'.[71] This is not simply information about the resources but also the growth of knowledge perceived as specialist and expert within a social distance.[72] As Melling and Turner have shown such 'social distance' is 'historically constructed', 'institutionally defined' and 'bounded by specific social and contractual relationships'.[73] It is argued here that 'local knowledge' concerning the asylums and more precisely, the dangerous lunatic certification procedures, 'filtered in an area' through attendance at the petty session hearings and through newspaper coverage allowing the asylum to become established within a 'social distance' and within late Victorian 'popular mentality'.

Indications of insanity?

Families in the southeast of Ireland not only gained a knowledge of the legal mechanisms involved in dangerous lunatic certification procedures, they also acquired an understanding of how to successfully present evidence of behaviour that medical and legal experts accepted as indications of mental illness.[74] The next section of this chapter will interrogate the medical and lay evidence recorded in the 340 dangerous lunatic certification warrants;[75] the size of the sample compares favourably with other studies.[76] Most certification warrants followed the format introduced in the 1840s, discussed in chapter three, which allowed for the inclusion of biographical and medical details. The certifying medical doctor's name, the date of examination and the details of the mental disorder were recorded. The lay witnesses' evidence of mental illness occupied the larger section on the form. This section detailed the name of the informant, their relationship to the defendant and their testimony. Finally, the warrants contained the signatures of the certifying magistrates.

These warrants are difficult sources and present historians of psychiatry with a series of methodological challenges.[77] Similar to asylum casebooks, certification warrants were mediated.[78] Lay testimony provided during hearings was filtered by bureaucratic language while witnesses and recording clerks selected, prioritised and reconfigured evidence deemed to be most relevant. This was particularly true with regard to incidences of violence and danger. The warrants also contained formulaic phrases: repeatedly witnesses describe themselves as being 'in dread and fear of his/her life' and there was a frequently expressed fear that the individual would do 'grievous bodily harm to him/herself and others if left at large'. These distortions of the testimony complicate the task of excavating the stories of these patients and their families. However, as the remainder of this chapter will suggest, the warrants can be rich sources[79] and here are mined to uncover the dynamics of familial relationships and emotions, lay aetiologies of mental illness and to trace the impact medical discourses had on lay testimony during hearings.[80]

The dynamics of the Irish family has generated an extensive litera-ture. Historians and demographers have argued that the consolidation of landholdings among middle-income farming classes, the high levels of emigration, hunger for land and Famine memories undermined familial 'affective' bonds. This produced a familial environment, it has been argued, that was devoid of emotional gratification. The emphasis families placed on land and inheritance suggests that economic considerations were the main determinants of the choice of marriage partner.[81] The 'match' gave parents 'considerable influence over their children's marriage' and scholars have concluded that the 'Irish were not raised in a society where emotional intimacy was seen as the primary reason for marriage'.[82] Many rejected marriage outright and the institution declined in popularity in the late nineteenth century. In addition, high levels of emigration ensured that a significant portion of young adults was raised in the expectation that their futures were abroad[83] producing, it has been argued, a familial environment that offered little affection for offspring and siblings.

The importance of emotional bonds amongst Irish families has received less attention. Guinnane has argued that the relatively strong sense of familial obligation in rural Ireland indicates that celibate farmers found emotional satisfaction in extended families. They operated as 'marriage substitutes' allowing those with property to avoid the risks of an unsuccessful marriage.[84] He also argued that offspring who did not inherit family farms were not necessarily badly treated. Instead, they received alternative inheritances, such as dowries, education or financial support to assist emigration. There was a 'clear place for the aged in households'.[85] This was secured by a written agreement, known as 'the writings', which 'spelled out the conditions of the farm's transfer to the younger genera-tion'.[86] These 'writings' ensured that heirs were required to provide for parents and siblings in the family home. The emotional 'leave-taking' known as emigrants' or 'American' wakes also testify to the presence of affectionate bonds within families and the recognition of loneliness amongst relatives remaining in Ireland.[87] Dangerous lunatic certification warrants – and the asylum casebooks and letters mined in chapter seven – attest to the presence of a range of familial emotional contexts. There was significant friction and tense relationships within families and the family could be a source of pathology from which an individual needed to be removed. As both Marland and Suzuki have argued, doctors stressed the importance of a stable and emotionally satisfying household for the preservation of mental health among bourgeois and pauper families. There was therefore a tension between the family as a site of emotional satisfaction, affection and support and as a site of violence, discord, stress and anxiety.[88] These apparently conflicting views of the family are evident in the assessment of dangerous lunatic certifications.

The disruptive presence of violent behaviour within a household and a community was repeatedly attested to in lay testimony during certifications. The connection between violence and mental disorder was not unique to Ireland or to dangerous lunatic certifications. In England, violence frequently featured in relatives' testimonies at Devon asylum in the late nineteenth century, and the manifestation of dangerousness often prompted the transfer of workhouse inmates to asylums.[89] It also featured among voluntary committals to Sainte-Anne asylum in Paris though committal procedures there did not require evidence of violent behaviour.[90] Writing of Sainte-Anne, Prestwich has suggested that 'families may have exaggerated the violence, either from fear or from an emotional need to justify their actions'.[91] The Irish lunacy inspectors certainly claimed that evidence of violence was embellished to secure certification, however Neilson Hancock, Professor of Political Economy and Jurisprudence, argued in 1879 that certification was delayed until violent behaviour erupted.[92] The indications of mental disorder contained in the certification warrants considered here repeatedly attest to mental disturbance that culminated in extreme violent outbreaks against both the community as a whole and individual households. In addition, in many warrants the presence of a 'fear of violence' was cited and these fears could be quite real. Finnane has shown that families used the legislation and asylums as defences, and physical violence directed against others was a key factor in the decision to commit.[93] Violence therefore emerged as a key element in lay cultural understandings of mental disorder and consequently the function of the asylum became intrinsically linked with 'dangerous insanity'.

Violence took on many forms and domestic violence between spouses featured frequently. Prestwich has suggested that 'wives appear to have used voluntary asylum admission as a means of defence' from physical abuse.[94] The evidence from this study indicates that abuse was not the sole preserve of either sex and there were similarities with late nineteenth-century domestic violence cases. C. A. Conley uncovered the presence of mutual violence where wives exhibited 'little or no deference to male authority'.[95] Responses among families and officials to evidence of violence among dangerous lunatic certifications were generally gendered.[96] Husbands' testimonies against their wives often evidenced an act of violence perpetrated against his person, but testimony was accompanied by additional indications of mental disorder. In February 1853, Ann F.'s husband ascribed the cause of her illness to a 'fever nearly thirty years ago, and [she] has been insane at intervals ever since.' He claimed that she had seized 'on a razor, opened the blade of it and rushed at [him]'. It required 'forcible resistance' to prevent her taking his life. Patrick K. swore that his wife, Maryanne, had on several occasions 'violently assaulted' him 'without any apparent cause'. Patrick had previously sought medical treatment, presumably from the dispensary doctor, but obviously felt this was no longer sufficient as he claimed, she 'used language towards said [him] denoting an intention of committing an indictable offence'.[97] Formulaic legal phraseology, drawn from the Dangerous Lunatic Act and probably included by clerks bookended the lay narratives contained in these warrants. The frequent incidence of spousal abuse indicates that certifying officials accepted it as a signifier of mental disturbance and that there were limitations to the toleration of domestic violence in nineteenth-century Ireland.

Domestic violence included other forms of familial abuse. Parents were reported as assaulting children and there is support for Suzuki's contention that a 'lack of parental affection was often regarded as a sign of insanity'.[98] Violent assaults by fathers and mothers perpetrated on male and female children were viewed as unnatural acts. Attacks on children often occurred while a spouse was being abused. In September 1854, Honor G.'s husband swore that she 'got out of bed, threw herself on the children, put her arms on theirs and tried to force salt into their mouths'. He stated that he 'had to make use of considerable violence to take her from them'.[99] Elizabeth Steiner-Scott has suggested that magistrates' responses to domestic violence cases that included attacks on children were gendered exhibiting a particularly harsh attitude towards women.[100] This is less evident among asylum certifications. Attacks on children featured more frequently in evidence sworn by wives against their husbands and these assaults tended to be more violent. The wife of Edward F. petitioned for his committal following a series of assaults against her and her daughter, which continued for four months. Eleanor F. stated that he had 'assaulted his wife and daughter in so violent [a] manner by striking them with a large stick and kicking them'. In the cases of Edward, Maryanne and others, families had tolerated irrational behaviour for some time. Prior to his violent assault on the family, Edward had exhibited signs of pyromania and had 'brought out a quantity of old books, paper and brushes and set them on fire under the eaves of his house'. He had 'frequently got a quantity of salt with which he rubs his person and puts it in his shoes and will get onions and garlic and will pound them and will put them in his ears and has frequently followed his wife with a spade and poker and threatened to take her life.'[101] The family had tolerated his behaviour for some time, and while families' motivations remain relatively obscure, it was often the manifestation of violence coupled with previous history of erratic behaviour that persuaded them to certify. Violence and dangerous behaviour was disruptive to all members of the household, not just the married couple, and placed the security of the family and the surrounding community at risk.

Kerby Miller and Bruce D. Boling have argued that generational tensions were common in Irish families and the warrants attest to the disruption and tensions caused by the presence of adult offspring within laterally extended households.[102] Parents and siblings expressed anxieties and fears that were prompted by the presence of violent adults, particularly men, within the household. Male and female adult offspring threatened relatives, though actual assaults were less frequent. The father of Thomas T. swore his adult son had 'raised stones and violently threatened him [the father] and endeavoured to break the door of the house and then smashed the window'.[103] The mother of Richard R. swore he had 'took up a stool and threatened' her; he had previously 'threatened to take his mother's and his own life'.[104] The threat of violence ensured that female relatives, particularly mothers, were disinclined to tolerate and manage male relatives in the household. Magistrates and officials concurred, as the threat of male violence against women was often sufficient to secure certification.

Adult offspring also perpetrated significant assaults on parents. Mothers certifying daughters testified to intensely violent assaults. Anne A. severely beat her mother, throwing her downstairs, and breaking furniture over her body.[105] Joseph A.'s father swore that his son had assaulted his mother and attempted to set fire to her bed with a candle. Joseph had a history of erratic behaviour and the family had endeavoured to confine him to the house. The assault on his mother occurred when he attempted escape.[106] Fathers were also targets of violent behaviour and, usually, a son was the perpetrator. John B.'s father swore that his son had assaulted him and his sister, Bridget.[107] When certifying daughters, fathers cited a range of behaviour that included violence and moral impropriety. Mary K.'s father swore that she had broken windows and torn her clothes 'to her nethermost garments.' She had also attempted to 'drown herself in a deep bog drain.'[108] Officials and families were less anxious about daughters' violence and certification to an asylum usually occurred when violence became more severe or threatened property.

The presence of several adults in a household also produced tensions among siblings though relatively few siblings initiated certifications. Parents remained important figures of authority in the household when initiating certifications. Usually, siblings worked on the family holding, and were co-resident when a crisis occurred.[109] In the case of the certification of a male sibling by another an assault that occurred when brothers were labouring was cited. Martin E. swore his brother, William, assaulted him with a pike and attacked another brother with a stone.[110] It was rare for brothers to swear evidence against sisters.[111] When a sister testified against a sister, severe violence was not cited, though frequent references were made to suicide attempts, erratic behaviour and minor assaults.[112]

In his study on commissions of lunacy, Suzuki found that families were particularly troubled by the public exposure of disruptive behaviour and this triggered the decision to seek institutional services.[113] Housing conditions among Irish labourers and small farmers, coupled with traditions of working on neighbours' holdings and patterns of social life, made the concealment of troublesome relatives difficult. Nonetheless, periods of domestic confinement were ended when a person was involved in public acts and became a physical danger to neighbours' property and person. In August 1855 a Wexford man swore information against his brother who, for two years, had exhibited various signs of mental derangement. He had thrown himself into the River Slaney, refused his food, and threatened to shoot his sister-in-law. His family had kept him confined in the house but he managed to escape by setting it on fire, destroying the adjoining houses.[114] While this event may not have been the neighbours' initial exposure to his mental disturbance, it may have been the first time he became a physical threat to those outside the domestic environment. This broader threat prompted the decision to certify.

Another form of public exposure occurred when neighbours witnessed altercations between individuals and their families. In contrast to Suzuki's finding that the 'mob' intervened in defence of the lunatic's rights, among cases studied here neighbours intervened to protect relatives from violent assaults and were sometimes the subject of assaults. For example, the neighbours of John C.'s family prevented him from seriously assaulting his relatives suggesting that the neighbours were aware that he could be difficult.[115] Public exposure of dangerous behaviour could also entail violence against property, often arson, a trend which Michael MacDonald found in his study of early modern certifications.[116] Arson was presented more frequently during female certifications.[117] One example was of a daughter who repeatedly tried to set her parents' house on fire 'by throwing fire into the bed'. She also assaulted her mother and father.[118]

Violence against property entailed damage to churches, workhouse property and the property of local landowners. Churches were often damaged when individuals sought refuge; for example, in March 1844, John O'B. damaged the chapel in Thomastown in county Kilkenny, breaking 'the lock and iron chain of the chapel gate' and 'three large panes of glass' when trying to gain access.[119] Other behaviour was more irreverent; in September 1863, John S. threw part of a fish at the altar during divine service, while Mary B. appeared in Ballinamona Chapel 'almost in a state of nudity'. There was also evidence that men and women tore and ripped clothing, sometimes stripping themselves. Houston has argued that among the middle- and upper-classes, the destruction of clothing represented the rejection of social position and a form of social suicide.[120] Among poorer socio-economic groups, it represented an incidence of irrationality and wastefulness, and this behaviour conformed to stereotypical images of mental illness. The destruction of workhouse clothing and attacks on workhouse property and staff represented a rejection of workhouse regimes. In some cases individuals were reported to have 'wandered abroad' and destroyed their clothing and were perceived to be a 'moral danger' to a community. Such behaviour was presented as evidence during seventeen cases and was usually one of a series of more worrying behavioural traits: Mary B. was brought before the justices when she attempted to stab her mother with a fork. She left her house 'for three or four days and came back with her clothes all torn.'[121] 'Wandering' was frequently evidenced during female certifications as it conflicted with nineteenth-century concepts of female respectability.

Evidence of an attempted suicide or a fear that individuals could harm themselves was frequently cited during certifications, suggesting that medical understandings of suicide influenced lay interpretations of such behaviour. During the eighteenth and early nineteenth centuries, traditional notions of suicide as a moral offence were replaced with more medicalised understandings. Suicide became 'retrospective evidence of disease' and those who attempted to commit suicide were sick.[122] However, during this time period, suicide was still an indictable crime and cases of suicide received extensive coverage in Irish and English newspapers. Police constables were advised that persons who attempted suicide were to be arrested and charged with an offence.[123] Although legal prosecutions occurred and religious authorities continued to condemn suicide, attempted suicide increasingly resulted in certification to an asylum. Lay witnesses variously described suicidal behaviour and some attempts were very determined. For example, in March 1867, Mary swore that her husband had 'cut his throat and windpipe with a razor.'[124] In April 1848, Margaret M. allegedly 'stabbed herself twice in the forehead with a scissors so that it bled and also threatened to do it twice more'. Mothers commented on suicidal behaviour more frequently when certifying sons than daughters. The mother of John N. claimed he 'broke out of the house through the window and went to the river Barrow and threw himself in and would have destroyed himself were it not that he was prevented'.[125] Spouses frequently claimed their partners displayed suicidal intentions, with husbands citing it more frequently.[126] The suicidal behaviour that wives reported when certifying husbands was more violent and determined. Mary W. claimed that for the previous two years, her husband, William, had attempted to drown himself and had taken poison.[127] This supports studies of nineteenth-century suicide in Britain, which indicate that male suicidal behaviour was violent.[128]

The warrants included evidence of families who maintained relatives in domestic environments, in spite of the financial and social difficulties. Scull has contended that capitalism and the emergence of asylums resulted in the replacement of traditional obligations to care for relatives in the community with incarceration in a 'specialised, bureaucratically organised state-supported asylum system'.[129] The families studied here appear to have endured relatives' disruptive behaviour for some time. During certification, families claimed relatives had behaved erratically for months, years, even decades. In 1866, John C. refused to eat for three months, while Mary W. lived in 'fear and dread of invisible objects' for a similar period. When providing medical evidence, doctors frequently stated that individuals had been ill for some time, specifying when they had been maintained at home or previously confined. The mentally ill were maintained at home for various reasons; domiciliary confinement facilitated concealing hereditary insanity but also allowed families to maintain contact with relatives. The conditions in which individuals were housed and familial treatment of them varied considerable. Suzuki has argued that the continued maintenance of the mentally ill at home allowed for the emergence of a 'domestic psychiatry' but there is little evidence of its development in Ireland.[130] Individuals were often locked in rooms, and physically restrained, confirming the lunacy inspectors' fears about domiciliary conditions. Families were, however, willing to go to some lengths to maintain a relative at home implying that they felt some familial obligation to care for them.[131] In 1905, John Dowling's sister paid a neighbour to care for him in her house.[132] In 1851, Mary J. testified that her brother, John, had inflicted violent assaults on the family and one sister was too badly injured to appear at the petty sessions hearing. One of his victims was her father, who was described as 'of unsound mind for the last two years'. Both father and son were cared in the domestic environment, though John was a significant danger to the whole family. However, when these arrangements could not be continued, it was the violent son who was certified, as he posed a threat to more vulnerable relatives. The family continued to maintain the father at home.

While violent behaviour was emphasised during dangerous lunatic certifications, it was often accompanied by additional indications of mental disorder. The interrogation of this additional evidence facilitates an assessment of lay understandings of mental illness and of the extent to which the 'rapid expansion of asylum populations' in Ireland was a product of 'the diffusion of medicine as a way of thinking about and acting on the body and mind'.[133] Mary E. Fissell and Nicholas Jewson have argued that the 'common-ground'[134] or in Jewson's phrase shared 'cosmology' which

had previously existed between doctors and their patients was disappearing by the eighteenth century. Eighteenth-century medical theories
fundamentally changed the doctor-patient relationship. Concomitantly,
vernacular medical knowledge was also changing in this period and as
Nancy Tomes identified, in Pennsylvania doctors and patrons 'shared
ideas about the nature of mental disease.'[135] The lay indications of insanity
studied here suggest that medical descriptions of mental disturbance had
become part of popular culture. By the first half of the nineteenth century,
the mentally ill were less frequently described as a 'madman' or 'out of his
mind' in the lay accounts, instead specific indications were referenced.[136]
The lay testimonies contained in dangerous lunatic warrants include references to individual's inability to exercise self-control, confirming Eigen's
suggestion that the concept of the 'will', and a failure to control it, 'had
taken on a curious life of its own'.[137] The loss of will was often expressed
as a form of violence against family or friends and violent behaviour
was contrasted with previous habits of frugality, stability and sobriety.[138]
'Incoherent' speech and actions were also cited; in August 1850 Peter L.
was reported to be 'in a state of excitement, speaking loudly and incoher-
ently in the public streets at New Ross'. Similar behaviour was cited in
lay testimony provided during Old Bailey criminal insanity trials.[139] The
negative impact passions had on the will was also attested to; in 1850
Catherine F.'s husband described her as being in a 'rage of passion' while
Eleanor F. in February 1851 claimed her husband Edward had a history of
'unguided passions'.[140] John Conolly argued that passions and emotions
subverted the individual's powers to control their will and as Eigen has
shown these 'passions' were presented as having 'autonomous power to
produce madness'.[141]

Families also reported a change in individuals' interior well-being,
a phenomenon Eigen argued emerged in nineteenth-century England,
and Catharine Coleborne observed in lay testimonies in late nineteenth-
century Australasian certifications.[142] Mary L.'s husband commented that
she had been 'depressed in spirits' before her attempted suicide in May
1847, while in October 1858, Bridget B.'s relatives described her as 'rather
melancholy' and 'uneasy'. Patients' 'fear' and paranoia were marshalled as
part of lay lexicons of insanity: in 1865 Mary W.'s relatives testified that
she was 'in dread and fear of invisible objects' while John C.'s relatives
stated that he accused his family of putting poison in his food. These fears
could focus on the disappearance of family members: Fanny C.'s husband

claimed she was convinced that 'people are coming to take away her children' while the schoolmaster, John C., insisted that his real wife and children had been 'taken away'. The belief that fairies 'took away' people was still popular in parts of nineteenth-century Ireland. Although fairies were not explicitly referenced in the warrants, the fear that relatives could be spirited away was evocative and informed reactions to certain behaviour. When Honor G. attempted to 'force salt into their [children's] mouths' and Edward's F. rubbed a 'quantity of salt' on 'his person and puts [sic] it in his shoes,' relatives could interpret this behaviour in a number of ways.[143] Salt was said to have curative powers but it was also believed that fairies had an aversion to it.[144] In her assessment of attitudes towards belief in fairies in the late nineteenth century, Angela Bourke has suggested that when fairy belief was discussed during serious criminal cases the courts sometimes treated the perpetrators leniently, pathologising their actions and sending them to local asylums.[145] However, responses could be harsher and other perpetrators were treated as criminals. As Bourke showed, the killers of Bridget Cleary were prosecuted. These mixed responses to fairy belief were not confined to medical doctors, magistrates and officials but shared by families who interpreted it as an indication of irrationality.

Between the 1840s and the 1860s, lay narratives of mental disorder were multilayered. While families frequently attested to violent and dangerous behaviour within households, such evidence was often accompanied by reports of 'unguided passions' and expressions of the 'wrong kinds of emotion' such as fear, anxiety and paranoia.[146] The 'stock eighteenth-century terminology' of mental illness was largely absent as lay testimonies included descriptions of people's interior worlds. Eigen identified a similar shift in language in his analysis of criminal insanity trials between 1800 and 1843. The emphasis on dangerous behaviour in lay testimony indicates that families were fully aware of certification requirements under the dangerous lunatic legislation and that, in the public mind, asylums were primarily associated with managing and containing 'danger', a point developed further in chapter six.

Lay or medical aetiologies of insanity?

Certification warrants can provide additional insights into evolving medical aetiologies of mental illness. As demonstrated in chapter three, from the 1840s local prison and dispensary medical officers examined defendants and signed medical certificates during dangerous lunatic certifications. Paid for these services from 1875, these duties formed part of the expanding field of nineteenth-century medical jurisprudence. In contrast to the mad-doctors Eigen studied in his assessment of the Old Bailey criminal trials, dispensary doctors in the southeast of Ireland seldom appeared as witnesses and were unlikely to be cross-examined during hearings.[147] Nor did Irish dispensary doctors claim to have particular expertise in identifying mental illness. They gained their experience from cases presented during routine practice in medical dispensaries and it was not until the late 1860s that informal educational classes on insanity were available in Ireland.[148] The medical evidence discussed here therefore represents local dispensary doctors' commentary on aetiologies of mental illness recorded between 1838 and 1868 while asylum superintendants' commentaries are explored in chapter seven.

Tomes and Suzuki have suggested that despite the protestations of influential alienists, medical practitioners were heavily dependent on middle-class families' lay testimony when providing evidence before commissions of lunacy in England.[149] Daily practice required practitioners to rely on family evidence and consequently lay testimony was central to the practice of certification.[150] Families had access to personal information unknown to practitioners. While John Conolly dismissed lay evidence as unreliable, George Man Burrows, J. C. Bucknill and D. H. Hack acknowledged that they were obliged to rely on it.[151] As Suzuki has argued, the incorporation of lay testimonies provided by middle-class and aristocratic clients may have been influenced by doctors' need to secure and maintain a lucrative client base. Medical practitioners signing dangerous lunatic certifications in Ireland were similarly dependent on familial and lay testimony though they were not influenced by the need to secure clients. Dispensary, workhouse and gaol doctors were particularly dependent on lay testimony when securing information on the causation and longevity of illness and on hereditary insanity. When reporting on causes of insanity in certification warrants, doctors referred to events that occurred several years previously, or to private family histories, suggesting that relatives and friends were important sources of information. While medical personnel may have guided families' responses and prioritised the evidence included in warrants, the narratives of causation contained in certification warrants were a blend of medical and lay aetiologies.

Local dispensary doctors admitted they depended upon family or other lay evidence. In 1851, William Thompson, the medical officer at Inistioge dispensary, county Kilkenny, certified that Edward H. was 'at present of unsound mind'. He had 'not seen him [Edward H.] committ [sic] any violence but [since] several witnesses have informed me of the fact I consider him a fit subject for confinement.'[152] In February 1847, Joseph Lalor, Kilkenny gaol physician who was subsequently appointed medical superintendent at Kilkenny asylum, reported that he depended on evidence provided by a fellow gaol inmate when certifying Anastasia D.[153] Highlighting that he had only limited direct contact with her – he had seen her twice – he recorded that the other inmate had known Anastasia for twenty-five years and informed him that she had been ill since her husband's death seventeen years earlier although there was no insanity in the family.[154] Most of Lalor's evidence was based on this testimony and it provided the basis of the case for institutional confinement.

Some medical officers were less confident about lay testimony and favoured their own examinations, visiting individuals several times before signing the medical certificate. George Lang, medical officer at Kilann dispensary, county Wexford, visited one woman for three consecutive days before concluding she was mentally ill, while another man was visited several times during a three-week period.[155] These doctors shared the unease that medical practitioners in Pennsylvania experienced when assessing cases of which they had no previous knowledge.[156] During examinations, dispensary medical officers tried to engage and converse with individuals.[157] George Weldon, medical officer at Gorey dispensary in county Wexford, claimed he had 'a lenghtened [sic] conversation with Thomas B.'. During it, Thomas talked of 'persons depriving him of his genitals' and referenced other 'improbable acts'. Based on this conversation, Weldon concluded he was insane.[158] Doctors also depended on their previous experiences of patients; Phillip R., confined in Kilkenny gaol in October 1849, was known to his physician 'for the last twelve years', and he considered Phillip to be 'insane at intervals'.[159] Likewise Henry Boxwell, the physician contracted to Wexford gaol, claimed to have known Edward T. 'for the last twenty years and consider[ed] that he labour[ed] under periodic attacks of insanity'.[160] Gaol physicians, who were simultaneously employed at local dispensaries, were sometimes consulted at the onset of symptoms. Thomas Elwood Linsey, medical officer at Broadway dispensary and Wexford gaol, attested that

Maryanne W. had 'for more than six years … frequently applied to me at my dispensary for advice. Her manner was odd, eccentric and particularly disagreeable. She frequently spoke of her sins and judgement to come, etc. on that theme she first showed insanity'.[161] In these cases, medical practitioners emphasised their own knowledge and experiences eschewing a dependence on lay testimony.

Most assessments represented a blend of medical and lay evidence. When certifying Fanny C. in 1864, and Mathew R. in 1863, dispensary doctors based their conclusions on personal examinations and on lay testimony.[162] Frederick Stock based his opinion of Margaret L. '[f]rom my examination of her as well as the evidence given before the magistrates'.[163] Stock acknowledged the importance of lay testimony but did not rely solely upon it. Nor did he dismiss it and privilege his own expertise. Finally, some practitioners provided evidence that was formulaic in form, suggesting they were indifferent and that they depended on lay evidence presented at court. In these cases, the person was usually described as being of 'unsound mind', a 'dangerous lunatic', 'requiring restraint' and a 'fit subject for the asylum'. The certifications were signed following a single examination of the person in either the gaol or the workhouse.

The causes of mental illness recorded in both lay and medical testimonies reflected generally held nineteenth-century medical theories. Physical causes dominated and included drink, fever, sunstroke, childbirth and head trauma.[164] In April 1860, one woman insisted her sister's disorder was caused by the birth of her first child.[165] Relatives provided information on attacks of fever, physical injuries, drinking habits and when pertinent, histories of institutionalisation. George Carpenter, medical officer, recorded that John W., a twenty-four year old labourer from Kilkenny, became ill when he fell into a coal-pit nine years previously.[166] Some of these events and behaviours occurred while the person was abroad and the medical officer relied on patient and/or family for information.[167] As Coleborne has shown, relatives also provided information on hereditary insanity and in Ireland, dispensary doctors and families frequently cited it in testimony.[168]

Dispensary doctors and families reported emotional and psychological pressures and disruptions to emotional well-being as causes of insanity.[169] These pressures and disruptions were not failures to control emotional expression as suggested by Norbet Elias but represented patients, families and doctors different understandings of the impact emotions had on the mind.[170] Marland has argued that in the first half of the nineteenth century, medical theories of puerperal insanity featured multiple and, at times, contradictory portrayals of emotions. Emotions could be disruptive and endangering, but also restorative for patients.[171]

Medical officers certifying patients in the southeast of Ireland also pathologised 'wrong' emotions – fear of poverty, anxiety caused by unemployment and changed circumstances were cited as causes of insanity. As Pamela Michael and Marland have argued, medical practitioners acknowledged the disruptive impact that broader social and economic conditions had upon mental and emotional well-being. Doctors reported the fear of Famine and destitution as causes among some patients; in 1850 one dispensary doctor recorded that one woman's illness was caused by 'the depression of the times and her family being reduced in circumstances'. While living conditions in Ireland improved after the 1850s, the spectre of Famine haunted the rural and urban poor. Labourers were still subject to the vagaries of bad harvests and the market. Nationally, wages and standards of living improved between 1850 and 1870, nonetheless the half-century after the Famine was punctuated by poor harvests in 1859 to 1864, 1879 to 1881 and 1894 to 1895.[172] Medical officers reported that fears about economic decline and potential ruin had a detrimental impact on patients' minds: Thomas H.'s illness was ascribed to the loss of his job at the local mill, while Anne M.'s illness was caused by 'loss of property and friends'. She was characterised as being 'middle class of life'. As discussed in chapter two, Tuke and Drapes also argued that financial worries had a detrimental influence on the mind. Suzuki identified similar evidence in his analysis of families' narratives of insanity among male patients at Hanwell Asylum.[173] Medical officers attributed male anxieties at failing to fulfil gendered economic roles as causes of insanity.[174] For example, in 1866 John C.'s inability to provide his family with 'assistance' – he was confined in gaol for debt – and their subsequent descent into a 'state of destitution' was reported to have 'prayed [sic] so much upon his mind that he became insane', while a shoemaker William W.'s dangerous insanity – he was said to have been 'weak-minded' – was precipitated by his failure to provide for his wife and the subsequent collapse of his marriage. Women's anxiety around poverty was not overtly linked with a failure to work or provide for a family.[175]

Instead, the root of mental anxiety among them was reported as being the inability to maintain appropriate standards of female respectability. In 1850, the cause of Anastasia Q.'s illness was assigned to 'Uneasiness [sic] of mind on account of some report against her character' while Margaret McC.'s 'mental anxiety' was a result of 'giving birth to a child the father of whom is unknown to her'.[176] Maura Cronin has argued that in post-Famine Ireland female 'respectability' within low-income social groups depended more on 'not disgracing oneself or one's family' than on economic status.[177]

Doctors and relatives observed that grief and other emotions associated with death and emigration impacted on mental stability. These featured frequently in both medical and lay evidence as causes of insanity. Elizabeth O'H.'s 'grief' at her parents' deaths was regarded as precipitating her illness, while Edward T., a farmer's son, 'took trouble at his mother's death'. Expressions of grief were associated with other forms of loss, including emigration. In nineteenth-century Ireland, emigration became a common feature of life, emerging as a 'family survival strategy'.[178] While emigration was firmly established before the Famine, it took on new dimensions in the 1840s and remained an important part of the Irish life cycle for the remainder of the century. Contemporaries and historians have argued that migration impacted on asylum admissions in various ways. Scull has argued that it was a significant factor in the increase in asylum admissions, however, Melling's study of admissions into Devon institutions indicates that migrants were less vulnerable to institutionalisation than settled families.[179] As discussed in chapter two, contemporaries argued that those who did not emigrate were often mentally enfeebled.[180] Tuke opined that the loss of breadwinners through emigration and the associated 'financial and social difficulties' caused significant 'mental strain' on those left behind.[181]

The impact that emigration had on the minds of those who were left behind in Ireland therefore remains unclear. As emigrants' wakes demonstrate, communities had embedded traditions that provided a mechanism or ritual that explicitly acknowledged the grief associated with emigration. When family members replied to emigrants' letters their responses were replete with expressions of loneliness. These letters attest to the emotional impact of emigration and to the fears families experienced when faced with the disintegration of households.[182] Dispensary doctors and families reported on these expressions of grief and loss in testimony during certification identifying them as causes of mental instability.[183] In 1852, when certifying his sixty year-old wife, one husband concluded she was driven to attempt suicide following the 'loss of her children who emigrated to America', while another man's illness was ascribed to the grief he suffered following his children's emigration to America.[184] For parents and others left in Ireland, uncertain as to whether they would see their relatives again, emigration meant the permanent fracturing and dispersal of families. A relative's emigration triggered additional emotional responses including jealousy and a sense of failure.[185] Henry Boxwell concluded that Michael B.'s illness emerged after 'two of his brothers went to America about a year since and his being left behind may have prayed [sic] on his mind.'[186] Similarly, Thomas Elwood Lindsey maintained that Maryanne W.'s malady was aggravated when some of the family went to America – 'sorrow for their loss, disappointment in not accompanying them hurried on the malady'.[187] These individuals were both twenty years old, members of the age group most likely to emigrate. Medical officers reported as causes of mental disturbance disappointment at being unable, or deemed unsuitable, to participate fully in what was increasingly understood to be the typical Irish life cycle.

Conclusion

Three general conclusions can be drawn from the close analysis of dangerous lunatic legal procedures and from the medical and lay testimonies recorded during petty session hearings. The certifications procedures, and newspaper reporting of them, ensured that lunatic asylums and the mechanisms of certifying people as dangerous lunatics became firmly established within Irish communities and formed what Geertz termed 'local knowledge'. This contributed to the significant rise in dangerous lunatic certifications later in the century and to the perception of asylums as sites for the containment of 'dangerous' insanity. It has also been argued that medical, legal and lay explanatory frameworks of mental illness intersected during these legal procedures and a shared language of mental illness emerged as lay definitions were incorporated into 'medical models'.[188] Moreover, the warrants tell us that when families and dispensary doctors presented evidence of violent behaviour or other aetiologies of mental illness, they did so in a gendered manner and that they reported and understood the emotional loss, loneliness and anxiety associated with death, emigration and financial worries as precipitating mental illness suggesting that concerns about the importance of stable and emotionally satisfying households extended to poorer families.

Notes

1   *Carlow Sentinel* (26 May 1849).
2   Eigen made a similar observation in relation to reports of criminal lunatic cases, see J. P. Eigen, *Witnessing Insanity. Madness and Mad-doctors in the English Court* (New Haven and London: Yale University Press, 1995), p. 6.
3   This does not include six individuals who were admitted between 1839 and 1846.
4   Eigen, *Witnessing Insanity*, p. 184.
5   J. Moran, 'The Signal and the Noise: the Historical Epidemiology of Insanity in Ante-Bellum New Jersey', *History of Psychiatry*, 14 (2003), 281–301; C. Coleborne, '"His Brain was Wrong, His Mind Astray": Families and the Language of Insanity in New South Wales, Queensland and New Zealand 1800–1920', *Journal of Family History*, 31:1 (2006), 45–65.
6   Finnane, 'Asylums, Families and the State', 143.
7   *Ibid.*, 141–143.
8   Melling and Forsythe, *The Politics of Madness*, pp. 107–108.
9   Wright, 'The Certification of Insanity', 268.
10 N. Tomes, 'The Anglo-American Asylum in Historical Perspective', in C. Smith and J. A. Giggs (eds), *Location and Stigma. Contemporary Perspectives on Mental Health and Mental Health Care* (Boston: Unwin Hyman, 1998), p. 14.
11 Wright, 'Family Strategies and Institutional Confinement of Idiot Children', 190–208; Finnane, *Insanity and the Insane*, pp. 175–220; Walton, 'Lunacy in the Industrial Revolution', 1–22.
12 H. Marland, *Dangerous Motherhood. Insanity and Childbirth in Victorian Britain* (Houndmills: Palgrave Macmillan, 2004), pp. 65–94.
13 H. Marland, 'Languages and Landscapes of Emotion: Motherhood and Puerperal Insanity in the Nineteenth Century', in Bound Alberti (ed.), *Medicine, Emotion and Disease*, pp. 53–78; Colborne, *Madness in the Family*, pp. 102–107; T. Dixon, 'Patients and Passions: Languages of Medicine and Emotion', in F. Bound Alberti (ed.), *Medicine, Emotion and Disease, 1700–1950* (Houndmills: Palgrave Macmillan, 2006), pp. 22–52.
14 R. McMahon, 'The Court of Petty Sessions and Society in pre-Famine Galway', in R. Gillespie (ed.), *The Remaking of Modern Ireland 1750–1950* (Dublin: Four Courts Press, 2004), pp. 101–137, p.129; P. Karsten, *Between Law and Custom. 'High' and 'Low' Legal Cultures in the Lands of the British Diaspora – The United States, Canada, Australia and New Zealand, 1600–1900* (Cambridge: Cambridge University Press, 2002).

15 McCabe, 'Open Court', p. 128.

16 *Ibid.*

17 *Ibid.*, p. 132.

18 Eigen, *Witnessing Insanity*, p. 9.

19 *Leinster Leader* (1 July 1905).

20 *Wexford Independent* (7 January 1860). For other cases, see *Carlow Sentinel* (3 September 1870); *Carlow Sentinel* (27 Aug 1870).

21 McCabe, 'Open Court', p. 137.

22 *Ibid.*

23 *Ibid.*, pp. 126–162.

24 McCabe, 'Open Court'; D. McCabe, 'Magistrates, Peasants and the Petty Sessions Courts, Mayo 1823–50', *Cáthair na Mart*, 5 (1985), 45–53; D. McCabe, 'Law, Conflict and Social Order in County Mayo, 1820–1845', (PhD dissertation, University College Dublin, 1991).

25 *Thom's Directory, 1850.*

26 Vaughan, 'Ireland, c.1870', p. 768.

27 N. Ó Cíosain, *Print and Popular Culture 1750–1850* (London: Macmillan Press, 1997), p. 29.

28 McCabe, 'Law, Conflict and Social Order in County Mayo, 1820–1845.'

29 P. Prior, *Madness and Murder. Gender, Crime and Mental Disorder in Nineteenth-Century Ireland* (Dublin: Irish Academic Press, 2008), p. 9.

30 See chapter five.

31 McCabe, 'Open Court', p. 155.

32 *Ibid.*, p. 150.

33 *Freeman's Journal* (15 March 1839).

34 Finnane, *Insanity and the Insane*, p. 113.

35 *Freeman's Journal* (7 April 1873); *Southern Star* (11 June 1892); *Irish Times* (16 May 1863).

36 *Freeman's Journal* (6 January 1862).

37 *Irish Times* (23 May 1862).

38 DDA, Archbishop Byrne's Papers, Charity Cases Box 2 (1922–26), James Brody, Parish Priest, to Fr Dunne, Secretary, Archbishop Byrne, 5 June 1923. Thanks to Dr Lindsey Earner-Byrne for this reference.

39 SPH, ELA, Letter from Father Cullen to Dr Drapes, 8 March 1906; Admission Register, 1902–1912.

40 *Twenty-second Report of Lunacy Inspectors*, H. C. 1873 [852] xxx, p. 9; *Eighteenth Report of Lunacy Inspectors*, H. C. 1868–69 [4181] xxvii, p. 5; *Eleventh Report of Lunacy Inspectors*, H. C. 1862 [2975] xxiii, p. 25.

41 *Fifth Report of Lunacy Inspectors*, H. C. 1851 [1387] xxiv, p. 6; *Twenty-third Report of Lunacy Inspectors*, H. C. 1874 [1004] xxvii, p. 11; *Eighteenth Report of Lunacy Inspectors*, H. C. 1868–69 [4181] xxvii, p. 5; *Eighth Report of Lunacy Inspectors*, H. C. 1857 session 2 [2253] xvii, p. 17; Scull, *The Most Solitary of Afflictions*, pp. 269–270.

42 DPH, CLA Minute Book, 20 March 1871.

43 *Leinster Leader* (22 July 1905).

44 McCandless, 'Liberty and Lunacy', p. 340.

45 Following his appointment to the asylum, White became a significant figure in the social and intellectual life of Carlow town. His social advancement can be mapped through commercial directories. In 1846 he was listed as a physician, surgeon and magistrate and by 1856 he was recorded as a member of the gentry, see *Thom's Directory, 1840–1866* and *Slater's National Commercial Directory*.

46 *Thirty-second Report of Lunacy Inspectors*, H. C. 1883 [C.3675] xxx, p. 7.

47 M. L. Legg, 'The Kilkenny Circulating Library-Society and the Growth of Reading Rooms in Nineteenth-century Ireland', in B. Cunningham and M. Kennedy (eds), *The Experience of Reading: Irish Historical Perspectives* (Dublin: Economic and Social History Society of Ireland, 1990), pp. 109–123.

48 *Carlow Sentinel* (June 1832).

49 *First Annual Report of the Carlow Mechanics' Institute* (Carlow 1853), p. 5.

50 E. Neswald, 'Science, Sociability and the Improvement of Ireland: The Galway Mechanics' Institute, 1826–1851', *British Journal for the History of Science*, 39:4 (2006), 503–534.

51 P. A. Townend, '"Academies of Nationality": the Reading Room and Irish National Movements, 1838–1905', in L. W. McBride (ed.), *Reading Irish Histories: Texts, Contexts and Memory in Modern Ireland* (Dublin: Four Courts Press, 2003), pp. 19–39.

52 *Journal of the Statistical and Social Inquiry Society in Ireland*, 73 (1893), n. p.

53 For examples see NAI, MFGS/58/399–402, County Carlow Petty Session Order Books, 1910–1922; NAI, MFGS 58/83–84, Athy Court County Kildare Petty Sessions Order Books, 1918–1919.

54 NAI CSPS1/3964 Rathangan Court Petty Sessions Order Books, 1869–1873.

55 Wright, 'The Certification of Insanity', 285; Melling and Forsythe, *The Politics of Madness*, p. 109.

56 P. Burke, *Social History of Knowledge, From Gutenberg to Diderot* (Oxford: Polity, 2000), p. 11.

57 For an example of an early case, see *Freeman's Journal* (15 March 1839).

58 Legg, 'Kilkenny Circulating Library Society', pp. 109–123; *Carlow Sentinel* (24 February 1849); (15 October 1870); (3 September 1870); *Irish Times* (22 October 1861).

59 *Nation* (3 August 1844); *Irish Times* (1 August 1862).

60 *Carlow Sentinel* (26 May 1849).

61 *Leinster Leader* (27 May 1905).

62 *Leinster Leader* (10 June 1905); (24 June 1905); (8 July 1905).

63 *Leinster Leader* (1 July 1905).

64 A. E. Kane, 'The Ritualization of Newspaper Reading and Political Consciousness: the Role of Newspapers in the Irish Land War', in L. W. McBride (ed.), *Reading Irish Histories: Texts, Contexts and Memory in Modern Ireland* (Dublin: Four Courts Press, 2003), pp. 40–62.

65 *Leinster Leader* (17 June 1905).

66 *Leinster Leader* (20 May 1905).

67 National Gallery of Ireland, *A Time and a Place: Two Centuries of Irish Social History* (Dublin: National Gallery of Ireland, 2007), pp. 128–30.

68 Legg, 'Kilkenny Circulating-Library Society', p. 117; M. L. Legg, *Newspapers and Nationalism. The Irish Provincial Press* (Dublin: Four Courts Press, 1999), p. 38.

69 Legg, *Newspapers and Nationalism*, p. 38; J. R. R. Adams, *The Printed Word and the Common Man: Popular Culture in Ulster 1700–1900* (Belfast: Institute of Irish Studies, 1987); Ó Cíosain, *Print and Popular Culture*; M. E. Daly and D. Dickson (eds), *The Origins of Popular Literacy in Ireland: Language Changes and Educational Development 1700–1920* (Dublin: Department of Modern History, Trinity College Dublin and Department of Modern Irish History, University College Dublin, 1990).

70 M. E. Daly, 'Literacy and Language Change in the Later Nineteenth and Early Twentieth Centuries', in Daly and Dickson (eds), *The Origins of Popular Literacy*, pp. 153–166.

71 Melling and Turner, 'The Road to the Asylum', 300.

72 Melling and Turner, 'The Road to the Asylum', 300; See also D. H. Alderman, 'Integrating Space into a Reactive Theory of the Asylum: Evidence from Post-Civil War Georgia', *Health and Place*, 3 (1997), 111–122; Hunter and Shannon, 'Jarvis Revisited', 296–302.

73 Melling and Turner, 'The Road to the Asylum', 300.

74 D. McLoughlin, 'Workhouses and Irish Female Paupers', in M. Luddy and C. Murphy (eds), *Women Surviving. Studies in Irish Women's History in the Nineteenth and Twentieth Centuries* (Dublin: Poolbeg Press, 1990), pp. 117–147; E. Dwyer, *Homes for the Mad: Life Inside Two Nineteenth-Century Asylums* (New Brunswick and London: Rutgers University Press, 1987), p. 87; Wright, 'Getting Out of the Asylum'; Prestwich, 'Family Strategies and Medical Power', 799–818.

75 Number of dangerous lunatic admissions to Carlow Asylum, 1856 to 1867.

Year	Annual Reports	Committal Warrants
1856	15	16
1857	7	9
1858	22	11
1859	11	16
1860	15	19
1861	17	17
1862	10	7
1863	6	5
1864	16	18
1865	13	14
1866	31	31
1867	17	16

76 Suzuki, *Madness at Home*, pp. 21–29.

77 Wright, 'The Certification of Insanity'; Andrews, 'Case Notes, Case Histories and the Patient's Experience of Insanity', 255–281.

78 Andrews, 'Case Notes, Case Histories'; G. Davis, 'The Historiography of Public Health Records in Research: A Critique of Case Notes', online publications, University of Edinburgh, (2002); F. Clondrau, 'The Patient's View Meets the Clinical Gaze', *Social History of Medicine*, 20:3 (2007), 525–540.

79   E. Malcolm's work on St Patrick's Hospital in Dublin examines patient committal for the earlier period, but this was a charitable institution, see E. Malcolm, *Swift's Hospital*. For studies of late nineteenth-century warrants, see also Finnane, *Insanity and the Insane*, pp. 129-1-74; Finnane, 'Asylums, Families and the State'; Walsh, 'Lunatic and Criminal Alliances'; Walsh, 'The Designs of Providence'.

80   M. Levine-Clark, 'Dysfunctional Domesticity: Female Insanity and Family Relationships among the West-Riding Poor in the Mid-Nineteenth Century', *Journal of Family History*, 25:3 (2000), 341–361.

81   Connell, *The Population of Ireland*; D. Fitzpatrick, 'Irish Farming Families before the First World War', 339–374; D. Fitzpatrick, 'Marriage in post-Famine Ireland', in A. Cosgrave (ed.), *Marriage in Ireland* (Dublin: College Press, 1985), pp. 116–131; D. Fitzpatrick, 'Divorce and Separation in Modern Irish history', *Past and Present*, 114:1 (1987), 172–196; T. Guinnane, *The Vanishing Irish: Households, Migration and the Rural Economy in Ireland, 1850–1914* (Princeton: Princeton University Press, 1997).

82   Guinnane, *The Vanishing Irish*, p. 93, p. 217; Fitzpatrick, 'Marriage in post-Famine Ireland,' pp. 116–131.

83   K. A. Miller, *Emigrants and Exiles. Ireland and the Irish Exodus to North America* (Oxford: Oxford University Press, 1988), pp. 353–426.

84   Guinnane, *The Vanishing Irish*, pp. 142–143, pp. 230–235.

85   *Ibid.*, p. 160.

86   *Ibid.*, p. 149.

87   Miller, *Emigrants and Exiles*, pp. 556–561.

88   Marland, *Dangerous Motherhood*, p. 93; Suzuki, *Madness at Home*, pp. 114–115; Tomes, *A Generous Confidence*, p. 127.

89   Melling, Forsythe and Adair, 'Families, Communities and the Legal Regulation of Lunacy in Victorian England', pp. 153–180; Scull, *The Most Solitary of Afflictions*, pp. 132–134.

90   Prestwich 'Family Strategies and Medical Power', 805.

91   *Ibid.*

92   W. Neilson Hancock, 'On the Report of the Irish Lunacy Inquiry Commissioners and the Policy of Extending the English Law for the Protection of Neglected Lunatics to Ireland', *Statistical and Social Inquiry Society of Ireland*, 7:6 (July 1879), 454–461.

93   O. Walsh has argued that this was not the case in all Irish asylums, O. Walsh unpublished conference paper 'A Perfectly Ordered Establishment: Liberal Asylum Administration in the West of Ireland, 1860–90' (Queen's University College, Belfast, 31 August, 2007); see Moran, 'The Signal and the Noise' for comparisons with New Jersey.

94   Prestwich, 'Family Strategies and Medical Power', 805.

95   C. A. Conley, 'Irish Criminal Records, 1865–1892', *Éire-Ireland* 28:1 (1993), 103; E. Steiner-Scott, '"To Bounce a Boot Off Her Now & Then": Domestic Violence in post-Famine Ireland', in M. Valulius and M. O'Dowd (eds), *Women and Irish History: Essays in Honour of Margaret MacCurtain* (Dublin: Wolfhound Press, 1997), p. 135; Levine-Clark identified similar patterns in West Riding Pauper Lunatic Asylum, see Levine-Clark, 'Dysfunctional Domesticity', 355.

96   Suzuki, *Madness at Home*, p. 149.

97 NAI, CSO CRF, Carlow 1865.
98 Suzuki, *Madness at Home*, p. 147.
99 NAI, CSO CRF, Wexford 1854.
100 Steiner-Scott, "'To Bounce a Boot Off Her Now & Then,'" p. 137.
101 NAI, CSO CRF, Wexford 1851.
102 K. Miller and B. D. Boling, '"Golden Street, Bitter Tears": the Irish Image of America during an Era of Mass Migration', *Journal of American Ethnic History*, 10: 1/2 (1990/91), 16–35.
103 NAI, CSO CRF, Carlow 1866.
104 NAI, CSO CRF, Wexford 1866.
105 NAI, CSO CRF, Wexford 1853.
106 NAI, CSO CRF, Kildare 1866.
107 NAI, CSO CRF, Kildare 1865.
108 NAI, CSO CRF, Kildare 1864.
109 NAI, CSO CRF, Wexford 1863.
110 NAI, CSO CRF, Wexford 1865.
111 NAI, CSO CRF, Kildare 1863.
112 NAI, CSO CRF, Wexford 1860; Wexford 1863.
113 Suzuki, *Madness at Home*, p. 121.
114 NAI, CSO CRF, Wexford 1855.
115 NAI, CSO CRF, Wexford 1852.
116 M. MacDonald, 'Lunacy in Seventeenth- and Eighteenth-Century England: Analysis of Quarter Sessions Records Part I', *History of Psychiatry*, 2:8 (1991), 437–456.
117 *Ibid.*
118 NAI, CSO CRF, Kildare 1856; Wexford 1866.
119 NAI, CSO CRF, Kilkenny 1844.
120 R. A. Houston, *Madness and Society in Eighteenth-Century Scotland* (Oxford: Oxford University Press, 2000).
121 NAI, CSO CRF, Wexford 1865.
122 M. MacDonald, 'Medicalization of Suicide in England: Laymen, Physicians and Cultural Change, 1500–1870', in C. E. Rosenberg and J. Golden (eds), *Framing Disease: Studies in Cultural History* (New Brunswick: Rutgers University Press, 1997), p. 85.
123 *The Constabulary Manual; or Guide to the Discharge of Police Duties* (Dublin: Thom, 1870), p. 45.
124 NAI, CSO CRF, Kildare 1867.
125 NAI, CSO CRF, Carlow 1859.
126 NAI, CSO CRF, Wexford 1866.
127 NAI, CSO CRF, Wexford 1865.
128 O. Anderson, *Suicide in Victorian and Edwardian England* (Oxford: Clarendon Press, 1987), pp. 148–190.
129 Scull, *Museums of Madness*, pp.13–14.
130 Suzuki, *Madness at Home.*, pp. 91–118; A. Suzuki, 'Framing Psychiatric Subjectivity: Doctor, Patient and Record-Keeping at Bethlem in the Nineteenth Century', in Melling and Forsythe (eds), *Insanity, Institutions and Society*, pp. 115–136; Marland,

Dangerous Motherhood; Marland, 'Destined to a Perfect Recovery', pp. 137–156; H. Marland, 'At Home with Puerperal Mania: the Domestic Treatment of the Insanity of Childbirth in the Nineteenth Century', in Bartlett and Wright (eds), *Outside the Walls of the Asylum* pp. 45–65; N. M. Theriot 'Negotiating Illness: Doctors, Patients, and Families in the Nineteenth Century', *Journal of the History of the Behavioural Sciences* 37:4 (2001), 349–368.

131   Wright, 'Family Strategies and the Institutional Confinement'; Suzuki, *Madness at Home*; Michael, *Care and Treatment of the Mentally Ill in North Wales*. For studies of other countries, see Prestwich, 'Family Strategies and Medical Power'; M. E. Kelm, 'Women, Families and the Provincial Hospital for the Insane, British Columbia, 1905–1915', *Journal of Family History*, 19 (1994), 177–193.

132   *Leinster Leader* (20 May 1905); (3 June 1905).

133   Finnane, 'Asylums, Families and the State', 143.

134   M. E. Fissell, 'The Disappearance of the Patient's Narrative and the Invention of Hospital Medicine', in R. French and A. Wear (eds), *British Medicine in the Age of Reform* (London and New York: Routledge, 1991), p. 93; N. D. Jewson, 'The Disappearance of the Sick-man from Medical Cosmology, 1770–1870', *Sociology*, 10 (1976), 225–244.

135   Tomes, *A Generous Confidence*, p. 122.

136   Eigen, *Witnessing Insanity*, p. 96.

137   *Ibid.*, p. 182.

138   NAI, CSO CRF, Kilkenny 1850.

139   Eigen, *Witnessing Insanity*, p. 87.

140   NAI, CSO CRF, Wexford 1850; Wexford, 1851.

141   Eigen, *Witnessing Insanity*, p. 77.

142   *Ibid.*, p. 184; Coleborne, *Madness in the Family*, p. 80.

143   NAI, CSO CRF, Wexford 1851; Wexford 1854.

144   S. O Súilleabháin, *A Handbook of Irish Folklore* (Detroit: Singing Tree Press, 1970), pp. 304–315. Thanks to Professor Ríonach Uí Ógáin for her assistance.

145   A. Bourke, *The Burning of Bridget Cleary. A True Story* (London: Plimlico, 1999), p. 34.

146   Marland, 'Languages and Landscape', p. 57.

147   Eigen, *Witnessing Insanity*, p. 6.

148   Finnane, 'Irish Psychiatry. Part 1', p. 308.

149   N. M. Theriot, 'Negotiating Illness: Doctors, Patients, and Families in the Nineteenth Century', *Journal of the History of the Behavioural Sciences*, 37:4 (2001), 349–368; Suzuki, 'Framing Psychiatric Subjectivity', in Melling and Forsythe (eds), *Insanity, Institutions and Society*, pp. 115–136.

150   Suzuki, *Madness at Home*, pp. 73–77.

151   *Ibid.*, pp. 39–64.

152   NAI, CSO CRF, Kilkenny 1851; Wexford 1852.

153   *Thom's Directory*, 1854.

154   NAI, CSO CRF, Kilkenny 1847.

155   NAI, CSO CRF, Wexford 1853; Kilkenny 1849.

156   Tomes, *A Generous Confidence*, p. 120.

157   Eigen, *Witnessing Insanity*, p. 131.

158 NAI, CSO CRF, Wexford 1866.
159 NAI, CSO CRF, Kilkenny 1849.
160 NAI, CSO CRF, Wexford 1847.
161 NAI, CSO CRF, Wexford 1851.
162 NAI, CSO CRF, Kildare 1864; Carlow 1863.
163 NAI, CSO CRF, Wexford 1865. Stock was the medical officer at Clonroche dispensary in county Wexford.
164 A. Digby, 'Women's Biological Straitjacket', in S. Mendus and J. Rendall (eds), *Sexuality and Subordination: Interdisciplinary Studies of Gender in the Nineteenth Century* (Cambridge: Cambridge University Press, 1994), pp. 192–220; V. Skultans, *Madness and Moral Ideas of Insanity in the Nineteenth Century* (London: Routledge, 1975), pp. 1–31.
165 NAI, CSO CRF, Wexford 1860.
166 NAI, CSO CRF, Kilkenny, 1851.
167 NAI, CSO CRF, Wexford 1860.
168 Coleborne, *Madness in the Family*, p. 58.
169 B. H. Rosenwein, 'Worrying about Emotions in History', *American Historical Review*, 107:3 (2002), 842.
170 Marland, 'Languages and Landscapes', p. 68; F. Bound Alberti, 'Introduction: Medical History and Emotional Theory', in Bound Alberti, *Medicine, Emotion and Disease*, p. xv.
171 Ray, 'Models of Madness', 229–264.
172 Ó Gráda, *Ireland. A New Economic History*, pp. 236–250.
173 A. Suzuki, 'Lunacy and Labouring Men: Narratives of Male Vulnerability in Mid-Victorian London', in R. Bivins and J. V. Pickstone (eds), *Medicine, Madness and Social History. Essays in Honour of Roy Porter* (Houndmills: Palgrave Macmillan, 2007), pp. 118–128, p. 122.
174 Suzuki, 'Lunacy and Labouring Men', p. 121.
175 M. Cronin, '"You'd be Disgraced!" Middle-Class Women and Respectability in post-Famine Ireland', in F. Lane (ed.), *Politics, Society and the Middle Class in Modern Ireland* (Houndmills: Palgrave Macmillan, 2010), pp. 107–129.
176 NAI, CSO CRF, Kildare 1861.
177 Cronin, '"You'd be Disgraced!"' p. 124.
178 M. E. Daly, *The Slow Failure: Population Decline and Independent Ireland, 1920–1973* (Madison: Wisconsin University Press, 2006), p. 14.
179 Melling and Forsythe, *The Politics of Madness*, p. 84.
180 Malcolm, '"The House of Strident Shadows"', p. 86.
181 Tuke, 'Increase of Insanity in Ireland', *JMS*, (October, 1894), 549–555.
182 D. Fitzpatrick, *Oceans of Consolation: Personal Accounts of Irish Migration to Australia* (Cork: Cork University Press, 1994); Miller, *Irish Immigrants in the Land of Canaan*.
183 T. Dixon, *From Passions to Emotions: The Creation of a Secular Psychological Category* (Cambridge: Cambridge University Press, 2003); Marland, *Dangerous Motherhood*; C. Coleborne, 'Families, Patients and Emotions: Asylums for the Insane in Colonial Australia and New Zealand, c.1880–1910', *Social History of Medicine*, 19:3 (2006), 425–442.

184   NAI, CSO CRF, Wexford 1852.
185   Miller and Boling, 'Golden Street, Bitter Tears'.
186   NAI, CSO CRF, Kilkenny 1851.
187   NAI, CSO CRF, Wexford 1851.
188   M. Jackson, 'It Begins with the Goose and Ends with the Goose': Medical Legal and
      Lay Understandings of Imbecility in *Ingram v Wyatt*, 1824–1832', *Social History of
      Medicine*, 11:3 (1998), 361–380.

5

Households and institutionalisation

Every child has a madman on their street:
The only trouble about our madman is that he's our father[1]

The certification of relatives into nineteenth-century Irish asylums occurred in the context of high levels of distress and anxiety for patients and families. As demonstrated in the previous chapter, violence and abusive behaviour perpetrated by, and on, the mentally ill, in addition to suicidal behaviour formed the backdrop to most asylum certifications. However, mental distress did not always result in admission to a specialist institution. Depending on the options available in the local institutional marketplace, people were admitted to workhouses, confined in prisons, housed in private institutions or maintained in households. The main concern of this chapter is to identify the groups in nineteenth-century Irish society most susceptible to admission into, and discharge from, asylums. Chapter six assesses the role of Irish workhouses.

Since the 1980s scholars have uncovered the subtle impact family and household structures had upon patterns of admission into nineteenth century asylums, however patterns of release have received less attention.[2] Writing in 1999, David Wright suggested that the focus on confinement, prompted by Michel Foucault's *Histoire de la folie à l'âge classique*, has resulted in a relative neglect of the 'area of discharge of pauper lunatics'.[3] John Walton's earlier work, which examined admissions to and discharges from Lancashire asylums, was an important exception.[4] While it is true that most work has focused on the social context of admissions, studies of asylums in Britain, America and elsewhere have shown that not only were most patients released from asylums, periods of confinement were not especially protracted and asylum managers and medical superintendents knew this was the case.[5] As Scull argued, 'a substantial fraction of those who entered an asylum in any twelve month period could expect to be discharged within the year'.[6] Finnane suggests that this was also true in Ireland, and in Carlow asylum most patients were discharged.[7] Historians have therefore challenged the assumption that 'through the incompetence of medical superintendents, individuals were incarcerated for very long periods'.[8] Nonetheless, the relative importance of familial, social and bureaucratic contexts of discharge and death has not been fully teased out. Jonathan Andrew's study of child-murderers discharged from Broadmoor and Perth criminal lunatic department, and Melling's and Forsythe's exploration of discharge procedures and patient deaths at Devon County and Wonford House asylums demonstrates that family and household structures were important for the release of patients. Nonetheless, asylum boards of visitors and the poor law authorities influenced procedures.[9] These works indicate that the sites of influence and power over patients' release differed between regions, and were dependent on administrative structures, as well as social and familial contexts.

This chapter will reflect on these questions through an examination of the social, familial and administrative contexts of admission, discharge and death at Carlow and Enniscorthy asylums from 1832 to 1922. During the time frame, the structure of Irish households and the population profile changed fundamentally. By the late nineteenth century, emigration had disrupted family structures and bonds of kinship. Celibacy became a common experience for a large proportion of the population, as an increasing number of individuals, particularly men, never married. Simultaneously, asylum authorities were constrained when managing high rates of admissions that overcrowded asylums.

Joan Busfield has argued that 'patient statistics do not provide objective, standardised levels of madness in different groups: rather they provide us first and foremost with information about who is processed by the asylum/mental health system.'[10] To explore the groups processed into Carlow asylum, the admission, discharge and death rates have been analysed in detail. This includes 5,517 admissions between 1832 and 1922. The data was derived from Carlow asylum admission, discharge and death registers, and through record linkage, it has been possible to track most patients who entered, left or died in the asylum. Patients' household structures have also been interrogated. It was not possible to link the asylum records with the individual nineteenth-century household census returns as these have been destroyed, however, the 1901 and 1911 returns were consulted.[11] To supplement these sources, Timothy Guinnane's and Kevin O'Neill's studies of nineteenth-century household structures have proved invaluable in overcoming the lacunae in census returns. The information recorded during dangerous lunatic certifications also contain details of household structures thereby providing information on patients' family circumstances from 1840 to 1867. Qualitative material has been derived from casebooks and letters from Carlow and Enniscorthy asylums.

The asylum population in Carlow asylum, 1832 to 1922

An accurate and nuanced assessment of those in society prone to asylum institutionalisation can only be established through a comprehensive analysis of asylum admission, discharge and death rates.[12] Finnane and Malcolm have demonstrated that in the post-Famine period, the Irish asylum population was predominantly single, male and relatively young, and most patients were certified as dangerous lunatics.[13] Carlow asylum population was similar in several respects; between 1832 and 1922 more men than women were confined – 55 per cent (3,000) of admissions were men – and men were more likely to be single. Between 1846 and 1922, 59 per cent (1550) of male and 48 per cent (1015) of female patients were single. Most patients spent less than six and a half months in the asylum and a significant proportion of these spent less than two months; 52.4 per cent (2886) of patients were discharged. This differs from Melling's and Forsythe's finding at Devon asylum where most patients died.[14] In Carlow asylum, the proportion of patients dying was 35.4 per cent (1931) between 1832 and 1922, a figure in excess of the mortality rate among the general population.[15] The mortality rate in Victorian asylums was usually higher than in the general population.[16]

This overview of Carlow's asylum population masks other patterns of susceptibility to confinement. Men did not form the majority of asylum admissions throughout the nineteenth century as some have argued,[17] while there were significant fluctuations in the male and female discharge and mortality rates and in the length of time patients spent in the asylum. To capture these changes, admission rates have been divided into two time frames and analysed separately: the first period covers the c1830s to the c1860s incorporating the Famine, and ends with the amendment to the dangerous lunatic legislation. The second time frame covers the

period from 1870 to 1921. The analysis of released patients' length of
stay has been divided into three periods: 1832 to 1855, 1856 to 1899 and
1900 to 1922. These timeframes coincide with the division of Carlow
asylum district and with the completion of extensions to Carlow asylum.
Throughout, the statistical significance of patterns was established using
a Student t-test or a Pearson t-test.[18] For the purposes of clarity and accessibility, the results have been presented as graphs.

During the 1960s and 1970s, scholars argued that women were
particularly vulnerable to institutionalisation and, consequently, asylums
were characterised as warehouses of female insanity.[19] A more nuanced
understanding of women's susceptibility to confinement that takes
account of class and mobility has emerged subsequently.[20] Scholars
acknowledge that while particular forms of mental illness were linked to
Victorian concepts of femininity and women, others were linked to 'men
and masculinity'.[21] Before the Famine, admission, discharge and death
patterns among female patients at the Carlow asylum differed from those
in the late nineteenth century. In the earlier period, the Carlow asylum
population was similar to later nineteenth-century English asylum populations. As figure 5.1 shows, before the Famine, men and women were
admitted into Carlow asylum in similar numbers and this reflected the
demographic profile of the region's population. Between 1832 and 1845,
291 women and 297 men were admitted and, while a greater number of
women were discharged from 1832 to 1855, both sexes spent an average
of twenty months in the asylum.[22] There were differences in the mortality
rates among male and female patients.[23] According to Finnane, in 1851
the national mortality rate in Irish asylums was 7.6 per cent among male
and 6.4 per cent among female patients. As figure 5.2 shows, before the
Famine the mortality rates at Carlow asylum were similar. There was a
small female advantage: 36.2 per cent of male and 34.5 per cent (840) of
female patients died. These pre-Famine patterns at Carlow asylum were
similar to patterns in English asylums in the late nineteenth century.
As Busfield has demonstrated, the higher male mortality rate, and the
'tendency to discharge women a little more quickly' coupled with the
small difference between male and female admission rates contributed
to the production of an asylum population with a small gender difference and an accumulation of female patients.[24] Similar, but not identical,
patterns were evident at Carlow asylum and produced a patient population with a small male majority.[25]

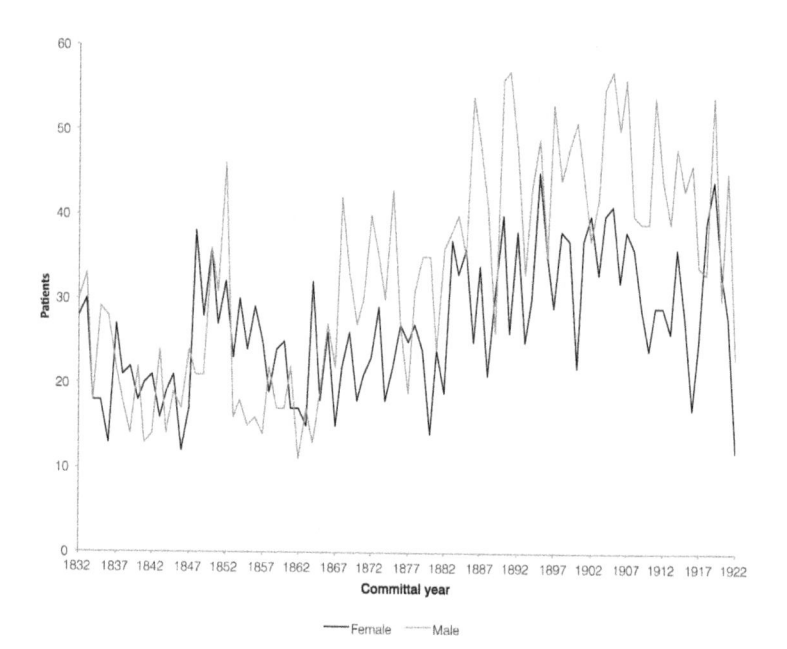

Figure 5.1   Male and female patients admitted to Carlow Asylum, 1832 to 1922

The Famine disrupted but did not fundamentally alter these patterns. As discussed in chapter two, there was an increase in admissions during the catastrophe, particularly among women. In contrast to Walsh's finding that male admissions accounted for 60 per cent of the 'surplus' Famine admissions at Ballinsaloe asylum, from 1848 to 1850, there were more female than male admissions at Carlow asylum.[26] Various factors influenced the increase in female admissions. There were more female lunatics maintained in the domestic environment in Carlow asylum district and they became vulnerable to institutionalisation as familial support mechanisms disintegrated due to emigration and death.[27] The increase also points to the introduction of gendered admission criteria that favoured women.[28] Ó Gráda and Guinnane have argued that such mechanisms were unsuccessful as it facilitated admissions into overcrowded, insanitary institutions and increased mortality rates.[29] This was the case at Carlow asylum; as figure 5.2 shows, female mortality rates exceeded male rates from 1848 to 1856, while women were also more likely to be discharged. From 1846, the number of women discharged climbed steadily and peaked in 1852. Among men, the increase in discharges occurred slightly later but it also peaked in 1852. Famine admissions caused significant overcrowding in the female wards from 1846, and by 1852 and 1853, both male and female wards were overcrowded. As the crisis brought on by the Famine abated, admission and discharge rates decreased.

The Famine did not have a long-term impact on the asylum and a more significant shift in admission, discharge and mortality rates among male and female patients occurred after the 1870s. As figure 5.1 clearly demonstrates, with the exception of the decade from 1910 to 1920, most admissions after 1870 were male. Men's susceptibility to confinement was partly a product of demographic changes. After the Famine, depopulation in the region and the division of Carlow asylum district ensured that by the 1861 census, there were more men living in the district. By 1911 they formed 55 per cent of the population. Nonetheless, as table 5.1 shows, male admissions were in excess of the size of the male population particularly after 1871.[30]

There appears to be a link between certification under the 1867 dangerous lunatic legislation and the increased susceptibility of men to institutionalisation. Dangerous lunatic admissions into Carlow asylum increased after 1867 and the application of the legislation was gendered. Prior to 1867, almost equal numbers of male (22.7 per cent – 173) and female patients (20.5 per cent – 168) were certified as dangerous lunatics. The asylum governors also certified male (60.3 per cent – 458) and female (63.5 per cent – 521) patients proportionately.[31] After 1867, each certification procedure was applied in significantly different ways. Between 1868

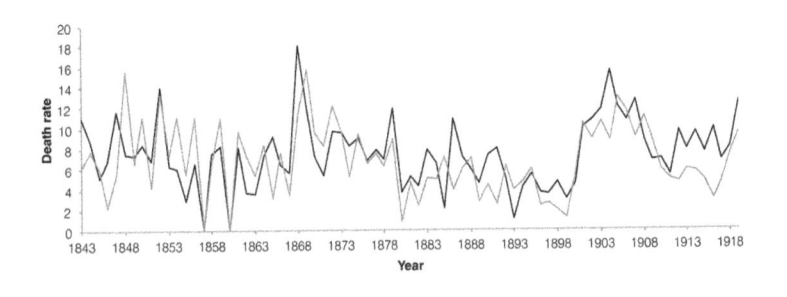

Figure 5.2   Mortality rates among male and female patients
in Carlow Asylum, 1840 to 1920

and 1922, 50 per cent (1127) of men were certified as dangerous lunatics compared with 37 per cent (599) of women while the governors certified 33 per cent (534) of women as opposed to 22.5 per cent (504) of men.[32]

Walsh has suggested that the high number of certifications among single, relatively young, men was caused by the emergence of impartible inheritance and male celibacy in post-Famine Ireland.[33] The rise in 'non-marriage' was more significant among families and in regions with substantial farm holdings.[34] However, patients with families with substantial farm holdings were a minority group in Carlow asylum, suggesting that changes in land inheritance had a limited impact upon certifications. Similarly, the argument that families' anxiety about potentially violent male relatives was aggravated by the agrarian outrages of the 1870s has limited traction for the Carlow asylum district.[35] Support for land agitation in nineteenth-century Ireland was sporadic and very localised and the Carlow asylum region was not at the forefront of agitation.

The increase in male susceptibility to institutionalisation undoubtedly occurred during a period in which communities became less tolerant of particular forms of male violence.[36] Recreational outlets that involved

Table 5.1   Per capita male and female admissions to Carlow Asylum, 1821 to 1911

Year	Pop. Male	Pop. Female	Pop. Total	Admissions per pop.		
				Male	Female	Total
1821	259,594	271,175	530,769			
1831	276,593	290,218	566,811	0.77	0.67	0.1
1841	297,490	307,679	605,169	0.69	0.74	−0.05
1851	244,975	257,732	502,707	0.87	1	−0.14
1861	146,203	145,834	292,037*	1.59	1.41	0.18
1871	134,609	133,321	267,930	2.41	1.73	0.69
1881	63,779	58,593	122,372**	6.26	5.12	1.14
1891	58,959	52,183	111,142	7.82	6.61	1.21
1901	53,712	47,602	101,314	8.56	7.35	1.21
1911	56,165	64,714	102,879	7.57	6.51	1.06
					t-value	3.133

*   After 1851, County Kilkenny is no longer included in the catchment area.
** After 1871 County Wexford is no longer included in the catchment area.

Source: W. E. Vaughan and A. J. Fitzpatrick (eds), *Irish Historical Statistics. Population 1821–1971* (Dublin: Royal Irish Academy, 1978), pp. 5–10

violence and culturally associated with men, such as faction fighting, and other non-formalised expressions of violence, were disappearing by the late nineteenth century. While women were involved in these events, participants were usually men. For example in Dublin, there was a campaign to abolish the notorious Donnybrook Fair while the Dublin Metropolitan Police were busy repressing wresting matches, prize fighting and adult street fighting.[37] There were attempts to abolish blood sports although these met with some resistance.[38] Popular sporting recreations, including most forms of football, were codified making them less violent while drinking was increasingly confined to specific spaces and events such as public houses and fair days.[39] In the same period, men were over-represented among general convictions for summary offences in the court system,[40] indicating that the increase in male susceptibility to asylum confinement through the judicial system was consistent with general nineteenth-century criminal statistics.

From 1846 to the mid-1870s, most patients admitted (65 per cent – 2613) into Carlow asylum were single; between 1846 and 1922, 48 per cent (1015) of female and 59 per cent (1550) of male patients were single. Single men were particularly vulnerable to institutionalisation after 1867 while married and widowed patients were usually female. The susceptibility of single people to institutionalisation pre-dates the emergence of large numbers of 'non-married' in Irish society. By 1911, 58.8 per cent of the Carlow district population was single, never having married, and most were men (58.4 per cent). Admissions among single patients were disproportionate to their presence in the population. Guinnane has argued that strong kinship networks gave single relatives some protection within extended Irish families, however, this may not have included the mentally ill.[41] Single patients were not particularly vulnerable to certification as dangerous lunatics highlighting again the impact families had on dangerous lunatic certifications. Prior to 1870s, married and single patients were admitted into Carlow asylum proportionately under each certification procedure.[42] After the 1870s, asylum governors certified more single than married patients (figures 5.3, 5.4, 5.5). Thus, the asylum population not only 'reflected the trend towards celibacy strongly evident in the general Irish population after the Famine'[43] but single people, particularly men, were also acutely vulnerable to incarceration – a pattern not unique to Ireland.

In terms of discharge from Carlow asylum, there were differences between male and female rates and these contrast with patterns Busfield,

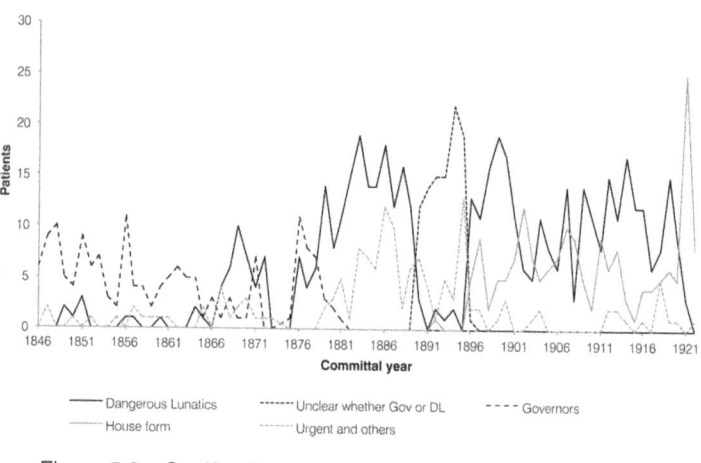

Figure 5.3   Certification of married patients to Carlow Asylum,
1846 to 1922

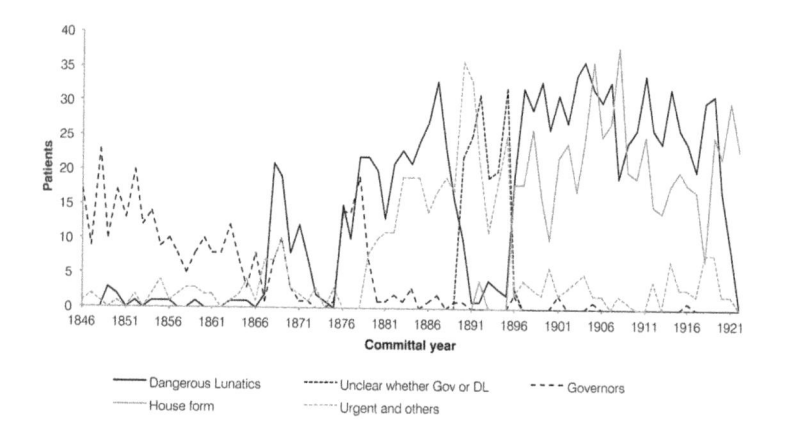

Figure 5.4   Certification of single patients to Carlow Asylum, 1846 to 1922

Melling and others found in English asylums. After 1868, there was an
overall increase in discharge rates from Carlow asylum and male rates
exceeded female. Most patients spent one year or less in the asylum. There
were some exceptions: there were a small number of patients confined
for four and even twelve years and these long-stay patients accumulated
in the asylum.[44] Among most long-stay patients in Carlow asylum the
average period spent in the asylum was three and half years and these

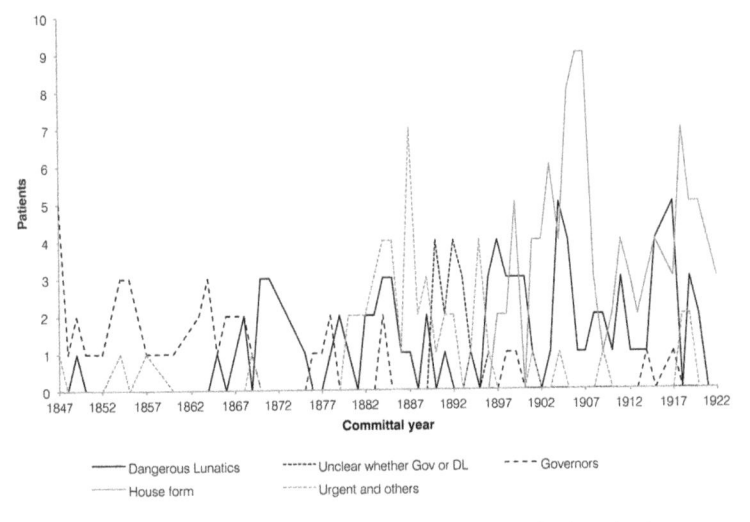

Figure 5.5   Certification of widowed patients to Carlow Asylum,
1846 to 1922

figures compare favourably with the discharge rates Scull, Melling and Forsythe, and Cherry identified in asylums in Devon and Norfolk.[45] There were significant differences in the length of time male and female patients were confined in Carlow asylum. From 1856 to 1899, men spent an average of fourteen months in the asylum while women spent twenty-one months.[46] The length of time patients spent in the asylum reduced during periods when rates of discharge increased. The variations in the length of time patients spent in the asylum were related to overcrowding within the institution. When accommodation was extended through internal rearrangements at Carlow asylum in 1837, in 1842, and in 1846,[47] there was a corresponding decline in discharge rates and an increase in the length of time patients spent in the asylum (figures 5.6 and 5.7). There was also an increase in discharge rates when new asylums were opened in the district. During phases of severe overcrowding, such as occurred during and after the Famine, the mean length of stay among discharged patients fell steadily.

Moreover, different discharge rates among male and female patients were related to levels of overcrowding in the separate wards. For example, from 1861 to 1874, the mean length of time women spent in the asylum increased dramatically at a time when there was space in the female wards. There was however severe overcrowding in the male wards throughout the

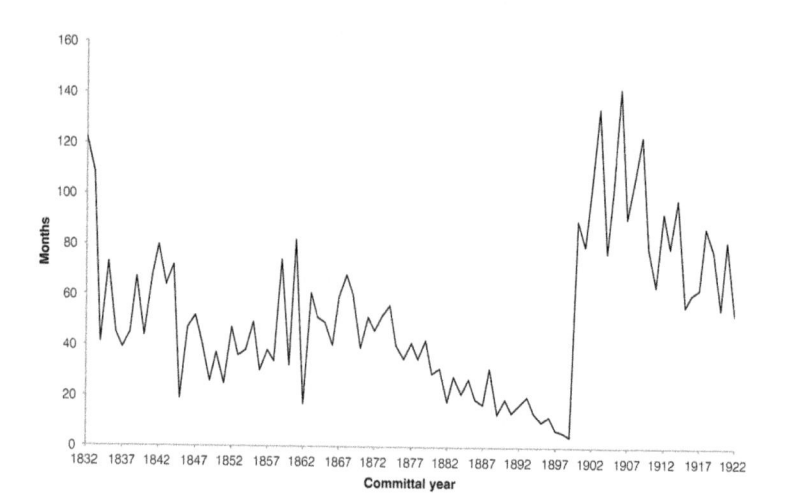

Figure 5.6   Mean length of stay for patients admitted to Carlow Asylum in each year from 1832 to 1922

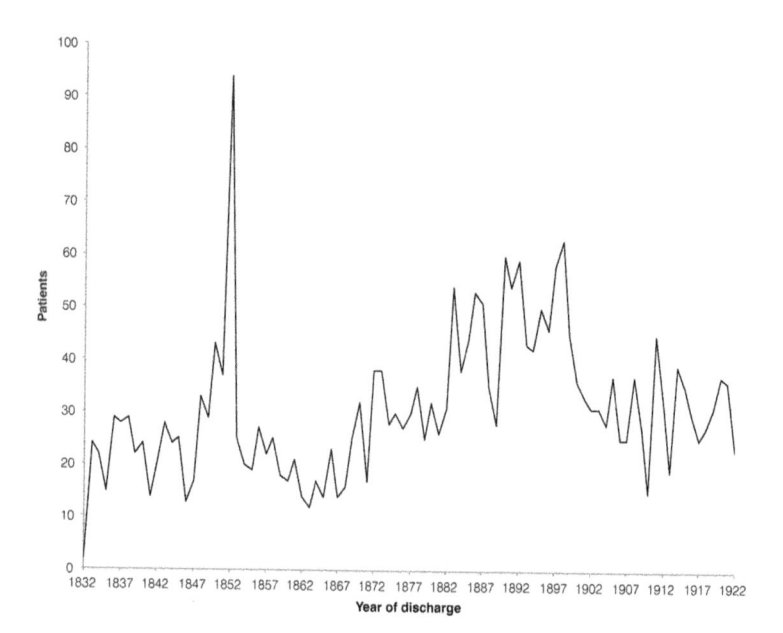

Figure 5.7   Number of patients discharged from Carlow Asylum, by year of recorded outcome, 1832 to 1922

1870s and 1880s, and as figure 5.8 highlights, from the 1870s men were discharged more quickly than women as asylum authorities discharged more patients when struggling to accommodate the surge in male admissions into cramped, and often dilapidated, wards.

Discharge rates from the asylum declined after 1900 and the average length of confinement among patients increased. There was also an increase in the number of long-stay patients. From 1900 to 1922 women were confined for longer periods – on average they spent twenty-eight months in the asylum while men spent nineteen months – as female discharge rates decreased.[48] The alleviation of overcrowding in the female wards as a result of renovations to the asylum therefore resulted in the confinement of women for longer periods. At the same time, overcrowding continued to be a problem on the male side of the asylum.

High admission rates into overcrowded and dilapidated buildings contributed to high mortality rates in late nineteenth-century asylums. Nationally, female mortality rates in asylums was lower than male though by 1901 the male rate was 6.3 per cent while the female rate had risen to 6.5 per cent.[49] In Carlow asylum, male mortality rates were higher than the female rates after 1880. There was severe overcrowding in the male wards in the 1880s and deterioration in living standards, resulting

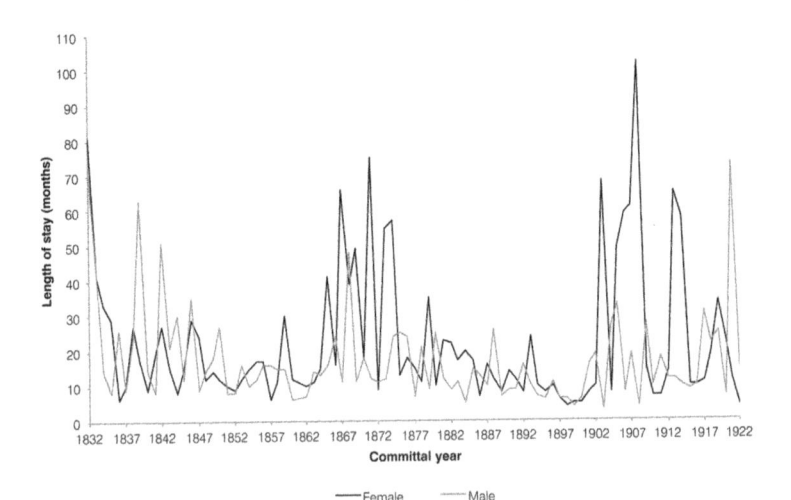

Figure 5.8 Mean length of stay among discharged male and female patients admitted to Carlow Asylum in each year from 1832 to 1922

in repeated outbreaks of dysentery. More male than female patients died from dysentery.[50] Male patients were also more susceptible to phthisis and tuberculosis and there was a slightly higher incidence of heart disease among male patients. Twice as many men died from epilepsy and the effects of syphilis. Women were more likely to die from 'senile decay' or 'senile debility'; these patients were usually fifty years and older when admitted and approximately half were confined for over eight years highlighting the link between senility and prolonged institutionalisation.

The social determinants that had the greatest impact on survival rates were gender and marital status. Patients' age at the time of certification was not particularly significant. Malcolm has noted that although the elderly were slightly overrepresented in asylums, the age structure was younger than that of workhouse inmates.[51] This was also true at Carlow asylum. In the forty years after the opening of the asylum, patients' mean age on admission was between thirty-four and thirty-six years old (figure 5.9). After the 1870s, the mean age of patients rose and by the 1910s, the average patient was in his or her early forties when admitted. From the mid-1870s onwards, the average woman committed to the asylum was older than her male counterpart (figure 5.9), although by 1911 there

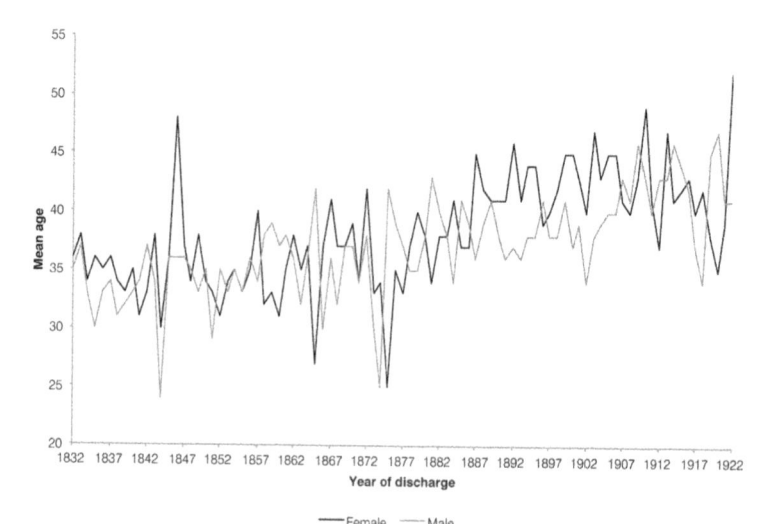

Figure 5.9   Mean age of male and female patients admitted to Carlow Asylum each year from 1832 to 1922

were more single men over forty-five in the general population. With some minor exceptions the mean age of male and female patients was similar when they discharged (figure 5.10).

In the early nineteenth century, patients who died in the asylum were relatively young both at the time of admission and death. The average man was between thirty-five and forty years at time of death, slightly older than female patients. During the Famine period the age of patients at time of death decreased significantly. As figure 5.11 demonstrates, the average age at the time of death rose throughout the nineteenth century reflecting the general increase in the admission of patients aged between thirty-five and fifty years. Patients were between forty and fifty years at death. The rise continued into the twentieth century when conditions in the asylum improved slightly. The death rate was high among patients aged over fifty years – a smaller cohort in the asylum – and most died following prolonged periods of confinement. Among this cohort of patients, female patients were sixty years at the time of death and were older than male patients.

Despite the lunacy inspectors' claims that families certified senile elderly relatives into lunatic asylums to rid themselves of them, there is little evidence of this behaviour.[52] There were relatively few admissions among

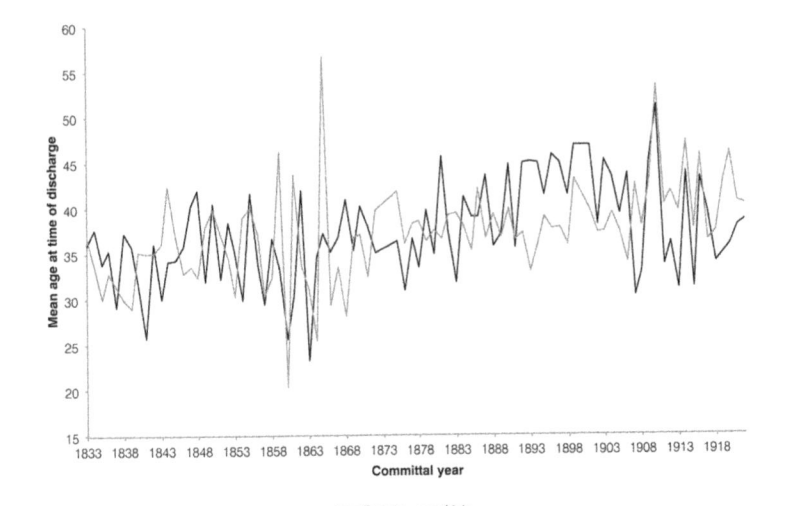

Figure 5.10   Mean age at time of discharge from Carlow Asylum in each year from 1832 to 1922 among male and female patients

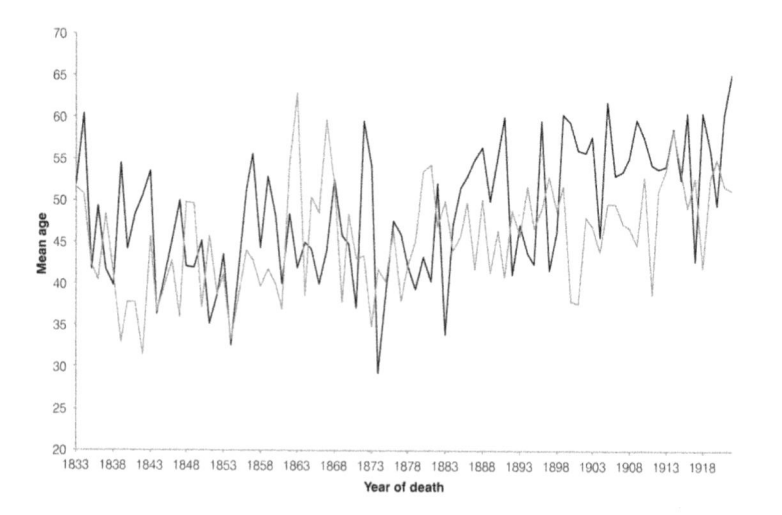

Figure 5.11   Mean age of male and female patients in Carlow Asylum at
time of death, 1832 to 1922

the elderly population of the district. While Guinnane has suggested that
living past fifty-seven years was rare in the nineteenth century and this
group represented the 'elderly in Irish society',[53] Pat Thane has demonstrated that reaching seventy years was generally accepted as 'old age' in
modern Europe.[54] Seventy years was also accepted as 'old age' under the
1908 Old Age Pension Act. Only 4 per cent of admissions into Carlow
asylum between 1832 and 1922 were seventy years and over. The numbers
did not decline after the introduction of the 1908 Old Age Pension Act.[55]
The pension was a substantial financial boost to poorer households in
Ireland providing an allowance of five shillings per week and Guinnane
found that its introduction resulted in a reduction in the number of
elderly in workhouses.

The statistical analysis of admission, discharge and death rates at
Carlow asylum studied here indicates that there were significant changes
in patterns during the nineteenth century. After the 1870s, single
men became the largest patient cohort as a result of gendered admission, discharge and mortality rates. The mandatory admission of male
dangerous lunatic patients ensured that asylum authorities were unable to
reduce admission rates, and instead, they introduced gendered discharge

policies that were partly determined by overcrowding in male and female wards, and were related to the governors' willingness to extend the asylum building. Overcrowding in wards could enhance male survival rates, as their length of stay in the asylum was relatively short, however, for those remaining in the asylum, it contributed to high rates of male mortality.

Families, households and asylums

As shown in chapter four, families were at the forefront of negotiations with medical and legal authorities and systems during certification procedures. Certification procedures under the dangerous lunatic legislation involved a variety of participants – familial, legal and medical – who had set a person 'on the road to the asylum.'[56] Michael MacDonald's assertion that 'insanity is defined by experts but discovered by laymen' was true in nineteenth-century Ireland.[57] Among dangerous lunatic admissions to Carlow asylum between 1840 and 1868, 82 per cent of the informants were close relatives, often members of the same household.[58] Additionally, household and family structures had a significant impact upon discharge. For example, Melling and Forsythe found that strong household ties among well-established, settled families were associated with higher levels of certification and discharge in Devon.[59] The next section of this chapter will explore the impact household structures, asylum governors and medical superintendents had on certification and discharge procedures.

Farming families with land holdings have preoccupied most demographic studies of nineteenth-century Irish households and these studies have identified the changing relationships between family members before and after the Famine. K. H. Connell's influential monograph posited that in pre-Famine Ireland, marriage took place at a younger age than the rest of Europe and produced larger families. This encouraged the sub-division of land holdings as younger families established separate households. Connell maintained that the Famine fundamentally altered these patterns and arranged marriages assumed a central position in marriage behaviour in post-Famine Ireland. There emerged 'a household system that limited marriage in Ireland to a single favoured son or daughter'.[60] When offspring married, parents remained as resented members of the household, while the young married couple took over the management of land holdings. Younger siblings usually left. Accordingly, farming households in post-Famine Ireland were typically 'stem' in structure, containing two married couples or at least a married couple and one widowed parent. Connell's thesis has since been revised.[61] Guinnane has suggested that it was not unusual for households to consist of extended families, containing 'someone related to the conjugal family unit other than the married couple and their children'.[62] The extended Irish family included siblings, grand-children, nieces and nephews and does not fit with either the stem-family or the nuclear family models.[63] Kevin O'Neill has analysed the structure of labouring households as well as small, middling and large farming families and identified similarities between them. He argued that labouring households 'show a high percentage of nuclearity, low lateral extension and relatively low overall extension'[64] suggesting that the 'high incidence of lateral extension' displayed by small farmers was 'a sign of increasing economic distress and self-exploitation'.[65]

Members of nuclear families featured as subjects and petitioners during dangerous lunatic certifications. Although certification warrants did not include details of informants' addresses, a close reading of relatives' testimony indicates that most patients were co-resident with the informant when certified. Heads of households – often parents (45.9 per cent) and spouses (32.9 per cent) – provided testimony of disturbed behaviour and mental distress. It was relatively unusual for siblings and adult children to certify relatives and members of the extended family – aunts, cousins and grandparents – did not feature. Adult offspring – often daughters – testified for the certification of senile parents in three cases, though not particularly elderly, two of these died in the asylum and one returned home.[66]

Parents who certified adult offspring as dangerous lunatics emerged from low laterally extended households. Parents were the primary carers and provided accommodation for adult offspring possibly in exchange for assistance in farm labour.[67] Most individuals certified by parents were single and in their twenties and this remained constant for most of the century. The 1901 and 1911 census household returns confirm that most patients emerged from domestic environments and were members of 'well-defined' nuclear families, though these varied in size.[68] Among patients identified in the 1901 census most were recorded as either heads of family (23 per cent) – male and female – or adult offspring – sons (23 per cent) and daughters (12 per cent). Only 7 per cent were wives who were not heads of households and a further 9 per cent were sisters. In 1911, just under half (45 per cent) the patients were heads of households – male and female – while an additional 10 per cent were married women who were not heads of households. Over a fifth (22 per cent) were adult sons while daughters formed only 6 per cent of patients. There were a small but relatively consistent number of patients who were boarders or servants when certified – 8 per cent in 1901 and 9 per cent in 1911. The presence of adult offspring, displaying signs of mental illness, in households indicates that relatives with 'some legal obligation' undertook a 'caring role' suggesting that mental illness was 'not the affliction of the most solitary householders in Victorian society'.[69] As discussed in chapter one, these patients were from poorer labouring classes among whom O'Neill found high levels of household nuclearity. Few patients emerged from multiple-family structures that were more common among non-Catholic families and were generally linked to wealth, particularly among farmers.[70]

Elderly patients were less likely to emerge from domestic contexts. For example, among the twelve patients aged seventy years and over admitted to Carlow asylum between 1911 and 1913, three came from nuclear families. Most were transferred from local workhouses though usually not as dangerous lunatics. Dangerous lunatic patients were younger than those certified through other procedures (figure 5.12) and only 7.7 per cent (22) were recorded as aged 55 years or over.[71] None were over seventy years of age. Initially, female dangerous lunatics were younger than their male counterparts but after 1870, they were marginally older than males (figure 5.13 and 5.14). Older patients were usually certified as 'ordinary' lunatics (figure 5.14). The susceptibility of the elderly to certification as 'ordinary' patients was often related to the disintegration of the nuclear family as those who had attained seventy years or more were more likely to have lost their immediate family – spouses and children – through death or migration.[72] Thus, widows – 8.8 per cent (186) of female admissions – were more likely to be certified by asylum governors.

The presence of mental illness in families had the potential to disrupt gendered domestic roles and boundaries that delineated household authority in Ireland. From 1843 to 1868, 51 per cent of patients certified as dangerous lunatics in counties Carlow, Kilkenny, Kildare and Wexford were men, and women frequently provided the evidence of mental disturbance. Female relatives provided testimony in 44.7 per cent of dangerous lunatic cases.[73] Among male dangerous lunatics, 63 per cent of witnesses were women while among female dangerous lunatics, 60 per cent of

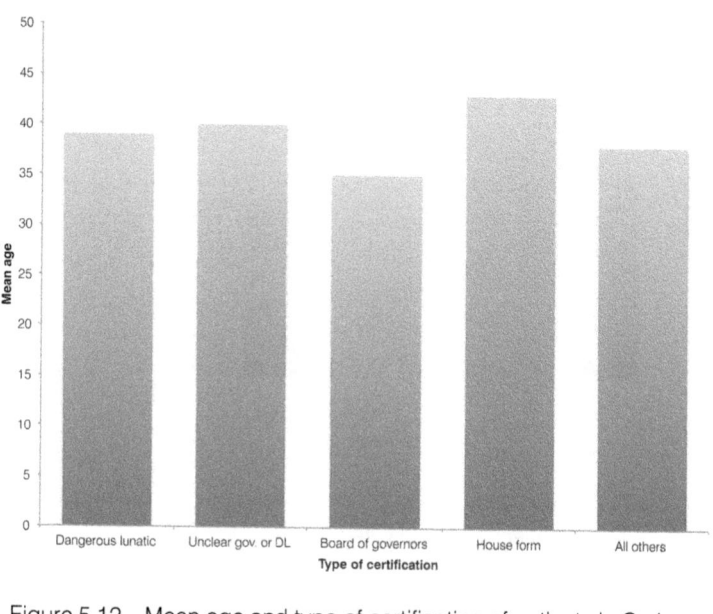

Figure 5.12   Mean age and type of certification of patients in Carlow
Asylum, 1832 to 1922

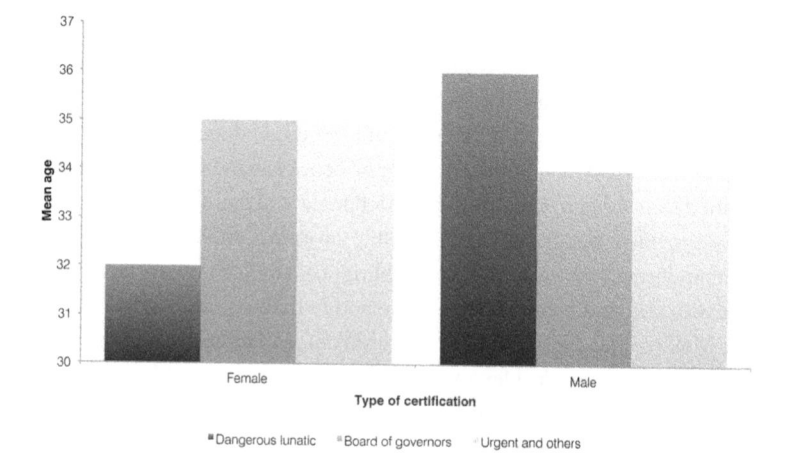

Figure 5.13   Mean age and type of certification among male and female
patients in Carlow Asylum, 1832 to 1867

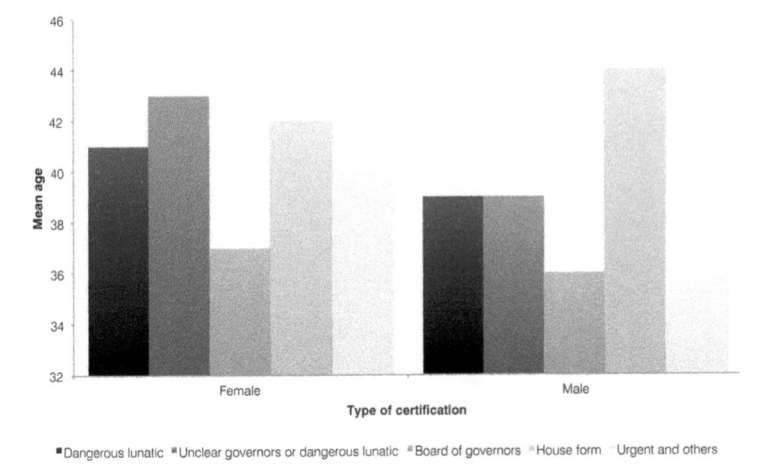

Figure 5.14   Mean age and type of certification among male and female
patients in Carlow Asylum, 1867 to 1922

witnesses were male. Women were not 'the victimised woman' subjected
to husbands, fathers and brothers' indiscriminate use of certification.[74]
However, husbands were more likely to commit spouses; 28.9 per cent of
female witnesses were wives certifying husbands, while 36.1 per cent of
male witnesses were husbands certifying wives.[75] The testimony of violent
behaviour male and female spouses provided during legal procedures
suggests that they used the asylum was as 'a temporary means of defence
from domestic violence'.[76] Women frequently certified adult offspring and
mothers were the largest cohort of female witnesses (44.7 per cent). They
attested to the presence of insanity among adult daughters more often
than fathers. Fathers comprised 58.8 per cent of male witnesses and they
certified sons more frequently. Thus both male and female heads of households provided testimony against adult offspring and usually against a
member of their own sex. Similarly, siblings usually committed members of
their own sex, and brothers were more active than sisters.[77] This contrasts
with Melling and Forsythe's findings at Wonford House asylum, a private
fee-based institution in Devon, where 'mothers and sisters figured rather
less prominently' among relatives authorising certifications.[78] The findings
at Carlow asylum indicate that the responsibility of caring for an insane
relative lay within the female domain and women were central in the adjudication of appropriate responses when the health and safety of the family

was in jeopardy.[79] When necessary, it was appropriate for women from low-income backgrounds to seek legal redress in the public courts. Poorer women therefore participated in the power nexus with state and medical authorities when determining the fate of male and female relatives both before and after the Famine.[80] Although the Famine had 'drastically weakened the position of women in Irish society' especially in terms of their economic power, women succeeded in maintaining influential positions in the home and developed a power base in the family.[81] These findings contrast with Elizabeth Steiner-Scott's observation that 'recourse to the courts was an uncommon occurrence for working class women' in post-Famine Ireland, particularly in instances of domestic abuse.[82]

Household structures also impacted on discharge rates, a subject largely neglected in the Irish context as scholars have paid relatively little attention to the social circumstances surrounding patients' discharge. Finnane has examined the regulatory frameworks that governed the discharge of patients, however, the application of these rules and the negotiations that occurred between asylum authorities, officials in other institutions and families during the process have not been explored.[83] Overall, 52.4 per cent (2886) of admissions to Carlow asylum between 1832 and 1922 were discharged under various categories; 'recovered' (42.8 per cent n=2361), 'relieved' (6.9 per cent n=359), 'relieved on trial' (0.8 per cent n=45) and 'not improved' (1 per cent n=53), while 0.3 per cent of patients (19) escaped from the asylum. The remaining patients were transferred from Carlow asylum to other public asylums, to local workhouses or they died.[84]

The regulations governing patients' release from asylums were determined by the different certification procedures. The 1838 Dangerous Lunatic Act specified that to discharge patients, two physicians were required to sign a medical certificate attesting to the patient's 'recovery'. This was then submitted to the Lord Lieutenant to secure a warrant allowing for legal release. In 1845 this was altered. From that date, it was no longer required that a patient be attested 'recovered' but simply no longer dangerous.[85] From 1846, dangerous lunatics, who were not criminal lunatics under the act, could be discharged without the Lord Lieutenant's warrant. They were to be treated and discharged 'as in the case of other Lunatic Poor.'[86] The 1843 privy council rules provided the framework that regulated the release of ordinary patients and under these patients were released when they ceased to be dangerous. Therefore from 1846, it appears that ordinary and dangerous lunatic patients were released on the basis of medical confirmation that they were no longer dangerous. Asylum governors formally authorised discharges while medical superintendents usually completed the necessary practical arrangements.

There were, however, problems with the procedures. In the 1830s, Carlow asylum authorities found that among patients admitted from other institutions, notably Richmond asylum, relatives had not been required to enter into a bond to accept patients on release. As a result, when patients recovered, relatives could not be found and some patients languished in the asylum, eventually dying there.[87] There was also ambiguity about the medical certificate. The fourteenth privy council rule did not specifically require physicians to sign medical certificates when releasing ordinary patients rather the rules indicated that: 'No patient shall be removed from the Asylum without the Manager first apprizing the Physician in order that he may state to the relatives his views of the case and his opinion on the subject'.[88] This was the case until 1862 when a revision to the privy council regulations specified that a medical certificate signed by both medical officers was mandatory when discharging a patient.[89] Moreover, the 1843 privy council rule implied that the family and not the physician decided whether a patient could be discharged. Matthew E. White, Carlow medical superintendent, complained in 1853 that families removed patients from the asylum 'prematurely' and against medical advice.[90] In 1862 the Irish Attorney General advised Richmond asylum that in cases when the medical officer considered an 'ordinary' patient unfit for discharge, the board could refuse to do so, even when in receipt of a request from family or friends. This was reiterated in the 1870 revision to the privy council rules, and a circular was subsequently issued to asylums.[91] Accordingly, asylum governors refused to release patients in spite of families' demands; in July 1868 a friend of John P. sought his discharge from Carlow asylum but, following an interview with the patient the board refused, considering him 'quite unfit to be entrusted to his friends'.[92] However, at Enniscorthy asylum in 1868, the new regulations were ignored and patients were discharged under the original 1843 privy council rules.[93]

From 1843, relatives and friends of ordinary lunatics were also required to enter legal bonds to accept patients on recovery.[94] The rate at which bonds were set was relatively high; Moses B.'s relatives entered into a £100 bond and provided two solvent securities of £50 each.[95] The lunacy inspectors and asylum authorities believed bonds safeguarded against the danger of the asylums being turned into a 'dumping ground for unwanted members of a community.'[96] However, governors sometimes refused to release patients whose families had not sworn bonds, as was the case in January 1877, when one woman's request for the release of her husband from Enniscorthy was refused on these grounds.[97]

The practice concerning the release of dangerous lunatic patients appeared to undermine the authority of medical superintendents. The 1867 dangerous lunatic amendment, in addition to ratifying existing discharge rules, required 'any relation or friend' to enter a recognisance in front of two magistrates guaranteeing the 'peaceable behaviour or safe conduct' of discharged patients.[98] This was interpreted as giving families the right to demand the discharge of relatives irrespective of the opinion of the asylum superintendents. It was amended in 1894, when the court of appeal ruled that the asylum superintendent had some discretion and could refuse to discharge dangerous lunatic patients whose family had entered a recognisance.[99]

Given the relative complexity of the regulations, asylum medical officers made errors and continued to use older regulations. On two occasions in 1883, Drapes at Enniscorthy asylum, wrote to the lunacy inspectors requesting sanction to release dangerous lunatic patients although this was unnecessary as the asylum board had approved them.[100] In December 1883, Nugent, in exasperation, referred him to the 1875 Lunatic Asylums (Ireland) Act and informed him that once the board had authorised the release, it was legal to discharge patients. In spite of this, in 1885 Drapes informed the asylum board that he had consulted the 1837 Dangerous Lunatic Act to clarify the discharge procedures when releasing a woman admitted earlier that year.[101] In the absence of clear enforceable regulations, families, governors, medical superintendents and in some cases, patients themselves struggled with the procedures.[102] Much depended upon the policies and attitudes of the medical superintendents. They, and asylum managers, identified patients suitable for release. For example, in September 1839, Patrick McCaffry at Carlow asylum contacted the relatives of patients 'deemed harmless' requesting they remove them.[103] Encouraged by Nugent, governors and medical superintendents systematically identified 'harmless' patients reviewing those suitable for transfer to workhouses.[104] O'Meara was particularly proactive in sending patients to neighbouring workhouses in the 1890s.[105]

When assessing patients, asylum medical staff sought specific changes in behaviour that demonstrated a patient was suitable to release. They found patients' resistance to work, either on the asylum farm or in the house, particularly troubling.[106] Failure to work could be a result of patients' poor physical condition as well as an objection to labour. While medical staff was tolerant of patients too debilitated to work, they interpreted refusals as symptoms of continuing 'poor mental condition'. James B., a male patient in Carlow asylum in 1906, suffered from delusions associated with work, particularly farm work, and believed that 'nobody works but horses and fools'. He worked 'fairly well in the division' but refused to engage in more appropriate work on the asylum farm believing 'his enemies would meet him there and attack him'.[107] Dr James J. Fitzgerald, Resident Medical Superintendent from 1903 to 1907, observed in the casebooks that his resistance to farm work encouraged his delusions. James remained in the asylum and was eventually transferred to the chronic ward. As outlined in more depth in chapter seven, work was integral to the asylum's therapeutic regime and was regarded as an indicator of a 'measure of normal functioning' and 'co-operation with asylum regimen'.[108] Patients' failure to work was interpreted as a refusal to join the ranks of the 'respectable' poor.[109]

The emphasis medical staff placed on patients' willingness to work sometimes overshadowed concerns for their mental state. A male patient admitted to Carlow asylum regularly worked on the farm and in the wards. His mental condition was poor; he was described as 'boisterous' and 'talkative' and he 'spent most of his night shouting and singing'. His behaviour did not change for six months. However, as soon as he demonstrated that he was capable of 'more rational' behaviour, he was quickly discharged. The key factor in the decision was his ability to approximate everyday activities in the form of labour.[110] Relatives outside the asylum displayed similar attitudes towards release. For example, in July 1860 Thomas D.'s father requested his son's 'liberation' as he needed his labour. He gave assurances that Thomas would be paid 'every care and attention' as the family was willing to employ a 'careful and competent person to look after him'.[111]

As Wright has demonstrated, the absence of 'dangerousness, suicidal intentionality, or violence towards others combined with the desire and ability of family members to care for and control an afflicted person' determined whether patients were released.[112] Medical staff honed in on patients' physical health, eating and sleeping habits, and their ability to interact with other patients during medical assessments. Patients that were excessively noisy or silent, refused to eat or work were causes of medical concern. The discharged patient was 'quiet and pleasant to deal with' 'goes out to work on the farm', 'takes his nourishment well', and essentially gave 'no trouble'.[113]

As the case of Thomas D. suggests the presence of relatives outside the asylum to enter into negotiations with authorities impacted on discharge rates; 57.6 per cent of married patients were discharged from Carlow asylum compared to 50.2 per cent of single patients and 42 per cent of widowed patients.[114] Patients were usually released into the care of spouses, fathers, brothers and sisters. Amongst released male patients, 51.2 per cent were single, 57 per cent were married and 44.2 per cent were widowed. The lower discharge rates among unmarried, single or widowed patients contributed to the creation of a predominantly single and male resident population. Single patients (36.1 per cent) were more likely than married patients (29.6 per cent) to die in the asylum.[115] Married men were more vulnerable than married women: 32 per cent (181) died in the asylum while 27 per cent (143) of married women died.[116] Male and female widows were particularly vulnerable; 49.8 per cent of male and 49.2 per cent of female (93) widows died there. Marriage therefore afforded patients some protection against dying in institutions.

Some families maintained contact with relatives in the asylum. As Andrews has highlighted, medical superintendents encouraged patients to maintain these contacts, although patients sometimes showed little interest or awareness of visits.[117] Relatives also wrote to asylum medical superintendents enquiring after patients' progress.[118] Relatives used visits to asylums as opportunities to request patients' release and they were generally aware of the legal procedures. The father of Patrick M., a twenty-one-year-old single man admitted to Carlow asylum in June 1906, visited his son weekly. After two and a half months he appeared before the asylum managing committee and successfully secured his release.[119] Relatives were often quite tenacious in pursuing cases and did not always accept asylum governors' refusals as final decisions; Luke R.'s father sought his son's release from Carlow asylum three times before finally securing it on the fourth attempt.[120] The lunacy inspectors claimed that families of dangerous lunatics abandoned relatives in the asylum,[121] however, requests and undertakings to assume responsibility for relatives came from families of 'ordinary' and 'dangerous' lunatics.[122] For example in March 1879, one dangerous lunatic, who had been 'quiet, harmless and well-conducted' since he entered Carlow asylum, was brought before the governors. His relatives were anxious for his removal and were 'willing to give a guarantee that a careful supervision shall be exercised over him'.[123] Michael Howlett, the medical superintendent concurred and he was released.[124]

The absence of defined, settled, nuclear families willing and able to care for relatives was detrimental to patients' opportunities for release. When discharging patients, asylum authorities sometimes discovered that families had emigrated or their circumstances had changed and they were no longer able to support mentally ill relatives. When Patrick M. was admitted to Enniscorthy asylum in 1878 his cousin and his sister-in-law undertook to remove him on his release. Five years later he was ready to be discharged, but upon investigation it was discovered his sister-in-law had gone to America while his cousin could not house or support Patrick. He was transferred to the local workhouse.[125] The existence of families outside the asylum did not guarantee that patients would be removed. In spite of the introduction of the legal bond, governors continued to encounter problems as families refused to accept relatives back into the home.[126] In March 1843, two female patients were sent home from Carlow asylum and notice was served on their relatives who had defaulted on bonds.[127] The governors also attempted to force families to accept discharged patients. One man, admitted to Carlow asylum in 1839, had recovered by March 1843. His friends were notified but they did not collect him and the governors ordered that the patient be 'transmitted to the co. Wexford and left with his brother'.[128] Families' refusals to accept relatives were sometimes motivated by anxieties that difficult social behaviour would re-emerge. The mother of one young woman refused to accept her daughter until there had been 'a complete reformation' in her character and demanded a guarantee of her daughter's 'future good behaviour and that there would be 'no further trouble'.[129] Another mother refused to accept the return of her son – his repeated stays in Enniscorthy asylum were caused by alcohol – because he had entered into a marriage she deemed 'distasteful'.[130] Other letters of refusal conveyed a strong sense of desperation among relatives anxious about the return of fractious relatives.[131]

Such refusals to collect relatives from asylums caused medical superintendents considerable anxiety. They, rather than asylum governors, usually investigated cases. Generally, medical superintendents did not 'retard the discharge of patients' particularly during periods of overcrowding. They were sometimes sympathetic towards patients whose families did not collect them. Painful and upsetting letters containing relatives' justification of their actions were withheld from patients. Asylum medical superintendents were also concerned about the legality of not removing a recovered patient. Drapes became particularly irate with the wife of one patient; he had agreed to keep her husband in the asylum while she completed practical arrangements for his release. After a month she had failed to collect him and Drapes demanded she come immediately. He feared that keeping 'any person here against his will for so long a period as your husband has been perfectly sane, would be to expose myself for an action of false imprisonment'.[132] Medical superintendents were also sensitive to accusations that they were trying to reduce costs by ridding themselves of patients. While in correspondence with the Convent of St Catherine about a member of their community in Enniscorthy asylum, Joseph Edmundson, Drapes' predecessor, was accused of trying to save money by releasing the nun. Edmundson explained that the urgency in discharging her was caused by 'the fear there is of her getting a relapse from associating with the insane.'[133] Likewise, Drapes feared that continued confinement following recovery caused depression and had 'an unfavourable effect' on the mind. He attempted to negotiate the transfer of one woman to Wexford workhouse on the understanding that she would promptly leave as she was keen to 'earn her bread'.[134] Medical superintendents' fears that patients would relapse were less troubling than those Andrews identified in infanticide cases.[135] Nonetheless, the relapse of patients had serious consequences. Two months after his release from Enniscorthy asylum, Michael S. was summoned before a local magistrate for firing a revolver on the public road. Michael's godfather had entered into a recognisance for his good behaviour.[136]

On assuming responsibility for released patients, families were warned that relatives should be returned to the asylum if symptoms re-emerged. As a result contact between families and asylum medical superintendents sometimes continued after the release of patients as families wrote to medical superintendents requesting advice.[137]

'Follow-up' care was the families' responsibility, and governors and medical superintendents placed significant stress on the families' ability to monitor relatives' mental condition and provide practical support. Daniel W. was refused permission to return to his mother's house, because she could not provide 'sufficient guard', whereas Frank D. was granted permission to take his wife home on condition that he employed someone to take care of her.[138] The landlord of a recovered patient's brother engaged a man to take care of him.[139] Patients themselves were also expected to take responsibility. James M.'s release was conditional upon his mother Bridget finding him employment.[140] These assessments tended to focus on the families' ability to provide practical support and there was limited evidence of the moral 'judgmentalism' Andrews identified among infanticide cases. When it did impinge on assessments, the patient was sometimes the target. When discharging Patrick McD. from Carlow asylum in 1886, O'Meara, the medical superintendent, recorded that he was 'well-known to the police' and had spent time in jail. He was criticised for failing to display remorse about his past; allegedly, he 'calmly relate[d] his past history of jail and bad conduct'. After three weeks in the asylum, it was noted his 'real character' emerged; he was described as lazy, snappy and abusive.[141]

It is unclear whether relapse was common among released patients. Recent work on record linkage has shown that patients were sometimes given separate admission numbers on each admission hindering the identification of relapsed patients.[142] Between 1832 and 1922, only 468 (8.6 per cent) patients in Carlow asylum could be identified as readmissions from the admission registers.[143] This is significantly lower than the lunacy inspectors' national estimates, which indicates that the proportion of readmissions among male patients was between 19 to 21 per cent from 1861 to 1911.[144] Asylum casebooks suggest that there was a higher incidence of readmission and confirm Ray's finding that readmission into the asylum was relatively straightforward. Patients' previous exposure to the asylum's regime increased the likelihood of return, although levels of overcrowding could hinder the readmission process. Most patients were readmitted by the medical superintendents (20 per cent, n=95) or the governors (47.6 per cent, n=223) and this was straightforward when families maintained contact with asylum authorities. Fewer returned patients were certified as 'dangerous lunatics' (25 per cent, n=119) although the use of the dangerous lunatic certification to admit relapsed patients increased after 1870. However, after the 1890s asylum governors certified most relapsed patients. The lunacy inspectors were bemused at the number of readmissions, claiming that it was more common among patients who had been out of the asylums for '8 to 10 years'.[145] In 1874, they argued that relapse was more common among female patients 'in whom moral causes predominate.'[146] However, most patients were returned to Carlow asylum within months of discharge and more men were readmitted.[147]

Conclusion

This chapter has argued that the patient profile generally associated with the Irish asylum population emerged in the late nineteenth century. It was a product of demographic adjustments in the asylum district after the Famine, an increase in the certification of men as dangerous lunatics after the 1867 and asylum management strategies. The patients confined in Carlow asylum came from low-income, settled, nuclear families, whose members – male and female – approached legal authorities to secure certification when mental disorders became violent. Patients' household structures impacted on opportunities for release and the presence of a family in the local community gave patients some protection against prolonged periods of confinement in asylums or local workhouses. Asylum medical superintendents were central to negotiations about patients' release, particularly in the case of 'ordinary' patients. While governors formally authorised discharges, medical superintendents investigated families' social and economic circumstances, selected patients they considered suitable for discharge and brought them before the asylum governors. In the case of ordinary patients, families' applications for releases could be denied on medical grounds. While some superintendents were not always familiar with the legal procedures, generally they were under pressure to relieve overcrowding and discharge patients.[148] Moreover, the chapter has suggested that the readmission of relapsed patients into overcrowded asylums was facilitated when contacts between families and asylum medical superintendents were maintained and consequently certifications were authorised through asylum governors rather than the petty session hearings.

Notes

1   P. Durcan, 'Madman', *Life is a Dream. 40 Years Reading Poems 1967–2007* (London: Harvill Secker, 2009), p. 91.

2   Wright, 'Getting Out of the Asylum', 139; Wright, 'Family Strategies and the Institutional Confinement of "Idiot" Children', 190–208; Tomes, *A Generous Confidence*; Walton, 'Lunacy in the Industrial Revolution', 1–22; Prestwich, 'Family Strategies and Medical Power', 799–818.

3   Wright, 'The Discharge of Pauper Lunatics from County Asylums in Mid-Victorian England', p. 94.

4   J. K. Walton, 'Casting Out and Bringing Back in Victorian England: Pauper Lunatics, 1840–1870', in W. F. Bynum, R. Porter and M. Shepherd (eds), *The Anatomy of Madness. Essays in the History of Psychiatry*, II (London: Tavistock, 1985), pp. 132–146.

5   For example, see NAI, CSORP 1845/G3928.

6   Scull, *The Most Solitary of Afflictions*, p. 271.

7   Asylum officials were obliged to maintain admission, discharge, removal and death registers. These contained information about patient's name, date of death, discharge, date of last admission, outcome and medical notes. Discharge registers only survived for the period from February 1846 to June 1900. Additional information on the fate of patients was gleaned from admission registers. Through nominal record linkage, the admission registers and the death registers have been combined thereby creating a relatively complete narrative of each patient's period of incarceration. Only 12.6 per cent (696) of patients' outcome was not recorded.

8   Wright, 'Getting Out of the Asylum', 139. There were some examples of asylum doctors' 'incompetence' in releasing patients, see NAI, Department of Health, L19/26, Annie C.

9   J. Andrews, 'The Boundaries of Her Majesty's Pleasure: Discharging Child-Murderers from Broadmoor and Perth Criminal Lunatic Department, c. 1860–1920', in M. Jackson (ed.), *Infanticide. Historical Perspective on Child Murder and Concealment, 1550–2000* (Aldershot: Ashgate, 2002), pp. 216–248; Melling and Forsythe, *The Politics of Madness*, pp. 191–194.

10 J. Busfield, 'The Female Malady? Men, Women and Madness in Nineteenth-Century-Britain', *Sociology*, 28:1 (1994), 259–277, 262.

11 E. M. Crawford, *Counting the People. A Survey of Irish Censuses, 1813–1911* (Dublin: Four Courts Press, 2003). The 1901 and 1911 censuses have been accessed through the National Archives of Ireland website.

12 Busfield, 'The Female Malady?', 265.

13 Finnane, *Insanity and the Insane*, p.131; E. Malcolm, '"The House of Strident Shadows"', pp. 179–180; E. Malcolm, '"Ireland's Crowded Madhouses"', pp. 315–334.

14 Melling and Forsythe, *The Politics of Madness*, p. 192.

15 This does not include the mortality rate during the Famine.

16 Busfield, 'The Female Malady?', 265.

17 Walsh, 'Gender and Insanity in Nineteenth-Century Ireland', p. 72.

18 The independent measures 'Student t-test' were used to determine whether there is a genuine difference in the means of a quantity (such as age, length of stay, etc.) taken in two independent groups. Pearson t-test is used when testing the connection between two categorical variables, such as counts. The tests produce a value, denoted by the symbol t, which measures the difference between the means of the two groups. This calculation takes into account the sizes of the two groups. The measure t is a known random variable; that is to say, it is known just how probable or improbable it is to get a particular value. The usual way in which this is expressed is in terms of critical values; thus values are known such that the probability of getting a higher value of t is 5 per cent. This is the probability usually used in the social sciences and defines exactly what is meant by 'unlikely'. The result of the test is expressed in terms of the null hypothesis. This is the statement that the difference in the two means is due to random factors, and has no inherent significance. In the case of the Pearson t-test it implies that there is no connection and the two counts are in proportion. If the value of t obtained is sufficiently unlikely then the null hypothesis is rejected – the chances of getting such a value of t are so low that it cannot be just down to chance. There is therefore a real difference between the means.

19 P. Chesler, *Women and Madness* (New York: Avon, 1972); E. Showalter, *The Female Malady: Women, Madness and English Culture, 1830–1980* (London: Virago Press, 1991), p. 3.

20 Andrews and Digby (eds), *Sex and Seclusion, Class and Custody*; J. Oppenheim, *'Shattered Nerves': Doctors, Patients, and Depression in Victorian England* (Oxford: Oxford University Press, 1990).

21 Busfield, 'The Female Malady?', p. 259.

22 The low value of –0.11 accepts the null hypothesis indicating that there was no difference between the length of time men and women spent in the asylum prior to 1856.

23 The mortality rates were calculated by dividing the numbers dying as recorded in the Carlow lunatic asylum registers, 1832–1922, by the resident population at the end of each year in the asylum, as recorded in the *Annual Reports of Lunacy Inspectors*, 1843–1921.

24 Busfield, 'The Female Malady?', pp. 265–268.

25 For example see statistics for the resident population in *Report of Lunacy Inspectors*, 1845 [645] xxvi, p. 49.

26 O. Walsh, 'A Lightness of Mind', p. 163.

27 *Inquiry into the State of Lunatic Asylums and other Institutions*, pp. 96–97.

28 D. Fitzpatrick, 'Women and the Great Famine', in M. Kelleher and J. H. Murphy (eds), *Gender Perspectives in Nineteenth-Century Ireland: Public and Private Spheres* (Dublin: Irish Academic Press, 1997), pp. 50–69.

29 T. W. Guinnane and C. Ó Gráda, 'Mortality in the North Dublin Union during the Great Famine', *Economic History Review*, 55: 3 (2002), 487–506.

30 When a Pearson t-test is carried out on the per capita male and female admissions, the high value of 3.13 rejects a null hypothesis that there is no difference between male and female admission rates (the critical value for a significance of 0.01, for 8 degrees of freedom, is 2.896). Statistically, this is an unlikely result.

31   When a Pearson χ^2 test, at a significance level of 0.05, is carried out on these counts, the null hypothesis is accepted, suggesting that they are purely random.

32   When the Pearson test is applied to the counts for the post-1867 period, the null hypothesis is rejected, with a very high value of the Pearson χ^2 statistic of 98.41 (for four degrees of freedom, the critical value for a significance of 0.01 is 9.488).

33   Walsh, 'Gendering the Asylums'.

34   Guinnane, *The Vanishing Irish*, pp. 133–165, pp. 212–213.

35   Walsh, 'Gender and Insanity', p. 85.

36   J. J. Lee, *Modernisation of Irish Society 1848–1918* (Dublin: Clarendon Press, 1989), pp. 1–19.

37   F. A. D'Arcy, 'The Decline and Fall of Donnybrook Fair: Moral Reform and Social Control in Nineteenth-Century Dublin', *Saothar*, 13 (1987), 7–21; B. Griffin, '"Such Varmint". The Dublin Police and the Public, 1838–1913', *Irish Studies Review*, 13:4 (1995/6), 21–25.

38   N. Garnham, 'The Survival of Popular Blood Sports in Victorian Ulster', *Proceedings of the Royal Irish Academy*, 107C (2007), 107–126.

39   R. Holt, 'Ireland and the Birth of Modern Sport', in M. Cronin, W. Murphy and P. Rouse (eds), *The Gaelic Athletic Association, 1884–2009* (Dublin: Irish Academic Press, 2009), pp. 33–47; Malcolm, 'The Rise of the Pub', pp. 50–77.

40   M. Finnane, 'Irish Crime with the Outrage: the Statistics of Criminal Justice in the Later Nineteenth Century', in N. M. Dawson (ed.), *Reflections on Law and History* (Dublin: Four Courts Press, 2006), pp. 203–222.

41   Guinnane, *The Vanishing Irish*.

42   The application of a Pearson χ^2 test to a cross-tabulation of the different forms of admission and the marital status of the patients for each decade indicates that the use of the differing forms of committal to each marital status altered significantly after 1870s. In every decade to the 1870s the null hypothesis was accepted; the differing forms of committal were applied in proportion to each marital status group. The results from the Pearson χ^2 test for the later decades suggest that from the 1880s, the forms of committal were applied in different ways to people of different marital status.

43   Finnne, *Insanity and the Insane*, p. 180.

44   Malcolm identified a higher proportion of long-stay patients in Irish asylums see Malcolm, '"The House of Strident Shadows"', pp. 180–181.

45   Melling and Forsythe, *The Politics of Madness*, pp. 186–189; S. Cherry, *Mental Health Care in Modern England. The Norfolk Lunatic Asylum, St. Andrew's Hospital, 1810–1998* (Woodbridge: Boydell Press, 2003), p. 74.

46   When a *t*-test is carried out, the high value of 2.95 rejects the null hypothesis. This is an unlikely result confirming that women spent longer in the asylum during this period.

47   See chapter three.

48   This result is not as significant as it would seem, because it was heavily influenced by the disparity between the numbers of male and female patients in the asylum. The value of *t* variable, 1.6, is not significant at a significance level of 5 per cent.

49   Finnane, *Insanity and the Insane*, p. 234.

50   See chapter seven.

51 Malcolm '"The House of Strident Shadows"', p.180.

52 Scull, *Museums of Madness*, p. 252.

53 Guinnane, *The Vanishing Irish*, p. 121.

54 P. Thane, *Old Age in English History. Past Experiences and Present Issues* (Oxford: Oxford University Press, 2005), pp. 287–307.

55 Guinnane, *The Vanishing Irish*, p. 63.

56 Melling and Turner, 'The Road to the Asylum', 298–332.

57 M. MacDonald, *Mystical Bedlam: Madness, Anxiety and Healing in Seventeenth-Century England* (Cambridge: Cambridge University Press, 1981), p. 113.

58 The relationship is stated in 211 of the 340 surviving committal warrants sworn between 1838 and 1867. In 173 of these 211 warrants, a family member initiated proceedings.

59 Melling and Forsythe, *The Politics of Madness*, p. 98.

60 Guinnane, *The Vanishing Irish*, p. 134.

61 Guinnane, *The Vanishing Irish*, pp. 139–143; Fitzpatrick, 'Irish Farming Families before the First World War', 339–374; Boyle and Ó Gráda, 'Fertility Trends, Excess Mortality and the Great Irish Famine', 543–562.

62 Guinnane, *The Vanishing Irish*, pp. 139–143.

63 *Ibid.*, pp. 133–165.

64 O'Neill, *Family and Farm*, p. 161.

65 *Ibid.*, p.162.

66 NAI, CSO CRF Wexford 1851; Wexford 1863; Wexford 1860.

67 O'Neill, *Family and Farm*, p. 139; D. Hirst and P. Michael, 'Family Community and the Lunatic in Mid-Nineteenth-Century North Wales', in Bartlett and Wright (eds), *Outside the Walls of the Asylum*, p. 77.

68 Melling and Forsythe, *The Politics of Madness*, p. 104; Garton, *Medicine and Madness*; Coleborne, '"His Brain was Wrong, his Mind Astray"', 45–65.

69 Hirst and Michael, 'Family Community and the Lunatic', p. 77; Melling and Forsythe, *The Politics of Madness*, p. 84.

70 Guinnane, *The Vanishing Irish*.

71 *Eleventh Report of Lunacy Inspectors*, H. C. 1862 [2975] xxiii, p. 25.

72 T. R. Cole and C. Edwards, 'The 19th Century', in P. Thane (ed.) *The Long History of Old Age* (London: Thames and Hudson, 2005), pp. 211–262.

73 In the 1851 census women formed 51 per cent of the Carlow district population. By 1861 this had fallen to 49.9 per cent. Between 1832 and 1867, women testified in 44.7 per cent of the warrants and men were 55.3 per cent.

74 J. Andrews and A. Digby, 'Introduction: Gender and Class in the Historiography of British and Irish Psychiatry', Andrews and Digby (eds), *Sex and Seclusion, Class and Custody*, p. 24.

75 Husbands accounted for 36.1 per cent of the committals petitioned by male relatives.

76 Prestwich, 'Family Strategies and Medical Power', 805.

77 Among male relatives, brothers formed 12.7 per cent (6) of petitioners.

78 Melling and Forsythe, *The Politics of Madness*, p. 116.

79 J. Bourke, *Husbandry to Housewifery: Women, Economic Change and Housework in Ireland 1890–1914* (Oxford: Oxford University Press, 1993).

80   J. Bourke, '"The Best of all Home Rulers": The Economic Power of Women in Ireland, 1880–1914', *Irish Economic and Social History*, 13 (1991), 34–47; O. Walsh, 'Gendering the Asylums: Ireland and Scotland, 1847–1877', in T. Brotherstone, D. Simonton and O. Walsh (eds), *The Gendering of Scottish History: An International Approach* (Glasgow: Cruithne Press, 1999), p. 210.

81   J. J. Lee, 'Women and the Church since the Famine', in M. MacCurtain and D. Ó Corráin (eds), *Women in Society. The Historical Dimension* (Dublin: Greenwood Press, 1978), pp. 37–45; Bourke, '"The Best of all Home Rulers"'; C. Ó Gráda, *Ireland Before and After the Famine; Explorations in Economic History, 1808–1925* (Manchester: Manchester University Press, 1993); Breen, 'Dowry Payments and the Irish Case', 280–296.

82   Steiner-Scott, '"To Bounce a Boot Off Her Now &Then"', p.138.

83   Finnane, *Insanity and the Insane*, p. 115.

84   It is not possible to filter out patients who were transferred to Enniscorthy asylum, and so for the sake of consistency, the Kilkenny transfers are included. The remaining patients were transferred from Carlow to other public asylums. Between 1832 and 1852 1 per cent (53) was transferred to Kilkenny, to the old and new asylums.

85   8&9 Vict. c.107, s. 11 (1845).

86   9&10 Vict. c.115, s. 3 (1846).

87   DPH, CLA Minute Book, 3 February 1835.

88   *Twenty-first Report of Lunacy Inspectors*, H. C. 1843 [462] xxvii, pp. 94–99.

89   Finnane, *Insanity and the Insane*, p. 116.

90   'Twentieth Annual Report by Dr White of the Carlow District Hospital of the Insane Poor for the year ending 31 March 1853', *DQJMS*, 16 (August–November 1853), 391.

91   Finnane, *Insanity and the Insane*, p. 116.

92   DPH, CLA Minute Book, 20 July 1868.

93   SPH, ELA Letter Book, 6 August 1868.

94   *Eighth Report of Lunacy Inspectors*, H. C. 1857 session 2 [2253] xvii, p. 15.

95   SPH, ELA Letter Book, 21 March 1884.

96   *Eighth Report of Lunacy Inspectors*, H. C. 1857 session 2 [2253] xvii, p. 6.

97   SPH, ELA Minute Book, 18 January 1877.

98   30&31 Vict. c.118, s.10 (1867).

99   30&31 Vict. c.118, s.11 (1867); Finnane, *Insanity and the Insane*, p. 116.

100 SPH, ELA Letter Book, 20 July 1883, 8 December 1883.

101 *Ibid.*, 10 April 1885.

102 NAI, CSO CRF, Carlow 1845.

103 DPH, CLA Minute Book, 18 September 1839; see also 21 December 1841, 19 July 1848 and 10 October 1848.

104 DPH, CLA Minute Book, 12 March 1886.

105 *Forty-second Report of Lunacy Inspectors*, H. C. 1893–94 [C. 7125] xlvi, p. 97; Bartlett, *The Poor Law of Lunacy*.

106 Melling and Forsythe, *The Politics of Madness*, p. 192.

107 DPH, CLA Male Case Book, January 1906–January 1908, James B.

108 Ray, 'Models of Madness', 248, 256.

109 M. Foucault, 'Madness and the Absence of Work', *Critical Inquiry*, 21 (1995), 2 90–298.
110 Ray, 'Models of Madness, 244.
111 NAI, CSO CRF, Wexford, 1860; Wexford, 1853.
112 Wright, 'The Discharge of Pauper Lunatics'.
113 DPH, CLA Male Case Book, January 1906–January 1908, Peter M.
114 The marital status of patients was not recorded consistently and for the majority committed prior to 1846 – 1503 patients – it was not transcribed in the committal registers. The fate and marital status is known for 2066 of patients committed between 1832 and 1922.
115 Between 1846 and 1922, 60 per cent (1550) of single patients committed to the asylum were male. The proportion of single female admissions was 40 per cent (1036). The proportion of single patients dying in the asylum was high, 35.9 per cent (567) of single men died in the asylum while 36 per cent of single women died.
116 A larger portion of married men died in Devon asylum, see Melling and Forsythe, *The Politics of Madness*, pp.104–105.
117 Andrews, 'The Boundaries of Her Majesty's Pleasure', p. 243.
118 SPH, ELA, Letter to Thomas Drapes, 22 November 1902; n.d.
119 DPH, CLA Male Case Book, January 1906–January 1908, Patrick M.
120 DPH, CLA Minute Book, 13 June, 8 August, 12 September, 12 December 1884.
121 *Fortieth Report of Lunacy Inspectors*, H. C. 1890–91 [6503] xxxvi, p. 7.
122 DPH, CLA Minute Book, 19 August 1872.
123 *Ibid.*, 14 March 1879.
124 Dr Michael Patrick Howlett was Resident Medical Superintendent at Carlow asylum from 1866 to 1880, *Medical Press and Circular* (26 September 1880).
125 See also SPH, ELA Letter Book, 5 November 1883, 18 November 1883; 15 December 1883; 24 December 1884.
126 DPH, CLA Minute Book, 3 February 1835.
127 *Ibid.*,15 March 1843.
128 DPH, CLA Minute Book, 3 February 1835.
129 SPH, ELA Letter, 16 December 1926.
130 SPH, ELA Letter, 20 July 1877.
131 SPH, ELA Letter, n.d.
132 SPH, ELA Letter, n.d.
133 SPH, ELA Letter Book, 15 December 1878.
134 SPH, ELA Letter Book, 15 December 1883.
135 Andrews, 'The Boundaries of her Majesty's Pleasure'.
136 DPH, CLA Minute Book, 13 May 1881.
137 DPH, CLA Male Case Book, January 1906–January 1908, Patrick M; SPH, ELA Letter to Thomas Drapes, 27 August 1902; 1 April 1908; 28 February 1908; 18 April 1914; 22 April 1905.
138 DPH, CLA Minute Book, 9 October 1885, 14 December 1888.
139 SPH, ELA Minute Book, 20 September 1877, see also Letter, 11 August 1919.
140 SPH, ELA Minute Book, 9 May 1900.
141 DPH, CLA Male Case Book, January 1906–January 1908, Patrick McD.

142   Paper presented by Nicole Baur, University of Exeter, 'In Search of the Patient' at Wellcome Trust conference 'Research Resources in Medical History (Edinburgh, 12–14 December 2007).

143   In some instances, the admission number was not repeated and personal details were used to establish whether the patient was in the asylum on a previous occasion.

144   Finnane, *Insanity and the Insane*, p. 234.

145   *Thirty-first Report of Lunacy Inspectors*, H. C. 1882 [3356] xxxii, p. 6; *Eleventh Report of Lunacy Inspectors*, 1862 [2975] xxiii, p. 21.

146   *Twenty-fourth Report of Lunacy Inspectors*, H. C. 1875 [C. 1293] xxxiii, p. 13.

147   60 per cent (n=280) of second admissions were male.

148   Wright, 'The Discharge of Pauper Lunatics', p. 104.

6

Workhouses and the mentally ill

In July 1868, Terence B., a thirty-one-year-old married labourer from the Courtown estate in Gorey, county Wexford was discharged from Enniscorthy asylum. He had been admitted as a dangerous lunatic to Carlow asylum in December 1849 and when a new institution was opened in Enniscorthy town in 1868, Terence was transferred. He did not remain there long. In August 1868, the Enniscorthy governors decided that Terence was no longer dangerous and tried to discharge him. They discovered he had no surviving relatives living in the locality and so they transferred him to the 'idiot' wards in Gorey workhouse.[1] Ten years earlier, in June 1858, a fractious inmate of the 'idiot' ward in Enniscorthy workhouse, Bridget M. assaulted a woman – hammering her head on the ground – and broke several windowpanes. The workhouse officials brought her before the local petty session hearings and testified that she was a dangerous lunatic. She was confined to Wexford gaol and then transferred to Carlow asylum in January 1859. This was the second time she had been certified.[2] The patient histories of Terence and Bridget highlight the importance of Irish workhouses in the institutionalisation of mental illness. A substantial proportion of asylum patients came from workhouses and asylum officials transferred harmless patients to workhouses to relieve overcrowding or, as in the case of Terence, when there was no support outside the asylum.

In contrast to England, nineteenth-century legislative and regulatory frameworks ensured that poor law and lunacy administration in Ireland formally remained discrete entities. As Peter Bartlett has correctly observed, in comparison to England, 'Ireland had entirely different administrative structures and criteria for admission' into workhouses and there were only a handful of regulations affecting both workhouses and asylums.[3] Nonetheless, central administration at Dublin Castle believed asylums were part of pauper relief. The members appointed to the 1878–79 Select Committee on Poor Law Union and Lunacy Inquiry asserted that mental illness was 'essentially a part of the general pauperism of Ireland'.[4] Pauperisation was fundamental to the experience of institutional confine-ment of mental illness in Ireland. District asylums were repeatedly referred to as institutions for the reception of 'pauper' insanity and the language of pauperism pervaded prison and lunacy inspectors' reports.[5] When certifying relatives, families confirmed they were unable to afford private institutions while poor law dispensary doctors signed dangerous lunatic medical certificates. Although treated as paupers in most respects, unlike workhouse inmates, asylum patients were not required to be desti-tute and were regarded as more 'deserving' objects of assistance. As Elaine Murphy has shown, the architects of asylum systems were steeped in the 'evangelical ethos of a public duty to provide care and cure.'[6] Initially, the Irish inspectors believed mental illness was 'the most distressing visita-tion to which human nature is subjected'[7] and those afflicted were not as culpable as workhouses inmates. Though these attitudes would subse-quently change, in the 1840s there was no suggestion that patients would abuse asylum relief.[8]

Excepting Oonagh Walsh, scholars have largely ignored the rela-tionship between the poor law and the asylum systems in Ireland, focusing on the criminalisation of the mentally ill. This chapter assesses the interactions between workhouses and asylums when dealing with the mentally ill. It will demonstrate that workhouse lunatic wards expanded the 'institutional market-place' in asylum districts, though in contrast to England poor law unions did not enter formal contracts with private or public asylums. The involvement of workhouses in lunacy manage-ment prompted significant debate among lunacy inspectors, poor law commissioners and the Local Government Board, and three separate parliamentary inquiries examined the workhouses' role in relieving pauper lunacy.[9] The debate was driven by two key sometimes counter-vailing pressures: the pressure to relieve overcrowding in asylums and to provide appropriate medical facilities for the mentally ill. In the absence of a clearly defined integrated system that adequately responded to these pressures, the movement of people between institutions was managed and negotiated locally. To explore these issues, this chapter draws on

Carlow, Enniscorthy, Athy and Naas poor law union records, in addition to Carlow and Enniscorthy asylum records. While there were additional poor law unions in the asylum district, most patients were transferred from these union workhouses and there are excellent collections of Carlow, Naas and Enniscorthy poor law union minute books for the nineteenth century. The Athy poor law union minute books are less comprehensive. Unfortunately, many workhouse admission registers were destroyed though the Athy indoor register has survived.

*

The poor law was introduced to Ireland in 1838, nearly twenty years after the asylum system.[10] By that date, ten district asylums had opened with 1,309 beds.[11] The Irish poor law was modelled on the 1834 English Poor Law Act and newly constructed workhouses were central to the relief system. Ireland was divided into 130 poor law unions and by 1845 most workhouses were opened. Destitution was the main criteria for admission to the workhouse though the old and the infirm were entitled to relief.[12] The Irish legislation did not initially provide outdoor relief, however, this changed in 1847.[13] Officially, outdoor relief was discouraged in Ireland as it was believed to be expensive, open to abuse and detrimental to the industrious habits of the Irish peasantry. Nonetheless, some poor law guardians provided it.[14] By the 1850s there were thirteen workhouses in the Carlow asylum district.[15]

Asylums and workhouses were financed through separate forms of taxation thereby inhibiting the integration of asylum and workhouse relief. The asylums were financed through the county cess and the grand jury system.[16] Poor law taxation was raised through poor rates, which were levied on electoral divisions that comprised individual poor law unions. There were separate inspectorates with, at times, apparently overlapping responsibilities. Under the 1838 act, the poor law commissioners were empowered to inspect institutions in receipt of grand jury presentments and parliamentary grants.[17] Lunatic asylums were not, however, mentioned in the act and it is unclear if the commissioners inspected these. When established in 1847, the Irish poor law inspectorate assumed responsibility for monitoring workhouses but the lunacy inspectorate, established in 1845, inspected all institutions accommodating the insane, and this also included workhouse lunatic wards. The lunacy inspectorate did not have any real powers to intervene in workhouse business but they could make recommendations.

From the 1840s, most workhouses had separate lunatic wards and while individual wards were relatively small, collectively they housed substantial numbers. The mentally ill accumulated in workhouses through various mechanisms; some workhouse inmates developed mental disorders after admission, while idiots and the mentally ill were admitted on the grounds of destitution.[18] In these cases, the inmates' mental state did not entitle them to workhouse relief.[19] In 1862, destitution was removed as the criteria for admission to workhouse infirmaries and accordingly poor law medical officers were entitled to admit patients on the basis of medical needs, but this was not extended to the insane.[20] The criteria for asylum and dispensary relief differed from workhouses. The 1851 Medical Charities Act specified that 'poor persons' were entitled to indoor and outdoor dispensary relief; they were not required to be destitute. Similarly, asylum patients were expected to be poor not destitute. The differences between these entitlement criteria created problems. For example, when asylums were overcrowded, poor law dispensary doctors could not send mentally ill patients to workhouses to await transfer to asylums, as they were not necessarily destitute. As a Celbridge guardian observed when discussing one woman's situation 'so far as the law stands at present, the only hope of getting this woman admitted to an asylum is to get her to beat somebody up' and then certify her as a dangerous lunatic.[21]

Nonetheless, the mentally ill accumulated in workhouse lunatic wards throughout Carlow asylum district. County Wexford workhouses, particularly New Ross workhouse, housed the largest number.[22] Among Kildare workhouses, Naas workhouse accommodated the greatest amount while Carlow workhouse housed relatively few though the number rose in the twentieth century.[23] Lunatic wards were not included in the original workhouse architectural designs, but were added subsequently. In his evidence to the 1857–58 Inquiry into the State of Lunatic Asylums, the workhouse architect, George Wilkinson, remarked that these wards were 'intended to relieve the other inmates of a disagreeable class of persons ... It was never thought they were proper places for them. They were however the only places. There was no room in any other institution.'[24] The accommodation was generally inappropriate and ad hoc, and the small lunatic wards were often overcrowded. As a result, classification of general workhouse inmates became difficult as workhouse lunatics spilled into the main body of the institution where other inmates watched over them. The workhouse medical officer provided medical treatment. The workhouse diet was often inferior to the asylum diet and there were few therapeutic activities.

Concern for the welfare of the mentally ill in workhouses emerged at an early stage. Francis White, arguing that they should be transferred to asylums, provided a bleak picture of conditions in lunatic wards in his annual reports. Similarly, in 1848, Denis Phelan, Assistant Poor Law Commissioner, reported that the inmates slept on straw-beds in badly ventilated cells, and were barefoot and badly nourished.[25] While the commissioners encouraged poor law guardians to ensure these inmates were cared for, cases of neglect were uncovered during the 1857–58 Inquiry into the State of Lunatic Asylums.[26] The worst conditions were in unions with relatively few inmates in lunatic wards and the members of the inquiry were generally opposed to the dispersal of lunatics in small numbers in the various workhouses in the country. The lunacy inspectors' criticism of workhouse conditions focused on the failure to provide indoor and outdoor therapeutic pursuits and to segregate the mentally ill: 'the same crowded apartments being indiscriminately used for patients under every type of disease'.[27] Unlike English commissioners in lunacy, the Irish inspectors did not approve specific workhouses as suitable for the mentally ill.[28]

It is doubtful whether the inspectors' visits to workhouse wards had a radical impact upon conditions but they did take place. For example, in 1856 they visited the workhouses in Athy, Carlow, Naas and Wexford poor law unions twice while Hatchell and Nugent inspected wards attached to Ennsicorthy, Gorey and Wexford workhouses in the 1870s. The inspectors sometimes made recommendations for improvements. For example, Nugent requested the Carlow and Enniscorthy poor law guardians make specific improvements to the lunatic wards in 1884.[29] However, according to a 1896 special commission that investigated nursing facilities in Irish workhouses and infirmaries, conditions in these workhouses were inadequate. Reporting on Athy workhouse infirmary in county Kildare, the commission found six inmates housed in three cells that were bolted at night. There was no day room and instead a corridor was used for recreation. The lunatic wards were 'clean, but unspeakably dreary and cheerless' and had the appearance of 'prison cells (6 feet by 10 feet) with small grated lights high in the walls'. Workhouse inmates watched over the lunatic wards although at the time nuns were permitted to nurse other inmates in the infirmary.[30] By the 1900s, the lunacy inspectors again criticised workhouse conditions; O'Farrell and Courteney described the wards as 'overcrowded, dark and dreary, almost devoid of furniture and articles of comfort or interest'.[31] O'Farrell and Courteney were particularly critical of the absence of specialised medical care, arguing that as a result mentally ill inmates were unlikely to recover. In common with others, they adhered to the view that asylums were the most suitable institutions for managing and caring for the mentally ill.[32] The members of the 1857–58 Inquiry had made similar points.

While this debate was ongoing, the Irish lunacy administration struggled to cope with the accumulation of 'incurable' or chronic patients in asylums. In spite of John Leslie Foster's confidence in 1817 that there would be no need for separate institutions for this patient group, chronic patients were a problem from an early stage. In 1817 James Cleghorn, physician attached to Swift's Hospital, had anticipated that asylums would be populated with 'incurable' patients. Initially, their admission into asylums was discouraged.[33] During the 1820s and 1830s, the prison inspectors criticised gaol superintendents who transferred prisoners into the asylums for these reasons.[34] Simultaneously, however, and in apparent contradiction of this, the inspectors called for provision for chronic patients, stressing that this should be within existing asylums.[35] This reflected the more sympathetic attitude toward incurable patients of administrators and policymakers, like Thomas Jackson.[36] In accordance with White's view that both curable and chronic patients should be cared for in asylums,[37] the 1843 privy council rules removed the ban on the admission of 'incurables' and accordingly there was an increase in the numbers in asylums.[38]

The number of chronic patients in asylums rapidly increased, as the new admissions joined existing long-stay patients accumulated in asylums. By the end of 1842, it was estimated that 102 of the 169 patients in Carlow asylum were incurable.[39] By 1856, the inspectors observed that three-quarters of the national asylum population were 'incurable' and by 1878, it was estimated that 2,656 of the 3,824 residents in asylums were 'probable incurable'.[40] This was not a problem for Ireland alone. In 1876, the inspectors estimated that chronic cases were now in excess of 'hopeful' cases in asylums across Europe and America where they accounted for four-fifths of the asylum population.[41]

The inspectors beseeched managers of asylums not to allow the asylums to degenerate 'into domiciles for incurable lunatics to the exclusion and serious detriment of acute cases'.[42] However, their own policy of encouraging the transfer of workhouse inmates into asylums put pressure on overcrowded institutions and increased the number of chronic patients. From 1861 to 1891, workhouse admissions increased steadily and while the rate subsequently declined, as table 6.1 shows, large numbers in the asylums came from workhouses.[43] Moreover, the numbers of lunatics in Irish workhouses continued to increase rising from 2,292 in March 1851 to 4,087 in December 1901.

Due to the pressure on overcrowded asylums, by the second half of the nineteenth century asylum governors and the lunacy administration increasingly turned to the workhouses to assist in the management of chronic patients. This shift in attitude coincided with changes in lunacy administration in England. As Bartlett has observed, in the 1860s there was an emphasis on the 'manageability' of mentally ill workhouse inmates and, from 1862 local asylum authorities in England were authorised to remove chronic patients to workhouses approved by the lunacy commissioners.[44] This change in attitude culminated in the 1867 Metropolitan Poor Act.[45] In Ireland, Francis White departed from the lunacy inspectorate in 1856 and by 1861 Nugent and Hatchell were more muted in their criticisms of conditions in workhouses, arguing these had improved as 'a more considerate system of treatment has been adopted.'[46] The members

Table 6.1   Proportion of patients admitted from workhouses into asylums, 1890 to 1900

	Total no. of Admissions	% of workhouse admissions
1890	3,095	12.79
1891	3,010	12.66
1892	3,181	13.3
1893	3,207	13.66
1894	3,229	14.25
1895	3,216	15.17
1896	3,329	16.46
1897	3,285	16.62
1898	3,469	18.28
1899	3,549	18.79
1900	3,546	20.47

Source: *Fiftieth Report on District, Local and Private Lunatic Asylums in Ireland, H. C. 1901* [Cd. 760] xxviii, p. xiv.

of the 1878–79 Select Committee on Poor Law Union and Lunacy Inquiry subsequently disagreed with them, questioning the frequency with which they visited workhouses and claiming that both men had 'imperfect knowledge' of workhouses.[47] Nugent and Hatchell argued that transferring 'incurable' and 'harmless' patients from the asylums to workhouses would create much needed space in asylums.[48] From the 1870s, they actively encouraged workhouse officials to admit chronic and harmless patients from asylums, insisting that they received little benefit from the asylums as most were 'born idiots' and epileptics, 'who between them constitute the lowest intelligence in the human family.'[49] They also stressed that accommodating chronic patients in workhouses reduced the financial burden to the ratepayer, and would halt the expansion of asylumdom.[50] The estimated annual cost of housing a patient in an asylum was twenty-three pounds per head, while pauper lunatics cost eleven pounds in workhouses.[51] There was, however, no system whereby the inspectors approved workhouses as suitable for the care of the mentally ill and, while advocating the transfer of the 'harmless' patients, the inspectors repeatedly stressed that conditions in workhouse lunatic wards needed improvement. Some inroads were made; at the request of local asylum governors, separate accommodation and improved wards were provided at Kilkenny, Waterford and Limerick workhouses and, in 1866, the inspectors introduced a system to pay attendants to care for mentally ill in the workhouses. However, as O'Farrell and Courteney found, by the 1900s little had changed.

Local negotiations

Most poor law guardians steadfastly objected to the presence of mentally ill inmates in workhouses and were reluctant to accept them.[52] Accommodating the mentally ill was problematic. The classification systems operating in workhouses were undermined; for example in Carlow workhouse overcrowding in the lunatic wards resulted in insane inmates being housed in the general wards where they required careful supervision.[53] This usually involved an increase in number of keepers rather than the employment of nurses.[54] Their presence also resulted in workhouses being subjected to additional inspection by the lunacy inspectors and mentally ill inmates disrupted workhouse regimes. When difficult behaviour escalated, some officials attempted to transfer them to the asylum.

Melling and Forsythe have argued that there were financial burdens associated with transferring inmates to the aylum.[55] From 1843, poor law guardians in Ireland paid the cost of transporting workhouse inmates to the asylum.[56] However, the 1843 act only applied to workhouse inmates and was not extended to recipients of relief under the 1851 Medical Charities Act. As dispensary doctors discovered, the cost of transporting patients directly to asylums from home was not covered. Instead, doctors were obliged to admit patients to workhouses first and then guardians would pay the cost of transferring them to asylums.[57] Once transferred, asylums assumed responsibility for maintenance costs. The cost of transporting workhouse inmates to the asylum was a short-term expense that allowed guardians to shed long-term costs. The 1874 grant-in-aid also moved the expense of maintaining workhouse lunatics to the county at large.[58]

Scull has observed that 'the order and discipline of the whole workhouse was threatened by the presence of a madman'[59] and disruption 'was the language of negotiation' between workhouses and asylums. Workhouse officials often removed inmates following assaults on staff or attacks on property. For example, Mary M. was accused of 'assaulting an inmate [Margaret M.] breaking the windows of the workhouse and also breaking the vessels in which her food has been conveyed to her'.[60] When asylums were overcrowded, workhouse officials experienced difficulties transferring inmates and, in some cases, they had them certified as dangerous lunatics. However, this was not encouraged and was to be used 'as a last resort'.[61] Workhouse masters, matrons and porters often testified during these cases, highlighting the impact workhouse staff had upon patients' care. At Carlow asylum relatively few patients from workhouses were certified as dangerous lunatics and this occurred most frequently when the asylum was severely overcrowded. For example, between 1847 and 1851, 11 per cent of dangerous lunatics were workhouse paupers and this declined after 1851. Among these cases, there was little evidence of violence.[62] While several Kilkenny patients were described as 'wild', 'incoherent' and 'restless' they were not violent.[63] Clearly, poor law guardians were removing difficult inmates from severely overcrowded workhouses during the Famine.

Transfers continued after the Famine and in these cases the inmates were reported to have damaged workhouse property and attacked other inmates and workhouse staff. Poor law guardians were fearful of the dangers involved in maintaining mentally ill inmates in workhouses.

During the 1905 inquiry into the violent deaths at Naas workhouse, discussed in chapter four, it emerged that while in the workhouse, other inmates had watched over Dowling and the consequent laxity in supervision was believed to be pivotal to the tragedy. The inquiry into Dowling's actions received significant press coverage, highlighting the risks involved in keeping lunatics in workhouses.[64] After the incident, neighbouring poor law guardians became more resolute in attempting to remove lunatic inmates to asylums. The number of transfers from local workhouses to Carlow asylum rose for several years.[65] The master at Baltinglass workhouse was worried that a 'refractory' inmate, Henry Neale 'will do something like that fellow in Naas.'[66] The Dowling tragedy was not an isolated incident of violence, leading some poor law guardians to conclude that 'there were three classes of lunatics which should not be kept in a workhouse viz. dangerous, curable and those not cleanly in their habits'.[67] The asylums were clearly associated with containing danger rather than curable forms of insanity in public lay commentary. As N. J. Synnott, the chairman of Naas poor law union, explicitly stated 'the existing [Carlow] asylum was chiefly for dangerous lunatics'.[68]

Despite these problems and anxieties, guardians did not always remove inmates to asylums and they were not compelled to do so, as was the case in England.[69] Poor law guardians differed in their attitudes towards maintaining mentally ill inmates in workhouses.[70] For example, Enniscorthy workhouse officials had accepted dangerous lunatic inmates shortly before the new asylum in the town was opened, and they were anxious to transfer them to the asylum as soon as possible.[71] They were less certain of the advantages in clearing workhouse 'idiot' wards. Early in 1868, twenty-seven people were accommodated in Enniscorthy workhouse lunatic wards. When the new asylum governors approached the poor law guardians to organise their transfer to the asylum, the guardians refused arguing that the cost of maintaining 'idiot' paupers in the asylum was prohibitive and not in the interests of the county ratepayers.[72] Enniscorthy workhouse continued to maintain paupers in the 'idiot' wards and in 1911 there were forty-three inmates confined in the workhouse 'idiot' wards.

The profile of inmates transferred from workhouses to asylums varied between institutions. David Durnin's study of the South Dublin Union workhouse inmates transferred to Richmond asylum between 1880 and 1911 shows that in an urban context there were similarities between the asylum population and the population of the workhouse lunatic wards.[73] This was not the case in rural contexts. Between 1853 and 1916, 618 patients were transferred from local workhouses to Carlow asylum. Initially, only a few inmates were transferred per decade, however after 1879, the numbers increased – in 1884, twelve inmates were transferred and by 1904 this had increased to twenty-five. The numbers peaked at thirty-nine in 1905.[74] In contrast to Richmond asylum, where most of the workhouse inmates transferred from South Dublin Union workhouse were women, approximately equal numbers of male (310) and female (307) patients were transferred to Carlow asylum. The majority – 84 per cent – were single. Among patients whose fate was recorded, approximately a half died in the asylum indicating that workhouse asylum patients were significantly more vulnerable than other patients. Most were described as suffering from forms of illness that involved disruptive behaviour such as epilepsy (41), forms of mania (218), delusions (15), while only three were described as suicidal. A large number were diagnosed as suffering from forms of dementia (96) or were categorised as congenital imbeciles, mental defects, idiots and melancholics (111).

Poor law guardians intending to transfer workhouses inmates often encountered difficulties when asylums were overcrowded. As discussed above, to overcome this, some officials brought inmates before the magistrates. However, asylum governors certified the admission of most workhouse inmates and to achieve this, the poor law guardians established good working relationships with asylum officials.[75] As reported during the 1857–58 Inquiry into the State of Lunatic Asylums, the transfer of work-house inmates was facilitated by cooperation between workhouse and asylum personnel. This was made easier when there was an overlap in staff. Personnel were not required to perform specific functions in both the poor law and lunacy services. Nonetheless, in Ireland, as there were fewer resident landlords and gentry in particular counties, and doctors guarded appointments in welfare institutions jealously, there was often an overlap between workhouse, poor law dispensary and asylum staff and other personnel. From 1850 to 1890 at least one senior Carlow poor law officer regularly attended meetings of Carlow asylum governors. As shown in chapter one, Henry Bruen, Thomas Butler and Robert Clayton Browne (all governors) were chairman, vice-chairman and deputy vice-chairman of Carlow board of guardians.[76] While serving as Carlow governors, Hugh Faulkner was an ex-officio Carlow guardian, and Samuel and Thomas

Haughton were elected poor law guardians. Likewise, senior Athy poor law guardians, including William Caulfield, vice-chairman, and John Butler, deputy vice chairman,[77] were active Carlow governors. Staff employed in workhouses, dispensaries and asylums often worked in these institutions simultaneously or moved between them. Visiting physicians at Enniscorthy asylum, Drs Thomas G. Cranfield and Nicholas Furlong, were both local poor law dispensary medical officers, and Furlong was the workhouse medical officer.[78] Drapes, appointed visiting physician at Enniscorthy in March 1872 acted as *locum* at Enniscorthy dispensary in August 1878.[79] At Carlow asylum, the visiting physician was Dr Charles William McDowell, also a local dispensary doctor, while Dr Thomas B. Kynsey, an active Carlow asylum governor in the early 1870s, was the Athy workhouse medical officer.

These connections are reflected in the different numbers admitted from each workhouse. For example, at Carlow asylum most workhouse patients were transferred from Carlow (267), Athy (178) and Naas (177) workhouses between the 1870s and 1916 although the numbers from Naas workhouses declined during these years. Indeed, in 1902, Naas poor law guardians complained that they no longer had sufficient representation on the Carlow asylum board to secure transfers between institutions.[80] Other large unions in the district such as Wexford, whose guardians were not active on the board failed to establish a similar relationship, and this was reflected in the low number of transfers before 1868. Wexford guardians looked forward to transferring twenty-one male and female lunatics, idiots and epileptics upon the opening of Enniscorthy asylum.[81]

Medical officers were required to make the practical arrangements for these transfers. When transferring an inmate, they contacted the asylum medical superintendent some of whom were more cooperative than others.[82] Following Thomas O'Meara's appointment to Carlow asylum in 1880 the number of both admissions from, and discharges to, workhouses rose. The medical officers at Carlow, Athy and Naas workhouses cooperated with O'Meara to secure admissions. For example, P. L. O'Neill, medical officer at Athy workhouse, regularly identified inmates more suitable for the asylum at the point of entry into the workhouse and transferred them within days.[83] Athy guardians actively discharged inmates they believed were not entitled to relief.[84] The chairman of Naas guardians, P. J. Doyle, who had been a Carlow asylum governor, claimed in 1905 that through the cooperation of Dr James J. Fitzgerald, Resident

Medical Superintendent at Carlow asylum from 1903 to 1907, and the Naas workhouse medical officer, Dr F. J. Falkiner,[85] Naas guardians were able to transfer patients to Carlow asylum.[86] During Fitzgerald's four years at the asylum there was an increase in admissions from Naas workhouse. Family connections also helped. Although not a local dispensary doctor or workhouse medical officer, Carlow guardians paid Dr William H. O'Meara to certify workhouse lunatics; he was related to Thomas O'Meara.[87] In contrast, Shiell and Drapes at Enniscorthy asylum refused to admit 'idiots' and harmless workhouse inmates claiming they were prioritising dangerous and urgent admissions.[88] Drapes believed that the increase in workhouse admissions to asylums after the 1860s exacerbated overcrowding and contributed to the perception that mental illness was increasing.[89] In 1909, Thomas A. Greene, Resident Medical Superintendent at Carlow asylum from 1908, requested that Naas guardians stop transferring harmless lunatics and pointed out that the asylum management committee would be obliged to expand the institution further unless transfers ceased.[90]

Simultaneously, asylum medical superintendents were discharging 'harmless' patients to workhouses, including recovered patients without families to support them after release. The Carlow governors adopted this policy in 1842.[91] However, poor law guardians were often reluctant to admit asylum patients. On the recommendation of Nugent, Shiell at Enniscorthy asylum attempted to transfer harmless patients into Wexford, Gorey and New Ross workhouses in 1870. While Wexford and New Ross complied, Gorey union refused to accept them.[92] The 1875 Lunatic Asylums (Ireland) Act encouraged the transfer of asylum patients to workhouses by allowing 'harmless' lunatics to be moved with the consent of the Local Government Board and the lunacy inspectors. Under the act, the lunacy authorities continued to pay maintenance costs and asylum medical officers certified that patients were suitable for the workhouse.[93] The act also specified that asylum patients admitted from workhouses were to be returned to that workhouse on recovery.[94] The 1875 act had the potential to ease overcrowding in asylums and allow the admission of 'curable' patients. It was also cheaper to maintain harmless patients in workhouses and ensured the asylum superintendent retained control over the selection of patients. The act however was flawed; technically, accepting patients into workhouses should not have had any financial consequences for guardians. However, guardians encountered difficulties when they sought payments from asylum authorities. Richmond asylum

tried to avoid costs by discharging patients completely and then directing
them to the South Dublin Union workhouse. As these patients were not
transferred, the asylum insisted they were not liable for the maintenance
costs.[95]

The key weakness of the legislation was that guardians were not
obliged to accept patients and they frequently refused to do so. For
example, in 1881 O'Meara at Carlow asylum requested Celbridge, Naas
and Carlow unions accept 'hopeless, utterly demented and tranquil
patients to the individual unions'.[96] They refused, insisting there was
no room in the lunatic wards of the workhouses.[97] The asylum officials
contacted the lunacy inspectors questioning the legality of these refusals.[98]
Guardians refused to accept patients on various other grounds.[99] They
argued that some asylum patients were not destitute and therefore not
entitled to relief; this was a particular problem among paying patients.
The amounts families paid towards the upkeep of relatives were usually
derisory, but guardians presented them as evidence that patients were
not destitute. Workhouse officials also refused to accept patients who
had not originated in the union.[100] In some cases, asylum patients,
who had no relatives to support them on release – they had often
emigrated – and could not be transferred to the workhouses, were
allowed to remain in the asylum.[101] On the other hand, some poor law
guardians cooperated; O'Meara managed to persuade the Athy workhouse to accept transfers and, in August 1892, the Carlow guardians
announced that they intended to extend the workhouse accommodation
for the sick and the mentally ill.[102] In the early 1880s, several local boards
of guardians proposed that instead of transferring chronic patients to
workhouses, district asylums should construct extensions to accommodate harmless lunatics including workhouses inmates. The lunacy
inspectors opposed this, arguing that it was an expensive proposal and
would provide inferior care.[103]

The 1875 act was regarded as a failure and two years after its introduction, the lunacy inspectors commented that relatively few asylum patients
had been transferred to workhouses. They held the asylum governors
responsible for the failure.[104] However, the fact that destitution was used
as workhouse admission criteria for patients discharged from the asylum
was a significant obstacle. It limited the effectiveness of the legislation and
guardians used it as a means of refusing patients. When negotiating with
poor law guardians, asylum governors stressed that maintaining harmless

patients in asylums was more expensive to the ratepayers than housing them in workhouses, an argument guardians usually ignored and instead they focused on the union finances.

Auxiliary asylums?

Given the links between the poor law and asylum systems in Ireland, there was considerable demand for the integration of the two administrative systems and services. The commentary on the potential for reform went beyond condemning conditions in workhouse lunatic wards. A radical overhaul of legislation and administration, and the conversion of workhouses into auxiliary asylums for chronic patients, was recommended at various points during the nineteenth century. However, as will be demonstrated, these recommendations were seldom implemented and the interactions between the two welfare systems continued to be piecemeal and dependent on local interactions.

Inspectors and asylum governors had looked forward to the integration of the asylum and the poor law, under the 1838 act, and again, under the 1851 Medical Charities Act.[105] The inspectors delayed schemes alleviating overcrowding in asylums, anticipating that a clause forcing guardians to admit 'incurable' patients into workhouses would be introduced in 1838.[106] Their hopes were shared by asylum governors and at Carlow, in the immediate aftermath of the act's passing, further admissions to the overcrowded asylum were halted as 'impracticable' until the 'District Poorhouses, shall be opened and the idiots and harmless incurables now in this asylum [are] removed thereto'.[107] The anticipated innovation was not introduced although the proposal was resurrected on several occasions.[108] The 1843 House of Lords Select Committee consulted the influential English alienist John Conolly at Hanwell asylum, who suggested that the workhouses should be used.[109] However, George Nicholls, the poor law commissioner, disagreed and reminded the Select Committee that the main criteria for admission into workhouses was destitution not medical need.[110] Nicholls suggested adding chronic wards to existing asylums. The arrival and impact of the Famine further inhibited any potential for legislative change. Guardians who had been inclined to accept chronic patients in the initial years were less likely to do so by the 1840s.

From the 1850s, three parliamentary inquiries examined the relationship between the poor law and the asylum systems, and the available institutional provision for the mentally ill. Each inquiry inspected the numerous institutions that housed patients and agreed that the Irish lunacy legislation was flawed. The parliamentary inquiries were also tasked with the job of considering whether accommodation in Irish workhouses could be appropriated to contain the 'harmless insane'.[111] The 1857–58 Inquiry into the State of Lunatic Asylums focused more explicitly on asylums and identified many of the problems encountered in day-to-day management. The investigation uncovered examples of poor legislation and regulation, and instances of staff ignoring regulations due to a lack of knowledge and information. The inquiry also examined conditions in workhouses where pauper lunatics were accommodated and concluded that they were unsuitable environments. The members proposed that where accommodation was available, workhouses should be renovated and made suitable for 'quiet cases of imbecility and idiocy'.[112] While critical of the cramped lunatic wards, they supported the establishment of purpose built facilities, an important distinction. The ensuing report proposed that in each asylum district, partially vacant workhouses should be converted into auxiliary asylums and then certified as 'fit for purpose'. Asylum governors and physicians would retain control over the selection of patients suitable for admission. However, the members encountered difficulties when devising a management structure for 'auxiliary asylums'. To overcome the difficulties that separate mechanisms of funding posed to the integration of the two systems, it was proposed that the primary managers would be local asylum governors while the poor law guardians would be entitled to visit and inspect the auxiliary asylums. The two managing bodies would agree on financial liability based on patients' settlement.[113]

This proposal, along with the other recommendations of the 1857–58 Inquiry into the State of Lunatic Asylums, was never realised. Lord Naas incorporated some of the recommendations in his failed lunacy bill of 1859.[114] The lunacy inspectors, and in particular White, opposed the establishment of auxiliary workhouse asylums. In his evidence to the Inquiry he insisted that workhouses were not suitable for the insane.[115] By the 1860s, however, the asylums were once again overcrowded, as the 1850s expansion programme had not provided enough accommodation and, as discussed above, Hatchell's appointment as White's replacement on the lunacy inspectorate resulted in a shift in attitude. In their 1862 report, the lunacy inspectors argued that chronic patients did not require specialist accommodation in asylums. Supervision of tranquil patients could be successfully carried out in any institution. They suggested that the Lord Lieutenant nominate two or three workhouses in each county for the 'chronic, epileptic and idiot' patients. The costs would be charged to the union as a whole, rather than to individual electoral divisions.[116] The lunacy inspectors repeated these suggestions in subsequent reports and insisted that asylums should be reserved for curable patients.[117] While they acknowledged that workhouse lunatic wards were inadequate and offered 'indifferent assistance', they insisted that, renovated workhouses with appropriate facilities could be used.[118]

The inspectors' change in attitude was, however, largely superficial and this became evident during the hearings of the Select Committee on Poor Law Union and Lunacy Inquiry which was established to examine workhouse accommodation in 1878. Although lunacy legislation and accommodation were not the main concerns of this inquiry, these were investigated. By the 1870s there was a commonly held belief among administrators that the extremes of Irish poverty, particularly the Famine, had produced an excess of workhouse accommodation. It was argued that these facilities could be appropriated successfully as hospitals and asylums.[119] During the inquiry, the members visited several asylums and workhouse lunatic wards and consulted asylum superintendents and the lunacy inspectors. They concluded that there was not an excess of workhouse accommodation arguing that the existing internal architectural design of the workhouses – based on a system of classification – coupled with the changing character of workhouse inmates was at the root of many problems. A large number of inmates were aged and infirm, and the sick. In workhouses with classification systems, infirmaries, lunatic wards and other departments were overcrowded with the aged, the infirm and the sick, while other parts of the institution had spare accommodation. Nonetheless, there was general disapproval of abandoning classification systems to alleviate localised overcrowding.[120]

During the inquiry, it was noted that, according to the Central Criminal Lunatic Asylum (Ireland) Act, 1845, the Lord Lieutenant was entitled to erect and reclassify existing asylums as 'provincial' asylums for specific patient groups and the legislation explicitly referred to the chronic patients.[121] In spite of Nugent's earlier support of auxiliary asylums, in evidence to the Select Committee on Poor Law Union and Lunacy Inquiry, the inspectors admitted that they had never used the legislation to request the establishment of provincial asylums.[122] The committee's members caustically observed that the lunacy inspectors 'have constantly recommended "plain substantial buildings" for chronic cases; but the Lunacy Department has invariably insisted upon the erection of costly asylums instead'.[123] In his evidence, Hatchell insisted that the medical community would object to separate institutions for chronic patients on the grounds that they were inferior to asylums and that they would lower the professional status of medical officers employed in them.[124] Also, tranquil patients worked in the asylums, often watching over other patients.[125] He insisted that asylum governors and not poor law guardians should manage the new institutions while asylum superintendents should distribute patients between the institutions. Thus, the inspectors' objections were founded on a desire to protect the medical profession's status and an insistence that asylum administrators would be the gatekeepers of these institutions. The asylum administration, and not the Local Government Board, was to be in the ascendency.

The Select Committee on Poor Law Union and Lunacy Inquiry's final recommendations were comprehensive. Having reviewed workhouse architectural design and internal classification systems, the members proposed that three groups of institutions be established. A portion of the existing twenty-two lunatic asylums would be reclassified as curative hospitals catering for patients from every social class. It was hoped this would remove the stigma of pauperism attached to asylums and encourage the admission of paying-patients.[126] The remaining asylums would be appropriated for chronic patients, including epileptics. Workhouses would accommodate quiet and harmless patients. In the Carlow asylum district, it was proposed that sections of Enniscorthy, Gorey and Shillelagh workhouses would be used. The members insisted the workhouses would be renovated to render them suitable.[127] The inmates scattered throughout the small lunatic wards in workhouses would then be transferred to these auxiliary facilities. The members of the inquiry avoided developing detailed arrangements for the management of these institutions leaving it up to 'whatever department maybe ultimately charged with the lunacy administration of this country'.[128] The Local Government Board, responsible for workhouses after 1871, was not particularly enthusiastic, arguing that, while not technically illegal, the recommendations were not 'in accordance with the intention of the legislature'.[129] The Board was concerned that it did not have authority over lunacy administration and asylums in Ireland, but conceded that 'So long as there is no interference with the existing arrangements of workhouses' the Board would allow the appropriation of workhouses as auxiliary asylums.[130] Despite this concession, the inquiry recognised that in the event of auxiliary asylums being established, the Local Government Board 'must necessarily exercise authority over the management of them'. This would require transferring the central administration of lunacy to the Local Government Board.[131]

The report of the 1890–91 Committee appointed by the Lord Lieutenant of Ireland on Lunacy Administration echoed many of the 1878–9 Select Committee on Poor Law Union and Lunacy Inquiry's recommendations, however, there was little will to change the law relating to lunacy administration in Ireland. The 1890–91 Committee focused on the relationship between workhouses and asylums and, again, it was suggested that unoccupied workhouses be converted into auxiliary or provincial asylums. The Committee opposed initiating another wave of asylum building and concluded that the laws concerned with lunacy administration in Ireland required consolidation, as they did not 'sufficiently guarantee the proper treatment of the insane nor do they adequately safeguard the public against unnecessary detention in the asylums'. In particular, members found fault with the failure to clearly define the relationship between asylums and workhouses.[132] A key recommendation was to transfer the administration of asylums to the Local Government Board.[133] Although the recommendations of this committee were not acted upon immediately,[134] its influence can be seen in the 1898 Local Government Act which allowed for 'workhouses or other suitable buildings' to be set apart for the 'incurable insane'.[135]

Relatively few asylum districts implemented this provision of the 1898 Local Government Act. The financial arrangements ensured that the establishment of auxiliary asylums was not attractive to the county councils and there was confusion around how to initiate the process. In 1899, the Carlow governors attempted to locate a building in the district that could be converted into an auxiliary asylum. They did not, however, consider the local workhouses. The initiative received a mixed reaction from poor law guardians and there was tension over the location of the proposed auxiliary asylum. Naas guardians insisted that the auxiliary asylum be located in county Kildare, arguing that establishment of a second asylum in county Carlow had obvious, mainly financial, benefits for that county but it was less beneficial for residents of county Kildare. County Kildare ratepayers would continue to pay the cost of transporting patients to Carlow asylum while families visiting relatives would endure hardships of travel.[136] Consequently, suitable buildings that could accommodate sixty patients were sought in county Kildare and one of the first identified was the old gaol in Naas.[137] The county surveyor's estimated cost of converting the building into an asylum was £4,000, although the lunacy inspector quoted a much higher figure of £12,000. The gaol was sited in Athy rural district and the council was opposed to the development 'on account of expense and unsuitability'.[138] The next proposal was to convert the old Lock hospital in Kildare town.[139] This was also rejected and Naas gaol was considered a second time. However, the momentum behind the establishment of an auxiliary asylum in county Kildare dissipated, partly because of difficulties with interpreting the legislation: for example, it was unclear whether a resident medical superintendent would be appointed. The Carlow asylum governors insisted that one should be appointed but the Naas guardians saw this as an attempt to establish a 'lunatic asylum proper'.[140] The Naas guardians also felt that they were entitled to greater representation on Carlow asylum management committee, arguing that the establishment of an auxiliary asylum had financial repercussions for the union. They resented the fact that Carlow asylum management committee could make decisions on the management of the proposed auxiliary asylum without the guardian's approval.[141] The ongoing squabbles ensured that the matter dragged on, and in the absence of an alternative, Carlow asylum was expanded.[142]

Conclusion

Peter Bartlett has argued that in England the poor law unions were the primary administrative bodies responsible for the confinement of pauper lunatics. Although Melling and Forsythe have suggested that the relationship between the two systems was weaker in Devon, links between the English county asylums and the poor law can be located in patient groups and in the statutory framework, particularly the 1808 and 1863 Acts.[143] In

Ireland, it is accurate to state that the asylums 'remained formally outside the control of the Poor Law Commissioners.'[144] Nonetheless, a relationship evolved and workhouses were incorporated into welfare provision for pauper lunatics. Asylum, workhouse and poor law dispensary employees and management were often the same people and a significant proportion of patients emerged from workhouses.[145] However, there were significant obstacles to the use of workhouses. It was generally agreed that they required significant renovations before they could be accepted as part of the provision for lunacy accommodation and most poor law guardians completed only cosmetic changes.[146] The failure to standardise the entitlement criteria for workhouse, dispensary and asylum relief created barriers to the full integration of the services as did the decision not to compel poor law guardians to accept patients transferred from asylums. Guardians were generally anxious to reduce the expense of maintaining lunatics to the poor law unions as most were driven by local concerns, one of which was keeping the cost to the taxpayer at a minimum.[147] The attitude of the lunacy inspectors and asylum doctors towards accommodating the mentally ill in workhouses was apparently contradictory. At various stages, they insisted that all forms of mental illness should be treated in asylums while simultaneously they resented the transfer of workhouse inmates to their institutions as these inmates contributed to the silting-up of chronic patients in overcrowded asylums. The workhouses were simultaneously perceived to exacerbate, or offer solutions to, overcrowding in the asylums.

Notes

1   SPH, ELA Letter Book, Robert Henderson to Gorey Union, 27 July 1868; Robert Henderson to Thomas Tristram, Clerk, Gory Union, 6 August 1868.
2   NAI, CRF CSO, Carlow 1858.
3   Bartlett, *The Poor Law of Lunacy*, p. 2.
4   *Poor Law Union and Lunacy Inquiry*, p. lxxvii.
5   *Fourth Report of Prison Inspectors*, H. C. 1826 [173] xxiii, p. 8.
6   Murphy, 'The Lunacy Commissioners and the East London Guardian, 1845–67', 499.
7   *Nineteenth Report of Prison Inspectors*, H. C. 1841 [299] xi, p. 8.
8   Finnane, *Insanity and the Insane*, p. 29.
9   These were the Royal Commissioners of Inquiry into the State of Lunatic Asylums and other Institutions for the Custody and Treatment of the Insane in Ireland, 1857–58; the Select Committee on Poor Law Union and Lunacy Inquiry (Ireland), 1878–79; the

Committee appointed by the Lord Lieutenant of Ireland on Lunacy Administration (Ireland), 1890–91.

10 1&2 Vict. c. 56 (1838).

11 Finnane, *Insanity and the Insane*, appendix, table A.

12 1&2 Vict. c. 56, s.41 (1838).

13 10 Vic. c.31 (1847).

14 Crossman, *Politics, Pauperism and Power*, pp. 11–13.

15 *Thom's Directory, 1850–1870.*

16 See chapter one.

17 1&2 Vict. c.56, s.47 (1838).

18 *Leinster Leader* (27 November 1909).

19 *Leinster Leader* (17 June 1905).

20 *Leinster Leader* (20 December 1902); (27 November 1909).

21 *Leinster Leader* (17 June 1905).

22 *Thirteenth Report of Lunacy Inspectors*, H. C. 1864 [3369] xxiii, appendix A, p. 83 and *Forty-Seventh Report of Lunacy Inspectors*, H. C. 1898 [8969] xliii, appendix D, p. 92.

23 *Thirteenth Report of Lunacy Inspectors*, H. C. 1864 [3369] xxiii, p. 83 and *Forty-Seventh Report of Lunacy Inspectors*, H. C. 1898 [8969] xliii, p. 92; DPH, CLA Registers of Admissions, 1846–1922.

24 Cited in *Poor Law Union and Lunacy Inquiry*, p. lxxi.

25 *First Annual Report of the Commissioners of Irish Poor Laws*, H. C. 1847–48 [943], xxxiii, pp. 93–94.

26 *Thirteenth Annual Report of the Commissioners for Administrating Poor Relief in Ireland*, H. C. 1860 [2654] xxxvii, Poor Law Commissioner Circular, 3 November 1859, pp. 25–26.

27 *Tenth Report of Lunacy Inspectors*, H. C. 1861 [2901] xxvii, p. 7.

28 *Poor Law Union and Lunacy Inquiry*, p. xcviii–cxiv; Melling and Forsythe, *The Politics of Madness*, p. 14.

29 Carlow County Archives (hereafter CCA), BC50/A/73, Carlow Board of Guardians, Minute Book, 25 September 1884.

30 *British Journal of Medical Science*, 1 (April 1896), 981–982; *Leinster Leader*, (25 April 1896).

31 *Fifty-first Report of Lunacy Inspectors*, H. C. 1902 [1265] xl, p. xlvi.

32 *Fifth Report of Lunacy Inspectors*, H. C. 1851 [1387] xxiv, p. 7.

33 *Fourth Report of Prison Inspectors*, H. C. 1826 [173] xxiii, p. 8.

34 *Fifth Report of Prison Inspectors*, H. C. 1826–27 [471] xi, p. 6; *Eighth Report of Prison Inspectors*, H. C. 1830 [48] xxiv, p. 13.

35 *Ninth Report of Prison Inspectors*, H. C. 1830–31 [172] iv, p. 9.

36 *Sixth Report of Prison Inspectors*, H. C. 1828 [68] xii, p. 11; *Seventh Report of Prison Inspectors*, H. C. 1829 [10] xiii, pp. 12–14.

37 *Inquiry into the State of Lunatic Asylums and other Institutions*, p. 18.

38 *Report of Lunacy Inspectors*, H. C. 1845 [645] xxvi, p. 58.

39 *Twenty-first Report of Lunacy Inspectors*, H. C. 1843 [462] xxvii, p. 88.

40 *Poor Law Union and Lunacy Inquiry*, p. lxiii.

41 *Twenty-sixth Report of Lunacy Inspectors*, H. C. 1877 [1750] xli, p. 12.
42 *Ibid.* p. 23; *Fifth Report of Lunacy Inspectors*, H. C. 1851 [1387] xxiv, p. 6.
43 *Sixty-second Report of Lunacy Inspectors*, H. C. 1913 [Cd.6935] xxxiv, pp. 156–157.
44 Bartlett, *The Poor Law of Lunacy*, p. 181; Melling and Forsythe, *The Politics of Madness*, p. 26.
45 Murphy, 'The Lunacy Commissioners and East London Guardians', 509.
46 *Eleventh Report of Lunacy Inspectors*, H. C. 1862 [2975] xxiii, p. 24.
47 *Poor Law Union and Lunacy Inquiry*, p. xcv.
48 *Eleventh Report of Lunacy Inspectors*, H. C. 1862 [2975] xxiii, p. 22.
49 *Twenty-third Report of Lunacy Inspectors*, H. C. 1874 [C. 1004] xxvii, p. 102.
50 *Ibid.*, p. 28.
51 *Twenty-second Report of Lunacy Inspectors*, H. C. 1873 [852] xxx, p. 7.
52 *Thirteenth Report of Lunacy Inspectors*, H. C. 1864 [3369] xxiii, p. 9.
53 For example, see CCA, BG/50/A/54, Carlow Board of Guardians, Minute Book, 2 August 1845, BG50/A/1; 23 January 1875.
54 *British Journal of Medical Science*, 1 (April, 1896), 981–982.
55 Melling and Forsythe, *The Politics of Madness*, p. 111.
56 6&7 Vict. c.92. s.15 (1843).
57 For example, see *Leinster Leader* (17 June 1905); (22 July 1905).
58 Ellis,'The Asylum, the Poor Law', 56.
59 Scull, 'Madness and Segregative Control: The Rise of the Insane Asylum', 3.
60 NAI, CSO CRF, Kildare 1858.
61 *Fourteenth Report of Lunacy Inspectors*, H. C. 1865 [3556] xxi, p. 123.
62 NAI, CSO CRF, Kilkenny 1847.
63 NAI, CSO CRF, Kilkenny 1851.
64 *Leinster Leader* (20 May 1905); (3 June 1905); (22 July 1905); (12 August 1905); (26 August 1905).
65 DPH, CLA Registers of Admissions, 1900–16.
66 *Leinster Leader* (24 June 1905).
67 *Irish Times* (16 May 1862); *Leinster Leader* (18 October 1902).
68 *Leinster Leader* (24 November 1900); (24 March 1900); (31 March 1900); (27 May 1905); (24 June 1905).
69 Bartlett, *The Poor Law of Lunacy*.
70 Melling and Forsythe, *The Politics of Madness*, p. 32.
71 For examples of the type of headlines, see: 'The Lunacy Danger', *Leinster Leader* (1 July 1905); 'Lunatics in Workhouses. A Doctor's Complaint', *Freeman's Journal* (31 March 1919); 'Fatality at Mountmellick Workhouse', *Leinster Leader* (1 July 1905); WCA, WX/BG 87/1/1/41 Enniscorthy Board of Guardians, Minute Book, 4 April 1868, 11 April 1868, WX/BG 87/1/1/41, Enniscorthy Board of Guardians Minute Book, 23 May 1868.
72 WCA, WX/BG 87/1/1/42, Enniscorthy Board of Guardians, Minute Book, 1 July 1868.
73 D. Durnin, 'Intertwining Institutions: the Relationship between the South Dublin Union Workhouse and the Richmond Lunatic Asylum, 1880–1911', (MA dissertation, University College Dublin, 2010), pp. 32–43.
74 Melling and Forsythe, *The Politics of Madness*, p. 110.

75 *Leinster Leader* (18 October 1908).

76 *Thom's Directory, 1844–1880.*

77 *Thom's Directory, 1850–1880.*

78 *Wexford Lunatic Asylum. Returns of the Names of the Governors of the Wexford Lunatic Asylum*, H. C. 1867–68 [442] lv.

79 WCA, WX/BG 87/1/3/1, Enniscorthy Dispensary Minute Book, 6 August 1878; SHE, ELA Proceedings of the Governors and Directors of the Wexford District Lunatic Asylum, 21 March 1872.

80 *Leinster Leader* (18 October, 1902).

81 SPH, ELA Letter Book, Thomas Shiell to Wexford Union, 10 June 1868.

82 *Fourteenth Report of Lunacy Inspectors*, H. C. 1865 [3556] xxi, p. 123; *Leinster Leader* (8 July 1905).

83 Kildare Local Authority Archives (hereafter KLA), Athy Poor Law Union Indoor Relief Register, 13 October 1888 to 22 February 1890.

84 KLA, Athy Board of Guardians, Minute Book, 7 May 1888; Crossman, *Politics, Pauperism and Power*, pp. 87–92.

85 *Thom's Directory, 1884–1890.*

86 *Leinster Leader* (29 July 1905).

87 CCA, BG50/A/74 Carlow Board of Guardians, Minute Books, 27 November 1884; 8 January 1885; 5 February 1885.

88 SPH, ELA Letter Book, Thomas Shiell, 23 June 1870; Thomas Drapes to Shillelagh Workhouse, 6 October 1883.

89 Drapes, 'On the Alleged Increase of Insanity in Ireland', 525–526.

90 *Leinster Leader* (27 November 1909).

91 DPH, CLA Minute Book, 16 February 1842.

92 SPH, ELA Letter Book, Thomas Shiell to Gorey Union, 21 November 1870; Thomas Drapes to Enniscorthy Union, 27 November 1883.

93 38&39 Vict. c.67, s. 9 (1875); *Leinster Leader* (20 December 1902).

94 38&39 Vict. c.67 s.11 (1875).

95 Durnin, 'Intertwining Institutions', p. 30.

96 DPH, CLA Minute Book, 8 April 1881.

97 *Ibid.*

98 *Leinster Leader* (29 July 1905).

99 *Thirty-fourth Report of Lunacy Inspectors*, H. C. 1884–5 [4539] xxxvi, p. 14.

100 SPH, ELA Letter Book, Thomas Drapes to Lunacy Inspectors, 3 November 1883.

101 SPH, ELA Letter Book, Thomas Drapes to Lunacy Inspectors, 24 December 1884; 14 May 1885.

102 *Carlow Sentinel* (August 1892).

103 *Thirty-second Report of Lunacy Inspectors*, H. C. 1883 [3675] xxx, p. 13.

104 *Twenty-sixth Report of Lunacy Inspectors*, H. C. 1877 [1750] xli, p. 12.

105 Geary, *Medicine and Charity*, pp. 158–180.

106 *Ibid.*; *Eighteenth Report of Prison Inspectors*, H. C. 1840 [240] xxvi, p. 9; *Twenty-First Report of Prison Inspectors*, H. C. 1843 [462] xxvii, p. 7.

107 DPH, CLA Minute Book, 18 August 1841.

108 *Ibid.*; *Twenty-first Report of Prison Inspectors*, H. C. 1843 [462] xxvii, p. 7.

109   *Report from the Select Committee of the House of Lords appointed to Consider the State of the Lunatic Poor in Ireland*, H. C. 1843 [625] x, p. v.

110   *Ibid.*, p. 95.

111   *Inquiry into the State of Lunatic Asylums and other Institutions*, p. 19; *Poor Law Union and Lunacy Inquiry; Report and Minutes of Evidence of the Select Committee on Lunacy Law*, H. C. 1878 [113] xvi.

112   *Inquiry into the State of Lunatic Asylums and other Institutions*, p. 23.

113   *Ibid.*, p. 20.

114   Finnane, *Insanity and the Insane*, pp. 38–39.

115   *Inquiry into the State of Lunatic Asylums and other Institutions*, p. 24.

116   *Thirteenth Report of Lunacy Inspectors*, H. C. 1864 [3369] xxiii, p. 9.

117   *Twenty-eighth Report of Lunacy Inspectors*, H. C. 1878-9 [2346] xxxii, p. 13.

118   *Twentieth Report of Lunacy Inspectors*, H. C. 1871 [440] xxvi, p. 6; *Twenty-seventh Report of Lunacy Inspectors*, H. C. 1878 [2037] xxxix, p. 16.

119   *Poor Law Union and Lunacy Inquiry*, p. xv–xvi.

120   *Ibid.*, p. xx.

121   *Ibid.*, p. lxxviiii; 8&9 Vict. c.107, s.15 (1845).

122   *Poor Law Union and Lunacy Inquiry*, p. lxxix.

123   *Ibid.*, p. xc, p. lxiv.

124   *Ibid.*, p. ixxxiv.

125   *Ibid.*, p. 59.

126   *Ibid.*

127   *Ibid.*, p. lxxiv.

128   *Ibid.*, p. lxxxii.

129   *Ibid.*, p. lxxxv.

130   *Ibid.*, p. lxxvii.

131   *Ibid.*, p. ciii.

132   *Committee appointed on Lunacy Administration*, p. 2.

133   *Ibid.*, p. 3.

134   J. Robins, *Fools and Mad: A History of the Insane in Ireland* (Dublin: Institute of Public Administration, 1986), p. 147.

135   61&62 Vict. c.37, s.76 (1898).

136   *Leinster Leader* (24 March 1900).

137   DPH, CLA Minute Book, 13 September 1899.

138   DPH, CLA Minute Book, 11 October 1899; *Leinster Leader* (1 September 1900).

139   DPH, CLA Minute Book, 13 December 1899.

140   *Leinster Leader* (24 March); (31 March 1900).

141   *Leinster Leader* (24 March 1909).

142   *Leinster Leader* (25 August 1900); (3 April 1899).

143   Bartlett, 'The Asylum and the Poor Law'; Bartlett, 'The Asylum, the Workhouse and the Voice of the Insane Poor', 421–432; Wright, 'Getting Out of the Asylum', 137–155; Murphy, 'The Lunacy Commissioners and the East London Guardians, 1845–1897', 495–524; Ellis, 'The Asylum, the Poor Law', 55–73. Bartlett, *The Poor Law of Lunacy*, p. 50.

144   Walsh, 'Lunatic and Criminal Alliances', p. 134.

145   Bartlett, *The Poor Law of Lunacy*.

146   *Twenty-sixth Report of Lunacy Inspectors*, H. C. 1877 [1750] xli, p. 12.

147   K. T. Hoppen, *Elections, Politics and Society in Ireland 1832–1885* (Oxford: Clarendon
      Press, 1984); K. T. Hoppen, 'National Politics and Local Realities in mid-Nineteenth-
      Century Ireland', in A. Cosgrove and D. McCartney (eds), *Studies in Irish History
      presented to R. Dudley Edwards* (Dublin: University College Press, 1979), pp. 190–227.

7

Inside the asylums

On 30 January 1857, a single woman entered Carlow asylum and was diagnosed as suffering from 'mania'. She had become ill the previous November and the medical superintendent recorded that there was a history of insanity in her father's family. Religion, and specifically the 'late mission in the town', was recorded as the exciting cause of illness. She was discharged in May 1858. Her recovery was accredited to the 'general moral treatment of the establishment with attention to general health'.[1] She had been prescribed sedatives and a robust diet, supplemented with iron. While confined, she experienced the prosaic realities of asylum life, inhabiting overcrowded and insanitary dormitories, she was fed a dull monotonous diet and was required to do domestic work. This chapter provides some understanding of life in Enniscorthy and Carlow asylums for staff and patients by exploring the management and treatment regimes, although not claiming to provide what Roy Porter defined as the 'patient's view'.[2]

Whereas Carlow and Enniscorthy asylum minute books contained few references to patient care, asylum casebooks are particularly rich sources when exploring regimes of care and interactions between staff and patients. Jonathan Andrews and Gayle Davis have argued that casebooks and medical registers, as mediated sources, primarily represent the priorities and occupations of medical staff.[3] However, Wright has argued that the information in casebooks was a fusion of 'community-based lay and medical knowledge'.[4] Patients' medical and social histories were provided by families and medical staff and recorded in certification forms. As previously noted, this information was transferred subsequently into casebooks.

To this, medical asylum officers added their knowledge of patients' social and familial circumstances. Relatives, and sometimes patients themselves, provided additional information on arrival at the asylum or during an early visit. These statements often appeared in quotation marks in casebooks and while they lack contextual information, they are useful. As Hilary Marland has observed, patients, friends and relatives were allowed to speak through casebooks and ignoring these sources contributes towards silencing the patient.[5]

The Enniscorthy asylum casebooks interrogated here cover the period 1891 to 1904, whereas only one Carlow asylum casebook, covering 1906 to 1908, was accessible.[6] Detailed regulations governing asylum record keeping, and the format of casebooks, emerged slowly in Ireland, and when they were introduced asylum authorities were often unaware of, or ignored, the regulations. Replicating private lunatic asylum regulations introduced in 1842,[7] under the 1843 privy council rules asylum physicians were required to maintain casebooks and admission registers, in addition to certification warrants.[8] The lunacy inspectors published sample documents in their annual reports, outlining the expected format and questions. Further regulations were published in 1845.[9] In spite of this, there were variations in the type and format of medical records maintained at asylums, and by the late 1850s, it was clear that asylum authorities were ignoring regulations.[10] The 1862 and 1874 revisions to the privy council rules reiterated the stipulation that keeping patient records was mandatory. The 1874 revision specifically stressed the importance of patient casebooks. In 1900, the most detailed guidelines on record keeping at asylums were issued and the format of casebooks was also amended.[11] In 1903, William Dawson, medical superintendent at Farnhouse House, a private asylum in Finglas, Dublin, and Daniel F. Rambaut, of the Richmond asylum in Dublin, reviewed the casebooks in use in asylums and suggested further changes.

According to Dawson, by 1903, two types of casebook were used in Irish asylums and these were in use at Carlow and Enniscorthy asylums. The casebooks at Enniscorthy asylum contained twenty-one questions covering patients' social, biographical and medical histories. These sections were broken down into further sub-questions and included questions on family background, intended to aid medical officers in tracking 'heredity insanity'.[12] There were also questions on individual behaviour including alcohol consumption and on causes of illness. Medical officers were required to assess whether patients were dangerous and to record delusional behaviour. These questions occupied the first page of the clinical entry and the remainder, mainly free text, recorded the patient-doctor interviews. According to Dawson, asylum staff disliked these casebooks as they encouraged a 'mechanical and perfunctory manner of case-noting' that recorded 'unimportant facts' at the expense of more salient details. The format of the Carlow casebook differed, containing nine brief, mainly biographical, questions and the remainder of each record consisted of free text. Dawson dismissed these casebooks as worthless.[13]

While Carlow casebooks followed a different format from Enniscorthy casebooks, the clinical entries were similar in several respects. As Dawson argued, the value of these casebooks depended 'entirely on the experience of the writer.' From 1900, medical officers at both asylums followed the new 1900 lunacy inspectors' guidelines which had introduced headings recording the patient's clinical condition, including temperature and pulse. While the casebook format did not change, the content of the entries were in keeping with the new guidelines. Asylums were slow to purchase new casebooks. Thus, the assistant medical officer at Carlow asylum, Dr Edward McKenna, provided very detailed clinical histories similar to the entries in Enniscorthy casebooks and after 1900 described the patient's 'expression', iris colour, shape of head, temperature, pulse and heart sounds, and history of mental illness.[14] These details were also recorded in Enniscorthy casebooks after 1900. Therefore, while there were variations in casebooks' formats, by the end of the nineteenth century, the content converged in several respects.

Asylum staff

The influence asylum staff had upon patients' experiences in asylums clearly emerges from these sources. Asylum managers, medical and lay, fashioned institutional regimes of care. Lay managers were appointed to most of the Irish asylums constructed under the 1817 and 1821 Lunacy Acts. Managers held the most senior position and were responsible for day-to-day administration although they were accountable to the governors. They were pivotal to the implementation of successful curative regimes and were expected to have practical experience in treating mental illness.[15] In the

1830s, their duties were diverse and onerous. Managers were responsible for all administrative and medical matters and this included maintaining asylum records, which the lunacy inspectors were entitled to examine at any time.[16] They also had control over 'instruments of coercion' and were expected to be attentive to convalescent patients, providing sufficient stimulation through entertainment and work.[17] Visiting physicians and apothecaries assisted and in the early decades visiting physicians cared for the patients' physical well-being, not their mental state.[18]

The first lay manager at Carlow asylum was Francis Crofton, who died less than two years after the opening of the asylum.[19] Patrick McCaffry was appointed the following September.[20] He was selected over a local accoucheur and apothecary, Paul Cullen, who was supported by the county's Roman Catholic clergy and senior academics at Carlow College.[21] Supporters of lay management approved of McCaffry's appointment,[22] however, he proved to be a troublesome appointment.[23] On 22 September 1842 a special board meeting was held to investigate a charge brought by Thomas Keefe, the asylum gatekeeper, against McCaffry for raping his daughter Mary Keefe.[24] Mary subsequently gave birth in the asylum.[25] The Carlow governors and Francis White investigated the allegation and, subsequently, a public enquiry was held, which investigated the charges against McCaffry and the general management of the asylum.[26] The scandal quickly became politicised and allegations were made that it was part of an 'orange conspiracy' to remove McCaffry, a Roman Catholic, from his post.[27] Carlow town in this period was noted for heightened sectarian tensions.[28] The investigations concluded in November 1842 and McCaffry was dismissed, but there was no criminal prosecution.

Samuel Hitch, superintendent at Gloucester asylum and secretary to the Association of Medical Officers of Great Britain and Ireland, seized upon McCaffry's disgrace in his campaign to secure the position of asylum manger as a medical appointment.[29] As both Scull and Cooter have shown, asylum lay management was perceived to be a threat to the emerging field of medically trained alienists who were keen to establish medicine as pivotal in treatment.[30] They were hostile to the curative claims made for moral treatment. From the 1830s, the inspectors of asylums in Ireland made unfavourable comparisons between asylums run by lay and medical managers.[31] In his evidence to the 1843 House of Lords Select Committee, White stressed the need to expand medical involvement in asylums arguing that the absence of medical management contributed to low recovery rates.[32] As the main architect of the 1843 privy council rules, White's intervention was critical. When introduced, the rules demoted lay managers and entrusted patients' moral and medical treatment to visiting physicians.[33] After 1843 lay managers were required to 'superintend and regulate the whole of the establishment', maintain registers and other documentation, and oversee the domestic staff including the matron.[34] He was still required to report on patients to governors and the visiting physician but he had to defer to the physician with regard to patient treatment and care.

After 1843, medical men were usually appointed as asylum managers.[35] Although McCaffry's immediate replacement was another lay manager, William Parsons,[36] he was replaced by Dr Matthew Esmonde White in March 1848.[37] White had previously worked at Dublin's Rotunda Hospital. The lunacy inspectors and the general medical community welcomed his appointment.[38] By the late 1850s, medically trained men were firmly established as managers in most Irish asylums while the 1862 revision to the privy council rules formally instituted the post of resident medical superintendent.[39] Incumbents were required to be qualified physicians or surgeons.[40] They were responsible for medical and moral treatment of patients, and the domestic management of asylums.[41] The first Resident Medical Superintendent appointed at Carlow asylum in 1866, was Dr Michael Patrick Howlett, who replaced White. The position was relatively attractive as it offered financial stability. Salaries were graduated and in 1870, the lunacy inspectors delineated the rates according to asylum capacity. As table 7.1 shows, the medical superintendents at Carlow and Enniscorthy asylums were at the lower to middle end of the scale.

Table 7.1   Resident Medical Superintendent salary scales, 1870

Patient population size	RMS salary per annum
>250	£350
250–350	£400
350–500	£450
500–600	£500
600–800	£550

Source: *Twentieth Report on the District, Criminal and Private Lunatic Asylums in Ireland* appendix, H.C. 1871 [C. 440] xxvi, p. 164.

While the position of medical superintendents was strengthened, visiting physicians were criticised for encouraging irregular medical attendance.[42] There was considerable debate among the medical community on the usefulness of the post and a proposal to abolish it was considered in the 1850s.[43] This was rejected, though it was subsequently resurrected. Under the 1862 revision to asylum regulations, the post remained and the incumbent was directed to act under the direction of the medical superintendent. In the 1890s positions of visiting physician and apothecary were abolished when the post of assistant medical officer was created.[44]

Medical superintendents' knowledge and previous experience of managing asylums and treating the insane varied considerably. Only 'informal classes' on mental illness were taught in Dublin and Edinburgh from the 1860s and most medical superintendents gained experience while working in asylums.[45] The first medical superintendent at Enniscorthy Asylum, Dr Thomas W. Shiell, had been employed at the neighbouring Maryborough asylum before his appointment in 1868.[46] His successor, Dr Joseph Edmundson, appointed in 1874, had been medical superintendent at Castlebar asylum in county Mayo. Frequently, medical superintendents had held employments as asylum visiting physicians.[47] White and O'Meara at Carlow asylum and Drapes and Hugh Kennedy at Enniscorthy asylum were promoted from the post of visiting physician to medical superintendent within their own asylums. Few medical superintendents came directly from the ranks of workhouse medical staff, although there were exceptions.[48] Several medical superintendents employed in Carlow and Enniscorthy asylums spent time in Britain at some point in their careers. This type of medical migration between Britain and Ireland was commonplace in the post-Famine period.[49] For example, O'Meara, who was educated in Dublin, served as assistant house surgeon at the borough hospital in Birkenhead in England prior to his appointment at Carlow asylum in 1880. He remained until his death in 1903.

Visiting physicians frequently emerged from local poor law medical services, including the dispensaries, and often held poor law and asylum posts simultaneously. Visiting physicians and later, medical officers, were not guaranteed promotion to medical superintendent. Drs Thomas Cranfield, Nicholas Furlong and Charles McDowell were never appointed as medical superintendents at Enniscorthy or Carlow asylums, or elsewhere, while Dr Edward McKenna, who was assistant medical officer at Carlow asylum from 1903, did not replace Dr James J. Fitzgerald as medical superintendent on his departure in 1907.[50] Instead the post was left vacant until the arrival in 1908 of Dr Thomas Adrian Greene, who had been an assistant medical surgeon at Ennis Hospital.[51]

The career histories of senior medical staff at Carlow and Enniscorthy asylums generally conform to the profiles Finnane identified. A significant portion worked their way through the asylum system before being appointed as medical superintendents. Visiting physicians often had relatively little asylum experience when appointed and the time spent in the post was crucial for training purposes. They were expected to gain a thorough knowledge of asylum rules and regulations and an understanding of mental conditions while working. An incomplete training while working as visiting physicians ensured that when promoted to the post of medical superintendent, they were at a disadvantage. Although the Medico-Psychological Association insisted in the 1880s that medical superintendents should have previous service in an asylum, this provided limited assurance that appointees had sufficient experience.[52]

The medical superintendents and visiting physicians employed at Carlow and Enniscorthy asylums were typical of medical staff employed in smaller Irish asylums. The majority did not publish on psychiatry, although Drapes at Enniscorthy asylum was an important exception. He published several papers in the *Journal of Mental Science* and the *Dublin Journal of Medical Science*, while Fitzgerald at Carlow asylum identified the first case of beriberi in Ireland during his time at the Mater Miscericordiae Hospital. The asylum medical staff were influential and respected among their local communities. Scull has suggested that the working conditions of asylum superintendents and lay managers isolated them from their localities, but this was not true in either Carlow or Enniscorthy.[53] White and O'Meara were both magistrates and were members of local medical families, who had practices in neighbouring towns for several generations. Over the course of the century, the senior medical staff increasingly reflected the religious profile of the locality. In 1871, Catholics were under-represented in the medical profession; only 34 per cent of doctors were Catholic while 'just over three-quarters of the Irish population were Catholics'.[54] The sectarianism that emerged during the McCaffry controversy in the 1840s highlighted the distrust of Catholics among elites in small Irish towns. Later in the century, however, Catholic doctors were appointed to posts at Carlow asylum including Fitzgerald and Greene. The O'Mearas – Thomas, Thomas Patrick and William – were members of a local Catholic medical family and were typical of the Catholic professional middle-classes that emerged in this period. Drapes was a prominent member of the Enniscorthy Church of Ireland community. He represented Enniscorthy in the Diocesan Synod, and was a member of the Diocesan Council, the Board of Education and the General Synod.[55]

Inside the asylums, the staff members in most regular contact with patients were the keepers – later known as attendants and nurses – and the matron. The matron was the most senior member of the female staff. She oversaw the work of female servants and nurses and was responsible for domestic matters. By March 1851, the matron at Carlow was paid one hundred pounds a year.[56] Matrons had enjoyed some autonomy under lay management regimes but by the middle of the century, this had been eroded and they reported to the medical managers about female patients and domestic activities.[57] Asylum attendants interacted with patients on a daily basis and patients' experiences of asylum life were mediated through them. The attendants' and keepers' duties were quite onerous. Keepers were usually in charge of male patients. They were responsible for several patients and were required to keep them under constant observation. Nurses were in charge of female patients. The nurses and keepers cleaned, dressed and transferred patients to and from dayrooms and work areas several times each day. They were not permitted to restrain patients, but reported to the manager those they believed required restraint. Nurses had additional domestic duties including cleaning patients' dormitories and dayrooms. Convalescent and quiet patients, and assistant nurses, helped them in these duties. Given the onerous burden of work, there were tensions between attendants' and keepers' ability to run an efficient and disciplined institution, while simultaneously providing a humane system of care.

The ratio of staff to patients in asylums affected standards of care. In the 1840s, John Conolly believed there should be one staff member to oversee approximately fifteen to seventeen patients.[58] In 1832, the ratio at Carlow asylum was better – five keepers, five nurses and six assistant nurses were employed to care for 104 patients.[59] When the asylum expanded, the ratio remained quite good. By 1901, there were twenty male attendants and auxiliary male staff, including gardeners and a gate porter. There were twenty-four female nurses and auxiliary female staff, including kitchen maids and cooks. They cared for approximately 356 patients. This was a ratio of one staff member to every eight or nine patients, however these figures include staff members such as gardeners and maids who were not explicitly devoted to patient care. When auxiliary and night staff members are excluded, the ratio during the day deteriorates, nonetheless, they remain within Conolly's guidelines and were better than the ratios in larger asylums in Ireland and England.[60] There were specific periods of severe overcrowding when extra attendants were required. In 1846, the lunacy inspectors recommended that the Carlow governors employ an 'additional female servant to no7 & 8 wards' and governors repeatedly sought more staff.[61]

As Leonard D. Smith has noted, recruitment of asylum staff reflected 'the employment situation and the prevailing economic circumstances in the area.'[62] Due to the hard working conditions, asylum governors experienced difficulties in attracting staff.[63] There were, nonetheless, obvious benefits to the jobs. Staff members were provided with accommodation, fuel rations and, from 1856, a basic form of pension for long-serving employees.[64] Yet, in post-Famine Ireland, asylums struggled to keep staff, particularly female employees, due to the pull of emigration. The Carlow laundress Lucinda O'M., who had succeeded her mother to the post, emigrated when her working conditions did not improve. She had requested assistance in 1846 and two nurses were appointed but they promptly resigned.[65] They were not replaced and in September 1850, Lucinda emigrated to America.[66] These difficulties were not confined to the Famine period. In December 1899, Carlow asylum lost a nurse who had secured a position in the English prison service.[67] The asylum also faced problems when male attendants, who were members of the Army Reserve, were called up to active service.[68] Asylums regularly recruited male attendants with a military background, as they were believed to be familiar with disciplined working environments.[69]

Attendants used the threat of emigration as a bargaining tool when negotiating salary increases.[70] During the 1860s and 1870s attendants repeatedly complained that the conditions of employment and rates of remuneration were harsher than in England.[71] In a letter to the *Freeman's Journal*, one employee claimed that 'divisional attendants' in Prestwich asylum received sixty pounds per year while his counterpart in Ireland received twenty pounds.[72] The demands for increased wages led to the threat of strike at Richmond asylum in 1871.[73] It is, however, unclear whether the difference between salaries and conditions in England and Ireland were as extreme as portrayed. Generally in Ireland, there was a persistent rise in wages after the Famine, although wages outside the cities consistently lagged behind Britain until the twentieth century.[74] By 1869, the Carlow laundress was paid an annual wage of nine pounds with an allowance of sixteen pounds. A nurse was paid eight pounds and eight shillings with an allowance of fifteen pounds and ten shillings.[75] At the Richmond asylum a male attendant was paid eighteen pounds a year while a female was paid eleven pounds.[76] In addition, they were provided with accommodation, rations, clothing and fuel. While these wages were significantly lower than in English asylums,[77] they were higher than the income of unskilled and agricultural male labourers who, Vaughan estimated, earned fifteen pounds a year in 1867. Female staff members in asylums were in the same income category as lower skilled workers.[78] Cherry found that in the Norfolk asylum, the 'male attendant earned the same or less than a Norfolk farm labourer before 1870' while Melling found that attendants in Devon earned no more than agricultural labourers. Both male and female attendants in Ireland earned more than unskilled labourers, although less than skilled workers income, which Vaughan estimated to be forty-four pounds per annum in 1867.[79] Agitators for increases in Irish asylum wages sought the equivalent of skilled workers' wages.[80]

The timing of the demands for wage increases that emerged from the 1870s coincided with medical superintendents' efforts to raise the status of attendants more generally. In a letter to the *Freeman's Journal*, Dr Isaac Ashe, medical superintendent at the Dundrum Central Criminal Asylum, took umbrage when the editor described the 'under officials' in asylums as keepers, reminding him that the correct titles were attendants and nurses.[81] From the late 1870s, medical superintendents endeavoured to improve the calibre of asylum staff and through the Medico-Psychological Association, they attempted to provide more systematic training for them, introducing a handbook which attendants and nurses were encouraged to study.[82] The impetus behind this came from medical superintendents while asylum attendants remained focused on securing improved wages and conditions.[83] The two developments were related and by 1885 the Medico-Psychological Association had introduced an examination for asylum staff, and attendants who passed were entitled to a salary increase.[84]

The positions of asylum attendant and nurse were not particularly attractive. Life inside the asylum was very disciplined for both staff and patients. In addition to the onerous duties, the working day was extremely long. Although, the 1843 privy council rules did not specify the start and finishing time of employees' working day, patients' breakfast took place at eight o'clock in the morning. Sleeping-rooms were to be cleaned and ventilated before ten o'clock in the summer and eleven o'clock in the winter. Nurses and attendants rose between six o'clock and seven o'clock in the morning to carry out these tasks. In 1878, the attendants at Richmond Asylum claimed they worked sixteen hours a day.[85] By the twentieth century, attendants' working week could range from seventy to 100 hours.[86] Employees were obliged to live in the asylum, and governors and medical superintendents kept them under close observation and had significant influence on their lives. There was a hierarchy in the asylum between staff members and between staff and patients. All employees, including managers and medical superintendents, required the governors' permission to leave the institution, however briefly. Attendants were entitled to relatively few rest-days, they could not marry without the governors' permission, their diet was similar to patients and at times they were subjected to violent attacks from patients.[87]

Attendants' responsibilities included preventing patients from escaping and harming themselves or others. Asylum escapes were reported to the lunacy inspectors and were generally treated seriously. Patients often attempted to escape when they were engaged in therapeutic activities, such as playing billiards, attending religious service or working on the farm. Many escapees were found subsequently in family homes.[88] Investigations of attempted escapes were carried out to assess attendants' culpability and evidence of negligence could result in a fine or dismissal.[89] In most cases, attendants were just reprimanded or fined, particularly when patients were harmless or when families returned them to the asylum; attendants were seldom dismissed.[90] When the escapee was harmed, the matter was treated more seriously but still attendants were not always dismissed. Phillip D. escaped from Carlow asylum in July 1892 and was killed when crossing the nearby Dublin to Carlow railway line. At the time of his escape he had been working on the farm, under the supervision of an attendant. An inquest was held into the matter and, though reprimanded, the attendant was not found to be responsible.[91] Attendants' health was also undermined, as they were susceptible to the diseases in the asylum. Staff contracted, and occasionally died, from cholera, fevers and tuberculosis.[92] Some employees developed mental illness and, when families could not be located, they were admitted as patients.[93]

Given the workload and the difficult living conditions, it is unsurprising that rebellions against a highly disciplined regime occurred. The nature of these varied but included the development of personal and emotional relationships between staff members, which sometimes resulted in marriage. In 1878, two employees at Enniscorthy asylum, Moses Hickey and Hester Martin, married without informing the medical superintendent. On discovering the marriage, Edmundson suspended them both, however the governors' reaction was more gendered. They dismissed Martin while Hickey was reinstated after a 'severe reprimand'. The governors also resolved that in future cases both attendants would be dismissed.[94] There were also controversies when attendants left asylums at night without permission and this was viewed as particularly grave when female staff was involved. In the nineteenth century, nurses were not regarded as respectable, and female nurses wandering about at night were open to the accusation of immoral behaviour.[95] During the winter of 1899, several nurses in Carlow asylum dressed up as men and left the asylum during the night. When they were discovered, the governors held a special inquiry into the matter.[96]

The 1843 privy council rules insisted that attendants treat patients with humanity, and John Conolly went further suggesting they become 'companions of patients'.[97] Nonetheless, staff members maltreated patients and these abusive exchanges between patients and attendants were reported in asylum records. Other forms of interactions were largely absent. Allegations against attendants ranged from 'rough' treatment of patients to violent assaults.[98] In September 1885, a woman at Carlow sustained a fractured thigh while struggling with an attendant, who was bringing her to supper.[99] Asylum governors and medical superintendents were obliged to investigate these cases, and they were brought to the lunacy inspectors' attention. Attendants could be fined, dismissed or prosecuted, particularly when the patient died. For example, in June 1901 a male patient died in Carlow asylum. The post-mortem found two 'rents' in his intestines and lunacy inspectors held an investigation. It was unclear whether the tears were caused by an external injury or by the consumption of inedible articles; some 'foreign bodies' were found in his stomach. The inspectors established that an attendant had kicked the patient in the stomach the morning before his death. Although there was not enough evidence to bring the case to court with a 'reasonable hope of conviction'; the attendant was dismissed from the asylum.[100]

Attempts to improve the pay, working conditions and lives of asylum nurses continued into the twentieth century and the Carlow governors supported requests from staff for salary increases.[101] However, improvements were achieved through strike action rather than negotiations. In 1917 the Irish Asylum Workers' Union was founded and between 1918 and 1920 there was a wave of strikes in asylums across Ireland that focused almost exclusively on improving attendants' pay and conditions.[102] At times, the strike action became quite militant. Peadar O'Donnell, a leading Irish socialist, established a workplace soviet at Monaghan asylum between November and December 1918. Demands for improvements to attendants' training and educational requirements were largely absent from the striking workers' agenda. During the strikes, medical superintendents, hoping to improve the quality of asylum nursing staff, sought to make Medico-Psychological Association certificates in mental nursing mandatory for all attendants. The attendants and their union were opposed to these suggestions. The strikes were partially successful and culminated in a national agreement in 1920 that gave staff shorter working hours and improved pay. Some asylums did not adhere to the agreement and the changing Irish political and economic context in the 1920s ensured that the union's successes did not last.[103]

Patients and therapy

Asylum staff – medical superintendants, nurses and attendants – delivered the asylums' therapeutic regimes and central to the optimism that was associated with the foundation of the new system in the 1810s was moral treatment and management.[104] During the 1817 Select Committee hearings, Thomas Spring Rice and John Leslie Foster alluded to the work of the Tukes at the York Retreat and Phillippe Pinel in Paris, and advocated that a similar regime be implemented in a separate asylum system in Ireland.[105] Various forms of moral treatment had been initiated in several institutions in the eighteenth century but following its description in 1813 in Samuel Tuke's published treatise, it was generally associated with the York Retreat.[106] As Digby has argued, moral therapy was a flexible and, for some, a vague concept and its implementation varied between institutions.[107] It is 'broadly defined' as a treatment that focused on the 'rational and emotional rather than organic causes of insanity'.[108] The central objective was to assist patients in regaining self-discipline and self-control by focusing on individual will. Therapy focused on patients' psychological, moral, emotional and spiritual states. Physical forms of control such as medication and physical restraint were discouraged and sometimes wholly discounted. As part of the regime, asylum managers and staff were cast in the role of parents, while patients were children. Religious observance and work were encouraged ensuring that patients were re-socialised.[109] Digby has suggested that at the York Retreat the spiritual values of the Society of Friends imbued treatment with an 'ethical component'.[110]

In Ireland, moral treatment and management was associated with Thomas Jackson's system at the Richmond asylum and with William Saunders Hallaran (1765–1825), physician to the Cork house of industry and lunatic asylum, who also owned a private asylum, the Cittadella, in the city.[111] Jackson's work was explicitly praised before the 1817 Select Committee. However, the close relationship between the Irish asylum and prison systems ensured that contemporary penal theories influenced the management regimes devised for the Irish asylums. The prison inspectorate was particularly impressed by Hallaran's theories.[112] Although better known for his support of Mason Cox's 'circulating swing',[113] the prison inspectors approved of Hallaran's advocacy of patient classification and employment.[114] His classification system was based on patients' potential to recover and, similar to the 'work-discipline' associated with the York Retreat, and later, with John Conolly and John Bucknill, Hallaran advocated employing patients.[115] Under these systems, work was gendered; male patients were employed in 'horticulture' while women were engaged in needlework and domestic tasks.[116]

Hallaran's theories influenced the management and therapeutic regimes introduced to the asylums in the 1820s and 1830s. The regime blended contemporary theories of penal and lunacy reform although it did acknowledge that the mentally ill could not be treated as prisoners. The prison inspectors supported moral and religious instruction, employment, classification, moral government and employing trained attending staff in asylums. They believed 'moral and religious instruction' subdued excited passions and controlled 'the imaginations of the insane'. They adopted a hygienic approach to treatment, separating patients from 'injurious communication' and classifying them.[117] The design of the new asylums and surrounding environment facilitated these regimes. Patients worked on farms attached to asylums and it was intended that chapels – Catholic and Protestant – would be constructed. Asylums were kept small allowing for frequent contact between staff and patients. Patients were accommodated in separate cells.

The use of restraint was not explicitly prohibited, though John Conolly's non-restraint movement forced a re-appraisal of the appropriateness of using physical methods when managing patients in Ireland.[118] In the 1840s, the lunacy inspectors expressed disapproval of physical restraint and monitored its use, praising Carlow asylum for avoiding it.[119] The inspectors and medical staff were obliged to justify instances when it was employed, but it is doubtful whether the surveillance was particularly effective. When White introduced the use of 'camisole, arm-strap and bed-strap' at Carlow asylum in the 1850s, he argued that it was 'much safer, less exciting and far less likely to be injurious' to patients. White also defended seclusion as a method of managing violent and disruptive patients.[120] These management strategies were used in Carlow and Enniscorthy asylums throughout the nineteenth century, particularly among patients showing verbal or physical signs of self-harm or an intention to escape.[121] Seclusion was employed more often than confinement with camisoles or straps.[122] At Enniscorthy asylum, the threat to transfer patients to refractory wards – 'amongst the wild ones' – was used to force them to exercise self-control, and in the case of Mary C. the medical officer believed it was very effective concluding that Mary 'evidently can control her excitement when she chooses'.[123]

The form of moral management introduced to Irish asylums did not exclude the use of 'medicalised' treatments although, initially, Irish asylum staff was sceptical of their efficacy. In 1846, the visiting physician at Carlow asylum insisted that medicine or drugs were of little use, except in extreme cases, arguing that 'the change of scene, the improved diet, clothing, and good air, joined with regularity and discipline of the institution, are of more importance than medical agents.'[124] Staff employed general humoural remedies and when applied, the intention was to stimulate or pacify patients, depending on the disorder. Purgatives such as castor oil were employed frequently and the use of blisters, bloodletting and emetics continued until the late 1870s.[125] Bloodletting was believed to be effective in cases of mania, although it was only to be used in 'the most urgent cases'.[126]

Opiates and other drugs were prescribed frequently. In 1856, White acknowledged that he used morphine and other drugs to calm patients in Carlow asylum.[127] One twenty-two-year-old woman committed in July 1857, diagnosed as suffering from mania, with religious delusions and a tendency to 'injure herself and others', was prescribed a purgative of castor oil on admission.[128] When her condition did not improve, she was given morphine and chloroform at bedtime, a means of encouraging sleep in maniacs.[129] By the second half of the century, opiates were prescribed for patients with agitated and nervous disorders. It is unclear whether this was for therapeutic or management purposes.[130] At Enniscorthy asylum, Drapes supported the use of hyoscine. From the 1890s, it was repeatedly administered to calm patients diagnosed with forms of mania – often described as 'wild' and 'excited' – and to induce sleep.[131] It was delivered through hypodermic needles and quickly calmed agitated patients.[132]

Dietary regime was an important component of asylum therapeutics and at times it was observed that it rendered medical intervention unnecessary.[133] The lunacy inspectors regarded malnourishment as contributing to high instances of mental disorder and most patients were placed on diets to improve nutritional intake.[134] Iron was administered to fortify patients further.[135] The lunacy inspectors insisted that the Irish asylum diet was both 'nutritious' and 'plentiful', and generally of good quality.[136] Finnane argued that while dull, asylum diets were better than workhouse food and often better than patients' nutritional intake outside an institution.[137] On admission, patients were placed on an 'ordinary' diet that was frequently supplemented with 'extras'. The ordinary diets differed between asylums and there were considerable variations in the amounts of meat provided.[138] At Carlow asylum in 1844, breakfast consisted of an oatmeal stir-about with a quart of milk while dinner consisted of potatoes and milk supplemented with a quarter pound of bacon and vegetables two days a week. The final meal of the day – supper – comprised bread and milk. The diet became more monotonous the following year, when one pound of beef and soup served once a week replaced the twice-weekly allowance of bacon and vegetables.[139] Meat was believed to be particularly restorative and when the Carlow physician complained in the 1840s that the governors had reduced the meat allowance, the inspectors suggested that it be increased to three days a week.[140] In 1844 there was no provision for meat in Armagh asylum.[141] Asylum diets were more diverse in later decades although the food's nutritional quality did not always improve. At Carlow asylum, dinner comprised of either bread and milk or bread with a quart of soup made from beef, ox-heads and vegetables. This replaced milk three days a week. For supper, cocoa was also introduced.

The inspectors' 1844 insistence that governors provide meat more frequently was ignored in some asylums and, as E. Maziere Courtenay noted in 1886, the asylum returns on diet did not record the portion of meat, bone and fat in ox-heads.[142] By 1862 Carlow medical staff were entitled to prescribe dietary 'extras', including stimulants such as tea, wine or porter.[143] At Enniscorthy asylum, most patients were given 'extras' – milk, eggs, beef tea – when initially admitted. Also some asylums, such as Kilkenny and Limerick, devised specific 'hospital' diets while others drew up lists of 'extras' such eggs, milk, beef tea and rice, which were prescribed to weaker patients. At Killarney asylum, extras were restricted to patients, particularly men, who were working.[144] At Enniscorthy asylum, withholding 'extras' was sometimes used as a punishment for refractory behaviour, including refusing to work.[145]

The systematic delineation of 'ordinary', 'extra' and 'hospital' diets in individual asylums, was more common after the 1860s and by 1880 nearly all asylums provided discrete dietaries.[146] The 'ordinary' diet remained fairly monotonous and soporific, consisting of large amounts of bread, rice, potatoes and milk. Courtenay observed that tea or coffee was frequently given for breakfast.[147] Asylum medical superintendents reported excessive tea consumption, along with tobacco and alcohol, as contributing to the apparent increase in mental illness in the Irish population in the 1890s. Courtenay recognised that tea was popular among patients and acted as a source of comfort on admission. He did not discourage providing it although at Carlow and Enniscorthy asylums, the provision of additional quantities of tea and coffee was closely monitored.

In devising asylum dietaries, the inspectors were keen that they resembled patients' diets outside the asylum. Courtenay, noting the loss of freedom and choice patients experienced on admission, argued that familiar diets assisted them in accepting the asylum's regimes.[148] It was also hoped that this would encourage patients with problems and delusions associated with food to eat and would reduce the incidence of food refusal. In the post-Famine period, the staples of Irish diet – potatoes and milk – were supplemented with 'tea, bread, butter, bacon and flesh meat'. In spite of Courtenay's recommendations, these changes were not reflected in asylum dietaries. He criticised the omission of butter and bacon and the inclusion of cocoa, which was not generally consumed. He was less critical of small amounts of meat arguing that the Irish people were 'more contented on a farinaceous regimen than on animal foods.[149] At Enniscorthy asylum, a patient, James K. insisted he was used to having meat in his breakfast and demanded eggs in compensation while other patients refused meat completely.[150]

Courtenay's main criticism of asylum diets was the lack of variety. His appointment to the inspectorate in 1890 ensured that dietaries were monitored more closely. In that year, Carlow asylum was criticised for over-dependence on milk and bread and in a subsequent report the inspectors characterised the Carlow diet as inferior to a prison diet. They submitted a new dietary that included meat – stew, beef, bacon – four times a week and greater variety of vegetables.[151] Its implementation was delayed while building work on the asylum kitchen was ongoing; the delay continued until 1899.[152] The new inspectors also monitored dining arrangements in asylums. In 1893, Carlow asylum was praised for allowing patients to use 'plates, bowls, knives and forks', suggesting that these were not in general use previously.[153] In 1899, the inspectors discovered that male patients were served dinner in the corridors due to building works and this caused considerable disorder.[154] Overcrowding and renovations undermined mealtime discipline and order.

Work, recreation and religion

As noted earlier, patients were expected to work while in the asylum and work was fundamental to therapeutic regimes and to Victorian concepts of respectability. It also represented continuity with daily life outside the asylum. As shown in chapter five, Carlow and Enniscorthy medical superintendents believed that patients' ability to, and acceptance of, work indicated a return to health.[155] Male patients usually worked at 'field labour' although they were also employed at 'weaving and other trades'.[156] Female patients were confined to domestic work, sewing, cleaning and working in the laundry. This gendered division of employment was common in most nineteenth-century asylums.[157] These boundaries were not completely rigid; male patients were employed in domestic tasks on the wards and there is no evidence to suggest that they were particularly resistant to ward work, sometimes preferring it.

In 1835, ninety of the 104 patients in Carlow asylum were employed at various tasks including 'gardening, trenching ground, trades, servants, etc.'.[158] There was insufficient land adjoining the asylum and this limited the expansion of the farm.[159] In 1837, there was only six acres of 'profitable land'; the remaining space was occupied by 'buildings and airing yards'.[160] The small farm size also limited the financial profit accrued from agricultural labour. In 1836, the six-acre farm made a £120 profit. The lunacy inspectors were keen to increase these profits and urged the governors to purchase additional land insisting that the asylum could become self-sufficient.[161] Additional land was acquired and in 1842 Carlow asylum stood 'in a healthy situation, with about 15 acres attached, partly laid out with handsome or ornamental plantations.' A portion of the ground was under tillage and there was a garden, which supplied vegetables.[162] Ten years later the governors rented land from Henry Bruen, at four pounds per acre and the inspectors suggested they purchase it.[163] Although they refused in this instance, by December 1915 the Carlow asylum farm was approximately 122 acres.

Convalescent and harmless patients worked on the wards monitoring other patients and performed domestic tasks such as polishing floors. The numbers employed on the wards fluctuated and were not recorded consistently. As Cherry observed of Norfolk, the growth of asylums ensured that work became 'regulated by the requirements of the asylum as a managed estate.'[164] These patients formed part of the workforce and a key objection to the proposed establishment of separate asylums for chronic patients, discussed in chapter six, was that this would deprive existing institutions of convalescent working patients. Employing patients prompted additional concerns. In early October 1895, during her third sojourn in Enniscorthy asylum, Ellen C. was set to work in the laundry. On one occasion, an attendant noticed she had not returned to the ward and on investigation, found her dangling her legs in a boiler of scalding water in the laundry. Ellen was badly blistered and sent to the asylum infirmary. Though she was frequently described as 'wild', Ellen did not have a recorded history of self-harm.[165] Her behaviour not only had serious consequences for her own health, but it had the potential to expose the attendant to an accusation of neglect, resulting in a fine or even dismissal. While employing patients had a therapeutic and financial rationale, it also brought the potential for further disruption.

Patients' activities in the asylum were not confined to work and provision was made for recreation, including sport. Not only were recreations intended to prevent patients indulging in 'gloomy sensations', by the second half of the nineteenth century 'an active participation in sport was widely regarded as an essential requirement for high standards of physical, mental and moral well-being'.[166] Asylum managers introduced various forms of modest recreational activities. In 1843, Parsons, the manager at Carlow asylum, spent five pounds on a 'small selection of books' for patients and there were other small initiatives later in the century.[167] The reading material was often morally uplifting; in 1849, thirty-five Roman Catholic and twelve Protestant prayer books were purchased.[168] In 1891, the governors furnished O'Meara with a budget to provide entertainment, including the purchase of a set of lawn tennis rackets, net and balls.[169] There were proposals to form a band at Carlow asylum, but the governors did not approve.[170] At Enniscorthy asylum, patients played billiards and a handball alley was built.[171] However, overcrowding in asylums resulted in dayrooms and exercise yards being converted into dormitories, limiting recreational pursuits.

While moral treatment emphasised patients' spiritual states, medical attitudes towards the relationship between religion and mental disorders were mixed. By the nineteenth century, the belief that 'being out of one's mind had its place within Christian values as a potentially positive phase of spirituality' was losing popularity.[172] Excessive religious enthusiasm was contradictory to rationality and was believed to disrupt 'distressed imaginations'.[173] The high number of admissions during the 1851 Ulster revival and the Revivalist movement in Wales seemed to confirm the link between extreme religious states and mental disorder.[174] Asylum admissions associated with religious excitement were not confined to specific events. Between 1832 and 1922, thirty-three patients in Carlow asylum were described as suffering from religious delusions, enthusiasm, depression, mania and zeal.

Religion was also felt to have the potential to influence the mind positively and religious services were provided as part of therapeutic regimes in Irish asylums. Generally, only convalescent patients were allowed to attend services although the inspectors acknowledged that the 'less convalescent, appeared to have derived some benefit from religious advice and instruction...'[175] The 1843 privy council rules stipulated that asylum governors ensure clergymen visited patients when requested and encouraged frequent visits from parochial clergy.[176] The rules also stipulated that Roman Catholic and Protestant religious services be provided.

Asylum physicians selected patients well enough to attend.[177] In 1843, it was estimated that thirty-one male patients and thirty-four female patients at Carlow Asylum were able to exercise sufficient control to attend religious services.[178] The regulations also specified that Roman Catholic and Church of Ireland chaplains and chapels be provided in asylums.[179] The provision of religious facilities in Irish asylums intersected with nineteenth-century anxieties about the vulnerability of institutional inmates to proselytising. While 'visits of the Parochial Clergy to the institution' were encouraged, the privy council regulations specified that clergymen confine visits to 'patients of their own persuasion.'[180] The 1853 amendment to the privy council rules reinforced this; governors were required to give patients access to 'religious instruction and consolation', 'according to their respective creeds'. Clergymen were advised to 'scrupulously' avoid 'controversial subjects both in public service and in private visitations.'[181]

There were a series of controversies surrounding the provision of religious facilities in asylums in Ireland. In the 1850s, Belfast asylum refused to appoint an asylum chaplain while the governors at Ballinasloe asylum were slow to construct a chapel.[182] There was friction between Carlow asylum staff and local clergymen. The Catholic clergymen in Carlow town alleged that there was a sectarian bias operating against Catholics within the poor law union and the workhouse.[183] In August 1845, the Roman Catholic parish priest, Marcus Dowling, appeared at Carlow asylum with three other clergymen, demanding he be permitted to inspect the building. The asylum manager, Parsons, insisted he chaperone the group. Dowling objected maintaining that as parish priest he was 'authorised to go through whenever I please to visit all the patients'.[184] Parsons informed him that according to the privy council rules this was not the case, as Dowling was not the asylum chaplain.[185] Dowling complained to the Roman Catholic Bishop, Haly, also an asylum governor. The governors were generally supportive of Parsons' stance and agreed that Dowling should have contacted the manager in advance. Nonetheless, Parsons was obliged to apologise for his inappropriate language.[186] The events highlight the Catholic clergy's anxieties about accessing their flock in institutions that they believed had the potential to become the domain of Protestant influence. The presence of Catholic clergy on the asylum board did not alleviate these fears sufficiently.

Due to the importance of religion in the asylums, it impacted on architecture of the building. However, chapels were slow to materialise and without them, religious services took place in the asylum. At Carlow five pounds was spent on 'furniture for the celebration of divine service'.[187] The delays in building chapels were due to financial constraints as well as religious tension and as a result Protestant patients experienced difficulties in fulfilling religious observances. A proposal to erect a 'suitable apartment for divine service' in Carlow asylum was initially tabled in August 1855.[188] However, its construction was linked to other structural repairs and consequently there were long delays. In 1874, the lunacy inspectors finally reported that the chapel was complete.[189] Designed by George Wilkinson, it was a Gothic structure. The plan included two chapels, one for Catholic and one for Protestant worship, each with a separate entrance. However, it was used for Catholic worship only and the proposed Protestant chapel was not built. This reluctance to provide facilities for Protestant services was partly due to the small number of Protestant patients in the asylum.[190] Although there were significant Protestant communities in some counties in the Carlow asylum district – 11.6 per cent of the population of county Carlow and 15.6 per cent in the case of county Kildare – few patients, only 10.5 per cent, were Protestant.[191] By 1911, this had decreased further, confirming Malcolm's contention that Protestant patients were under-represented in asylum populations.[192] The small number of Protestant patients ensured that some asylums did not build facilities for Protestant worship for most of the nineteenth century. In September 1892, the Protestant chaplain at Carlow asylum, Rev J. Finlay, reminded the governors and the board of control of 'the need for a place of worship for members of the Church of Ireland.'[193] At the time services were held in a dining room. Eventually, in November 1898 the enlargement of the Roman Catholic chapel and the construction of a separate Protestant chapel was authorised.

Medical encounters

Patients immediately encountered the 'medical gaze' of the asylum on admission, when they were medically assessed. This was often the first time they met asylum medical staff.[194] By the late nineteenth century, assistant medical officers usually completed these initial medical assessments[195] and, as Dawson argued the large number of questions in asylum casebooks guided these medical interviews compensating for the limited experience of assistant medical officers.[196] It is unclear how frequently patients encountered medical superintendents while in the asylum. When they were present or consulted during interviews, specific references were made in the casebooks suggesting it was not commonplace.[197] Nonetheless, patient correspondence indicates that they knew medical superintendents suggesting there was some contact. Overall it would appear that assistant medical officers were in regular contact with patients while medical superintendents visited them less frequently but were kept abreast of progress. Medical superintendents communicated with relatives and friends when seeking additional information, negotiating patients' discharge and informing them of deaths.

On admission, patients were often very confused, distressed and fretful. They were described as very excitable, and were sometimes dragged from cars into the building; they frequently refused to get into bed and to dress.[198] Others were reported to be 'quite cheerful', willing to converse with the medical officer, while some were extremely quiet and low.[199] Patients who had harmed themselves prior to admission were often admitted with severe physical wounds such as Anne B., who had eaten glass when a picture she was hanging on a wall broke.[200] In spite of being in such distressed states, patients sat in asylum waiting rooms before being examined and this could prove disruptive. Two attendants were obliged to hold one woman, Anne E., on the seat.[201] Occasionally, a patient arrived in a straitjacket, though it was usually removed immediately.

The focus on patients' bodies on admission drew attention to their physical condition. Both sets of casebooks are replete with descriptions of patients' poor clothing, and unkempt and under-nourished bodies, underlining the extreme poverty and harsh circumstances most of them endured before admission.[202] Patients at Carlow asylum were photographed on admission and the medical superintendent sometimes remarked that the photograph was an accurate depiction of the person and the illness.[203] During the first month following admission, patients were regularly assessed, often weekly. Once a regime of treatment was established, doctors examined them monthly. When hopes of recovery deteriorated, consultations were reduced further, initially to every six months while chronic patients were examined once a year. The clinical records of these examinations reflect the asylum medical staff's therapeutic preoccupations, but these also contain the patients' concerns and delusions. While medical staff focused on patients' diet, disruptive nature and willingness and ability to work, they also recorded the patients' demands to return home, their resistance to the asylum regime and persistent delusions. In their commentary, medical staff created a distance between themselves and patients, and this was extended to attendants and nurses. The space between the various protagonists in the asylum was constructed by the language of social and class difference as well as medical objectivity.

As contemporary medical theories emphasised the importance of food and diet to recovery, patients' eating habits were closely monitored. Delusions surrounding food and cases of food refusal quickly came to light. In 1858, Daniel H. Tuke categorised the causes of food refusal into five groups: dyspepsia, suicidal tendency, idiocy, organic lesion on the brain or a delusion associated with food and/or eating. In the asylums, food refusal was most frequently identified among patients with delusions and among patients who had attempted suicide. Food refusal accompanied by delusions was felt to be especially problematic. Tuke noted that while delusions could cause patients to refuse food, the prolonged deprivation of food could induce delusions and exacerbate the problem.[204] Some patients experienced paranoid delusions and believed their food was poisoned or contaminated.[205] Other common delusions surrounding food focused on the relationship between it, and work and religion. John N. was admitted to Carlow asylum in March 1906, following an illness of several months. He refused to eat following admission, stating that 'a man does not require nourishment unless he is working in a farm'. Eventually, McKenna force-fed John using a stomach pump. This was done on several occasions and the patient offered no resistance. After a week in the asylum, he began to take solid food voluntarily and to work on the asylum farm, slowly becoming interested in employment. There was little improvement in his mental state; John remained withdrawn and only spoke freely 'about hard labour in the fields increasing one's appetite'. John's explanation for his behaviour suggests a mechanised understanding of the relationship between food consumption and work. For another patient, the consumption of food was enmeshed in religious tropes. He described food, particularly vegetables, as being 'out of bounds' and that the 'authorities of the Catholic Church told him he was not to eat the bread at the Naas Union'. Fasting, usually abstaining from meat rather than vegetables, was a common practise among Roman Catholics as a means of obtaining absolution.[206]

As John. N.'s treatment shows, extreme and sustained cases of food refusal resulted in patients being force-fed. Tuke argued that the decision to force-feed a patient should not be delayed, claiming that he never waited more than four days. Delays resulted in the patient becoming exhausted through starvation.[207] In asylums, stomach pumps tended to be employed in more advanced stages of starvation and with limited success. Ellen B. was fed with a stomach pump but she died after a month in Carlow asylum.[208] The delay in deciding to force-feed patients reflected medical superintendents' and nineteenth-century alientists' ambivalence about the procedure, particularly when patients were violent and offered resistance. Tuke discounted suggestions that chloroform be administered, fearing the effect it had on debilitated patients.[209]

Asylum doctors feared that force-feeding patients using stomach pumps endangered lives and preferred to use other methods, including a gag and spoons.[210] Often in these circumstances, the stomach pump was kept within the patient's field of vision. Tuke disapproved of such practises insisting the stomach pump was a 'remedy and not a punishment'.[211] He also discouraged the indiscriminate application of force-feeding in all cases of food refusal, insisting that it should only be used as a 'last resource' and 'when all persuasion has failed'.[212] He outlined the most efficient and safe methods to be used in the asylum, distancing himself from older methods that included the use of 'gags, bits and screws'. These methods frequently injured patients and there was the risk of food entering the lungs. Tuke's method involved injecting food into the stomach through oesophageal tubes. He admitted his method did not eliminate every risk associated with the procedure but was confident that skilled asylum doctors could perform the procedure successfully.

Force-feeding was used relatively frequently in asylums to intervene in cases of sustained food refusal and was prescribed for both male and female patients. Medical superintendents did not employ it more frequently among female patients in Carlow and Enniscorthy asylums and they remained ambivalent about it. The methods used were a brutal form of intervention, particularly when patients resisted.[213] For asylum doctors, the employment of the stomach pump and feeding tubes presented them with difficult decisions. Allowing patients to refuse food for prolonged periods could result in death, leaving the asylum open to accusations of neglect and mismanagement. However, such an extreme form of physical intervention could also prove fatal and consequently doctors delayed employing the procedure.

The identification of cases of delusions and food refusal on admission was part of medical officers diagnostic assessments. The disease categories they used followed those of the Medico-Psychological Association and influenced patients' experiences in asylum. At Carlow asylum, 66 per cent of patients were ascribed diagnoses. These included melancholia, mania, idiocy, dementia and epilepsy.[214] There were subsets within these categories, such as acute and chronic manifestations of disorders, recurrent cases and delusional insanity. The most frequently assigned diagnosis was 'mania' (39 per cent (1681)) and its various forms including 'acute mania', 'chronic mania', 'monomania', 'recurring' and 'relapsing mania', 'senile mania' and 'puerperal insanity'. 'Mania' was marked by disruptive behavior and 'excited' symptoms that were challenging to moral management regimes that valued order. Only 19 per cent (843) of patients were diagnosed with melancholia and its different forms. These patterns of diagnosis are similar to those identified at Devon asylum between 1845 and 1914 and Ticehurst private asylum between 1885 and 1915.[215] At Carlow asylum there were small groups of epileptics (3 per cent (132)) and 'idiots' 'imbeciles' or 'congenitally deficient' (2.6 per cent (115)) patients. A further 7 per cent (312) of patients were diagnosed as suffering from dementia and senility. There were twenty-one patients for whom the diagnosis of mental illness was doubted. Only one of these patients was discharged within a month while the remainder were discharged after three months, suggesting that they were either kept under observation for a period or the asylum authorities experienced difficulties in locating families or workhouse authorities willing to accept them.

As demonstrated in chapter four, during the certification procedures dispensary medical officers speculated on aetiologies of mental illness and recorded moral, physical and hereditary causes. These were transcribed from certification forms into casebooks, where medical superintendents augmented, confirmed or altered them. Physical causes incorporated damage to the brain, physical ill health, childbirth and venereal disease. These also included epilepsy and alcoholism.[216] Moral causes included stress and disappointment related to over-work, love or anxiety. Grief over the death of parents, spouses or siblings was also included in this category. As noted in chapter two, by the late Victorian period, biological pathologies and medical theories of hereditary insanity had become part of the schema explaining the apparent rise in the incidence of mental illness.[217] In the late nineteenth century, Drapes and other medical superintendents at Enniscorthy and Carlow asylums frequently recorded the presence of biological pathologies of insanity such as hereditary influences and general paralysis among patients, although these did not eclipse moral causes.[218]

Carlow and Enniscorthy asylum medical officers reported high incidences of hereditary insanity among patients. Drapes at Enniscorthy asylum explicitly linked the rise in the number of Irish asylum patients with hereditary influences.[219] The Carlow medical officers attempted to identify hereditary tendencies among families and closely followed up family histories. For example, Thomas M. was certified in January 1906, having threatened to kill his mother. There was no evidence of hallucinations or delusions and his explanation for his threatening behaviour was that:

> his mother was constantly aggravating him and speaking unseemly things to him of which he could not make head or tail and that on this occasion he felt so ashamed of her that he threatened to kill her in order to frighten her.

On investigation, McKenna concluded that Thomas' mother was herself mentally ill. He also established that the man's cousin had shot his sister and then drowned himself, while an uncle had slit his throat. Confident that there was a 'strong hereditary tendency to insanity in this man's family', McKenna kept Thomas under observation in the asylum. Throughout, McKenna remained unconvinced of Thomas' mental illness describing him as 'an excellent worker' who 'enjoys good bodily health'. However, evidence of hereditary insanity resulted in Thomas spending five months in the asylum.[220]

In Carlow asylum, hereditary insanity, and the associated disorders of congenital insanity and epilepsy, were recorded as causes of insanity among 26.5 per cent (615) of patients, while other traits of degeneration such as drink accounted for 12.7 per cent (293). Epilepsy was recorded among 4.5 per cent (104) of patients while old age accounted for 6.7 per cent (156). Male patients were more frequently described as exhibiting hereditary insanity (58 per cent), 'congenital mental deficiency' (61 per cent) and epilepsy (74 per cent). The number of patients described as 'idiots' and as having 'congenital mental deficiency' rose after 1843 when the privy council rules removed the ban on their admission. Medical assessments of 'congenital idiots' focused on the patient's ability to relate where they were, the date, and included descriptions of their educational abilities. They were invariably described as 'dull', 'slow', 'stupid' or of weak 'intellect',[221] a lexicon Wright identified in Earlswood Asylum.[222] The clinical entries for these patients chart an increasing number of attacks that resulted in a decline in mental state. By the end of the century, medical assessments of epileptic patients were tinged with sympathy – patients were described as 'poor' or 'unfortunate', in contrast to other patients who were 'mischievous' or 'cunning'. There was a sense of hopelessness in the reports of these patients and a large number died in the asylum. One epileptic patient, John George C., was admitted to Carlow asylum in January 1906. He had suffered from epilepsy for the previous eight years and had received treatment in Dublin. Despite this, his condition had steadily deteriorated and, on admission, he was described as an 'epileptic dement'. During his stay, the number of epileptic fits rose and the asylum doctor could not control them. In the interval between his attacks, his mental condition was described as 'very clear' and 'fairly intelligent'.[223] The repeated attacks took their toll on the patient, and he eventually died in December 1907.[224]

Drunkenness and, to a lesser extent, the presence of general paralysis, both regarded as traits of a degenerate population, were recorded among patients in both asylums. By the late nineteenth century, drink and general paralysis were believed to be 'stumbling blocks' for an inferior mental constitution already weakened by hereditary tendencies. Drink and general paralysis were usually recorded among male patients: 82 per cent of patients with 'intemperance' and 'alcoholism' were male.[225] Syphilis and general paralysis were treated as distinct diseases.[226] Only ten patients were explicitly assigned 'syphilis' as a cause of insanity, while a further fourteen were diagnosed as suffering from general paralysis on admission. It appeared more frequently as a cause of death and forty-three patients, mostly men, were recorded as dying from it. The incidence of the disease in the Carlow district was related to the close proximity of an army barracks at the Curragh in county Kildare; most patients admitted with it were soldiers. The Curragh area was famous for the 'wrens', a group of women who operated as prostitutes in the locality, and there was also a Lock hospital in Kildare town.[227] In the 1860s, Irish asylum doctors insisted that the incidence of general paralysis and syphilis was much lower in Irish asylums, as they associated the diseases with industrialisation and urbanisation.[228] They continued this line of argument in the 1890s, insisting that the Irish had to travel to acquire it.[229]

Among female patients in Carlow asylum organic aetiologies were related to a range of disorders concerning the female reproductive life, variously described in the casebooks as 'after childbirth', 'childbearing', 'pregnancy', 'puerperal state' and 'puerperal fever'. As Digby and Theriot have demonstrated, nineteenth-century British and American medicine defined women's mental state in biological terms and family members shared these interpretations, citing childbirth as a cause of mental illness.[230] In the asylum, women's menstruation cycles were closely tracked and reported upon. However, as Marland has shown, not all physicians agreed that asylums were appropriate sites for the treatment of puerperal insanity and relatively few cases – thirty – were recorded among patients in Carlow asylum.[231] Biological aetiologies associated with life stages were not confined to female patients – 37 per cent (17) of patients assigned 'time of life' as a cause of illness were men. After the 1890s, adolescence was identified as a cause among twenty-three male patients. The first case that explicitly referred to masturbation among adolescents was recorded in Carlow asylum in January 1905 and in some cases it was reported in the testimony provided by the patient or the family.[232]

Asylum doctors acknowledged that poorer populations were vulnerable to emotional stresses that had a detrimental impact on mental states. Aetiologies assigned to patients in Carlow asylum included changes in familial, social and economic status (57) variously described as 'adverse circumstances' (11), domestic trouble (34), fright (22), 'disappointment in love' (8) and grief (25). Labouring men and women were reported as vulnerable to stresses associated with financial ruin, poverty and emotional loss. Drapes and Tuke argued that the stress associated with poverty and economic ruin acted as an exciting cause of insanity among a population whose nervous systems were compromised through hereditary influences. Among patients whose aetiology was described as 'domestic trouble', 46 per cent (25) were men, and 53 per cent of patients recorded as suffering from 'disappointment in love' were male. Jealousy was recorded more often among male patients, at 71 per cent (15). As Suzuki has suggested, anxieties surrounding poverty, the fear of ruin, and emotional loss featured beside the more familiar biological pathologies among labouring men. Thus class, identity and status, in addition to gender, determined the application of disease aetiologies.[233] Women – 80 per cent (36) – were more likely to be assigned grief or death of a relative as aetiologies. Forty-five patients were certified following the death of a family member, usually a spouse or a parent. Grief associated with the loss of relatives through emigration was also recorded as an exciting factor in patients' clinical history. For example, James S. was described as 'being grieved at the departure of some of his children to America'.[234] Maryanne W., a twenty-nine-year-old single woman from Wexford, was described as displaying signs of mental illness for six years. However, the departure of her family to America, and her inability to accompany them, was interpreted as 'hurrying on the malady', culminating in her confinement in May 1851.[235]

Patients expressed their mental distress in various ways. They frequently communicated delusions to medical staff or harmed themselves. As discussed in chapter four, relatives cited evidence of suicide or a stated intention to commit suicide as proof of mental illness during certification. However, only thirty-one patients were recorded as displaying suicidal tendencies in Carlow admission registers. On admission, suicidal patients and those who were inclined to self-harm were usually put on a 'caution'. Attendants watched over them and they were sometimes required to wear a straitjacket. In certain cases medication was prescribed. There were five successful suicides, all male patients, reported in Carlow asylum between 1832 and 1922.[236] While staff successfully limited the number of suicides, they did not always ensure that patients did not injure themselves. Patients frequently harmed themselves when escaping or when resisting the asylum regime. Two days after his admission, John W. threw himself through a glass door while an attendant was transferring him between dormitories. Another patient, Martin D., threw himself out the window, seriously injuring his legs.[237]

Asylum medical staff also monitored patients' delusions. By the nineteenth century alienists regarded delusions and insanity as synonymous.[238] Delusions were understood to be a manifestation of 'wrong beliefs' and consequently asylum doctors dismissed them as meaningless.[239] Although patients' delusions were recorded in asylum casebooks, the subject matter was treated as 'empty speech acts, whose informational content refers to neither world nor self.' They were not the 'symbolic expression of anything'.[240] Patients' delusions did act as a form of communication between patient and asylum doctor, however problematic. According to the Carlow admission registers 3.5 per cent (151) of patients assigned a diagnosis between 1832 and 1922 suffered from forms of delusions. A higher incidence of delusional utterances was recorded in Enniscorthy and Carlow casebooks. Delusions were typically part of the symptomology among patients with histories of 'intemperance' or drunkenness. Thomas Clouston, at the Royal Edinburgh Asylum, identified delirium tremens as one of the five forms of alcoholic insanity and symptoms included high levels of delusions.[241] By the late nineteenth and early twentieth century, patients whose symptomology included delusions were perceived to be paranoid.[242]

Among Carlow and Enniscorthy patients, most recorded delusions were 'speech acts',[243] which climaxed in violent behaviour when patients acted out delusions. Patients' delusions can be categorised into three overlapping groups – delusions associated with the devil and/or religion, with threats over land or personal safety and, as discussed above, delusions about food and/or its supply. Wright identified similar delusions among patients in Buckinghamshire.[244] Delusions connected with land, cattle and money featured regularly, reflecting the main economic activities of the locality. One forty-year-old patient, an owner of a thirty-acre farm, was obsessed with money and it was believed he had lodged 'seven or eight hundred pounds' in the bank. His love of money was diagnosed as amounting to a 'monomania'. His behaviour became a matter of concern to his family when his parsimony resulted in a refusal to purchase cattle fodder and consequently twenty-five head of cattle starved to death. Houston and Suzuki identified similar instances of poor and irresponsible household management of finances resulting in certification.[245] Patients whose delusions involved land often believed that neighbours intended to deprive them of farms and these delusions frequently culminated in an attack on hapless neighbours thus prompting certification.

More grandiose delusions – patients who believed they were royalty, or aristocracy – were rare, although some patients were recorded as possessing an exaggerated sense of their own dignity. Bridget D., admitted to Enniscorthy asylum in March 1891, believed William E. Gladstone had bequeathed her the asylum,[246] while Joseph McC., an army man, claimed people were 'firing at him because he is like Lord Roberts', a resemblance confirmed in the casebook. His own dislike of Roberts was said to add to his 'melancholic state'. Joseph McC. experienced a 'sense of persecution' that stemmed from his army days, maintaining that the punishment exacted on him for misdemeanours such as drunkenness was 'increased manifold because he was an Irishman.' While the asylum personnel dismissed Joseph McC.'s allegations as evidence of his 'irrationality',

Joanna Bourke found that Irish soldiers in the British army were at times treated quite harshly.[247]

Physical environment

Patients' physical environment was an important part of restorative and therapeutic regimes. In the late nineteenth century, the inspectors encouraged governors to provide 'a simple homely form of ornamentation, which was indicative in itself of domestic comfort'.[248] They emphasised the need to remove the institutional and often prison-like appearance of asylums, thereby reflecting late Victorian attempts to domesticate the public/private space that was the interior of an asylum.[249] Superficial improvements were introduced to brighten conditions. In 1861, Carlow asylum was reported to be 'losing much of its original gloominess and prison-like appearance'.[250] It was painted on a number of occasions and blinds were purchased for the day rooms.[251] However, there were limits to what could be achieved: financial constraints ensured that local workhouse contractors supplied furniture instead of domestic retailers and this created a very drab interior.[252] In 1864, the inspectors criticised conditions in Carlow asylum, noting that 'the walls of the corridors are bare, monotonous and cheerless'.[253] As late as 1906 several patients admitted to Carlow and Enniscorthy asylums believed that they were in prison and some refused to speak to the medical superintendent until a solicitor was made available. While these impressions may have stemmed from patients' experiences of certification through the petty session courts, the asylum environment clearly did not allay these fears.

Patients experienced asylums as overcrowded insanitary places that at times became sites of disease contagion. The near decrepit buildings and the high levels of overcrowding in the wards contributed to mortality rates. While medical superintendents stressed that the asylum isolated patients from negative influences, asylum walls did not insulate them. The movement of people into the building ensured asylum patients did not escape outbreaks of epidemic disease or the spread of contagious infections in the locality. Families and friends visited relatives, while contractors brought food and other supplies. The governors held meetings in boardrooms and one or two inspected buildings periodically. This movement of people, coupled with the overcrowded conditions and the repeated delays in renovating the building, affected the health of patients and staff, sometimes resulting in death.

Figure 5.2 shows the mortality rate in Carlow asylum between 1832 and 1922 (chapter 5). The proportion of patients who died in Carlow asylum was 35.4 per cent and it was higher among men.[254] Due to the disproportionate number of men admitted to the asylums, male wards were constantly overcrowded and this undoubtedly contributed to the higher mortality rate. The lunacy inspectors argued that the high mortality rates in asylums were a result of the vulnerability of dangerous lunatic patients. However, mortality rates were higher among patients committed through other methods to Carlow asylum. Among the 2068 patients certified as dangerous lunatics between 1832 and 1922, 34.5 per cent (714) died while 39.8 per cent (806) of 'ordinary' patients died. The inspectors specifically linked the pre-1867 practice of confining patients in gaols with high mortality rates but there is little evidence for this.[255] Prior to 1867, 33.8 per cent (116) of the 343 dangerous lunatic patients died while 31.9 per cent of the 981 'ordinary' patients died. After 1867, there was a greater survival rate among dangerous lunatic patients. Among 'ordinary' patients certified between 1867 and 1922, 47.1 per cent (493) died while 34.7 per cent (598) of dangerous lunatics died.

Fluctuations in mortality rates were connected with economic conditions outside the asylum and with outbreaks of disease within the asylum. For example, the mortality rate increased dramatically during the Famine and remained high immediately after it.[256] Between 1849 and 1850 the mortality rates peaked and this peaking was similar to the mortality rates in workhouses. The proportion of patients dying in Carlow asylum never returned to its pre-Famine level and subsequent spikes occurred when the asylum was particularly overcrowded. During the economic crisis of the 1870s, the pressure mounted again. In addition, there was an outbreak of cholera, which had appeared in the locality intermittently since 1866.[257] When the disease appeared in Carlow asylum in the 1870s, the medical superintendent, Howlett, denied the outbreak was linked with the overcrowded conditions.[258] The lunatic inspectors disagreed, connecting it with overcrowding and the spread of other diseases such as dysentery.[259] In the 1870s, deaths from phthisis and epilepsy also rose as asylum conditions provided an ideal environment for the spread of phthisis. In the first decade of the twentieth century, there was a high mortality rate from 'pulmonary tuberculosis'. Most patients dying from it, and its various forms, were in the asylum for several years and probably contracted it while there.[260]

Outbreaks of dysentery in the late 1880s and early 1890s were related to the asylum's water supply. Since its construction in 1832, Carlow asylum had experienced difficulties with its sewerage and water systems due to the asylum's low-lying position. Although alterations were carried out in the 1870s, the problems persisted, but the governors were unwilling to pay to improve it.[261] They hoped that the asylum would be supplied with clean water by the Carlow town commissioners. The commissioners developed a scheme that would supply the town with a system of water-works.[262] They were, however, slow to develop the system and the water supply at the asylum was not improved. In 1887, another proposal to supply the town's water from reservoirs in adjacent hills was developed and, in return for an annual fee, it was proposed that the asylum would be supplied. Once again, nothing was done and the asylum continued to experience significant problems with its water supply. This resulted in a 'mild' epidemic of diarrhoea in September 1886. Twenty-three patients and an attendant were affected.[263] A year later, dysentery 'of a rather fatal character' appeared resulting in several deaths. On 13 January 1888, O'Meara reported that there were thirteen deaths from dysentery during the preceding month. The outbreak affected staff as well as patients and, in February, a deputy nurse died. The drainage system was blamed and O'Meara had part of the sewerage system cleaned. He also travelled to Dublin to consult the lunacy inspectors. Fresh cases continued to occur among staff and patients, though they were not fatal. O'Meara employed additional staff to cope with the crisis. Although the outbreak had abated by March 1888, no permanent solution to the problem of an adequate water supply for Carlow town or asylum was developed. Neither the town commissioners nor the asylum governors were willing to engage in extensive and expensive works. At the asylum, short-term schemes were devised including the sinking of a new well and the improved mainte-nance of existing wells.[264] Mild outbreaks of dysentery continued to occur during the year.[265]

In December, the governors developed their own water scheme that consisted of a double supply.[266] The first supply would come from the river Barrow and would be used for washing and other sanitary purposes. A second supply, for drinking and cooking, would come from a deep spring well. Work on the second supply was postponed until the appropriate season. The decision to continue with the existing supply of water for drinking and cooking resulted in the re-appearance of dysentery in 1889.[267] Work on the new water supply continued throughout 1889, however, in November the board of control stopped it and drew up alternative, more expensive plans. As discussed in chapter two, the governors believed that the plans were too costly and not urgent.[268] Instead, they agreed to install water closets, and privy, bath and lavatory facilities in eight divisions of the asylum. Water closets and privies were installed in the airing yards and the hospital. It was estimated that the work would cost £10,000. The necessary funding was however slow to materialise.[269] In the meantime, the lunacy inspectors continued to criticise the governors for failing to improve sanitary conditions.[270] At this juncture, improving sanitation in Carlow asylum became part of the general improvements and additions to the building which resulted in a significant delay in improving the sanitary conditions.[271] This provided an ideal environment for the spread of contagious diseases, including the influenza pandemic of 1918, which had a dramatic impact on asylum mortality rates.[272]

Conclusion

The medical regimes in Carlow and Enniscorthy asylums were mapped onto contemporary formulations of moral management. Although Carlow and Enniscorthy were modest-sized asylums, financial and management problems, similar to those impacting upon larger institutions, adversely affected patient care and by the late nineteenth century the early optimism had evaporated. By the late Victorian period, Carlow and Enniscorthy asylum doctors, struggling with high rates of admissions, employed pessimistic theories of degeneracy and hereditary insanity when identifying aetiologies of insanity. They also noted the corrosive effects that emotional and economical anxieties had on mental well-being and frequently reported on the poor physical condition of patients entering the asylum.

In keeping with theories of moral management and the non-restraint movement, asylum officials were preoccupied with maintaining order and regularity in the asylum throughout the nineteenth century. Consequently, in buildings where patients' meals were served in corridors, kitchens were deemed ill-equipped to prepare nutritious diets and patients did not have access to a good water supply, disciplining both patients' and staff's behaviour and bodies became a defining management strategy. However, patients' experiences were heterogeneous and they interpreted the regime's focus on employment, work, religious observance and medical interventions variously as therapy, exploitation, punishment and danger.

Notes

1   DPH, CLA General Register, 1857–76.
2   R. Porter, 'The Patient's View: Doing Medical History from Below', *Theory and Society*, 14:2 (1985), 175–198.
3   Marland, *Dangerous Motherhood*, pp. 99–105; Andrews, 'Case Notes, Case Histories and the Patient's Experience of Insanity', 255–281; A. Beveridge, 'Life in the Asylum: Patient's Letters from Morningside, 1873–1908', *History of Psychiatry*, 9 (1998), 431–469; G. B. Risse and J. H. Warner, 'Reconstructing Clinical Activities: Patient Records in Medical History', *Social History of Medicine*, 5 (1992), 183–205; G. Davis, 'The Historiography of Public Health Records in Research: A Critique of Case Notes'; Clondrau, 'The Patient's View Meets the Clinical Gaze', 525–540.
4   Wright, 'Delusion of Gender?', 160.
5   Marland, *Dangerous Motherhood*, p. 101.
6   One Carlow asylum casebook is in St Canice's Hospital, Kilkenny but access was not granted.
7   5 & 6 Vict., c. 123 (1842).
8   *Report of Lunacy Inspectors*, H. C. 1844 [567] xxx, pp. 45–46.
9   8 & 9 Vict., c. 107 (1845).
10 *Inquiry into the State of Lunatic Asylums and other Institutions*, pp. 7–8.
11 *Fiftieth Report of Lunacy Inspectors*, H. C. 1901 [Cd.760] xxviii, p. 217.
12 Chapter two.
13 Dawson, 'Note on a New Case-Book Form', *JMS*, 49:205 (April, 1903), 267–271, 267.
14 *Fiftieth Report of Lunacy Inspectors*, H. C. 1901 [Cd.760] xxviii, p. 222; Dawson, 'Note on a New Case-book Form', 267.
15 Finnane, *Insanity and the Insane*, p. 177; *Copies of all Correspondence and Communication between the Home Office and the Irish Government during the year 1827, on the Subject of Public Lunatic Asylums*, H. C. 1828 [234] xxii, p. 23.
16 These included a general register of patients, visitors' book, provisions book and proceedings book; *Ibid.*
17 *Copies of all Correspondence and Communication between the Home Office and the Irish Government during the year 1827, on the Subject of Public Lunatic Asylums*, H. C. 1828 [234] xxii, p. 24.
18 See Finnane, *Insanity and the Insane*, pp. 39–47.
19 DPH, CLA Minute Book, 8 March 1832.
20 *Ibid.*, 2 September; 7 October 1834.

21 See also NAI, CSO, Official Papers (hereafter OP), 1835/346 and OP 1835/343, 344, 347, 348.

22 *Twelfth Report of Prison Inspectors*, H. C. 1834 [63] xl, p. 22; *Fourteenth Report of Prison Inspectors*, H. C. 1836 [118] xxxv, p. 32.

23 DPH, CLA Minute Book, 16 September 1840.

24 *Ibid.*, 22 September 1842.

25 *Ibid.*,15 February 1843.

26 NAI CSORP 1843/G/3954 'Carlow Lunatic Asylum'; *Carlow Sentinel* (15 October 1842).

27 *Carlow Sentinel* (29 October 1842).

28 Malcolm, 'The Reign of Terror in Carlow'.

29 NAI, CSORP, 1842/G/16744, Samuel Hatch to Sir James Graham, 8 December 1842.

30 Scull, *The Most Solitary of Afflictions*, p. 190; R. Cooter, 'Phrenology and British Alienists, 1825–45', *Medical History*, 20:1&2 (1976), 1–21, 135–151.

31 *Report of Lunacy Inspectors*, H. C. 1845 [645] xxvi, p. 59.

32 Finnane, *Insanity and the Insane*, p. 42.

33 *Ibid.*, p. 43.

34 *Ibid.*

35 The Irish medical managers joined an Association of Medical Officers of Hospitals for the Insane, see Finnane, 'Irish Psychiatry. Part 1'.

36 DPH, CLA Minute Book, 21 December 1842.

37 *Ibid.*, 28 March 1848.

38 *Fourth Report of Lunacy Inspectors*, H. C. 1849 [1054] xxiii, p .4; 'Recent Publications on Insanity', 421.

39 Finnane, *Insanity and the Insane*, p. 44.

40 *Fourteenth Report of Lunacy Inspectors*, H. C. 1865 [3556] xxi, p. 127.

41 Finnane, *Insanity and the Insane*, pp. 46–47.

42 Finnane, *Insanity and the Insane*, p. 44.

43 NAI Office of the Lunatic Asylums (hereafter OLA) 1, Minute Book of the Lunatic Asylums (Ireland) Commissioners, 1856–1860, letter from Dr. Corrigan to the Secretary to Lunatic Asylums Commissioners, 30 June 1858; J. Lalor, *Observations on the Offices of Resident and Visiting Physicians of District Lunatic Asylums in Ireland* (Dublin: J. M. O'Toole, 1860).

44 *Forty-second Report of Lunacy Inspectors*, H. C. 1893–94 [C. 7125] xlvi, p. 10.

45 Finnane, 'Irish Psychiatry. Part 1', p. 308.

46 *Wexford Lunatic Asylum. Returns of the Names of the Governors of the Wexford Lunatic Asylum*, H. C. 1867–68 [442] lv.

47 Finnane, 'Irish Psychiatry. Part 1', p. 311.

48 For example, Dr William Murphy, who was appointed to Killarney Lunatic Asylum in March 1871, had been the workhouse medical officer, see *Freeman's Journal* (13 March 1871).

49 G. Jones, '"Strike Out Boldly for the Prizes that are Available to You": Medical Emigration from Ireland 1860–1905', *Medical History*, 54:1 (2010), 55–74.

50 *Evening Herald* (4 December 1936); *Irish Press* (5 December 1936); *Irish Times* (7 December 1936).

51 *Irish Times* (3 July 1948); *Irish Independent* (28 June 1948).

52 Finnane, 'Irish Psychiatry. Part 1', p. 308.

53 Scull, *Most Solitary of Afflictions*, p. 249.

54 Vaughan, 'Ireland c.1870', p. 741.

55 *Irish Times* (16 October 1919).

56 *Sixth Report of Lunacy Inspectors*, H. C. 1852–3 [1653] xli, p. 29.

57 Finnane, *Insanity and the Insane*, p. 177.

58 J. Conolly, *On the Construction and Government of Lunatic Asylums* (London, Churchill, 1847), p. 83; A. Suzuki, 'The Politics and Ideology of Non-Restraint: the Case of the Hanwell Asylum', *Medical History*, 39 (1995), 1–17.

59 *Returns relating to District Lunatic Asylums in Ireland*, 1833 [695] xxxiv, p. 21.

60 Cherry, *Mental Health Care in Modern England*, p. 101; Melling and Forsythe, *The Politics of Madness*, p. 56.

61 DPH, CLA Minute Book, 21 October 1846.

62 L. D. Smith, 'Behind Closed Doors: Lunatic Asylum Keepers, 1800–1860', *Social History of Medicine*, 1 (1988), 301–328, 307.

63 Melling and Forsythe, *The Politics of Madness*, p. 57. For example, see DPH, CLA Minute Book, 9 January 1885.

64 19 &20 Vict. c.99 (1856).

65 DPH, CLA Minute Book, 13 January 1846; 18 November 1846.

66 *Ibid.*, 18 September 1850.

67 *Ibid.*, 13 December 1899.

68 *Ibid.*, 10 April 1885.

69 *Ibid.*, 9 January 1885, see also Melling and Forsythe, *The Politics of Madness*, p. 57.

70 *Fifteenth Report of Lunacy Inspectors*, H. C. 1866 [3721] xxxii, p. 8; *Freeman's Journal* (8 September 1871).

71 *Freeman's Journal* (9 January 1877); (14 September 1871).

72 *Freeman's Journal* (14 September 1871).

73 *Freeman's Journal* (17 November 1871).

74 Ó Gráda, *Ireland. A New Economic History*, pp. 236–237.

75 *Nineteenth Report of Lunacy Inspectors*, H. C. 1870 [202] xxxiv.

76 *Freeman's Journal* (8 June 1872); (7 June 1875).

77 Melling and Forsythe, *The Politics of Madness*, p. 57.

78 Vaughan, 'Ireland c.1870', p. 779

79 Cherry, *Mental Health Care in Modern England*, p. 102; Melling and Forsythe, *The Politics of Madness*, p. 57.

80 *Freeman's Journal* (18 June 1873).

81 *Freeman's Journal* (30 April 1877).

82 Finnane, *Insanity and the Insane*, p. 181.

83 D. Bates, 'Keepers to Nurses? A History of the Irish Asylum Workers' Trade Union 1917–1924' (MA dissertation, University College Dublin, 2010), pp. 31–38.

84 Finnane, 'Irish Psychiatry, Part 1', p. 309; DPH, CLA Minute Book, September 1898.

85 *Freeman's Journal* (18 March 1878).

86 D. Bates, 'Keepers to Nurses?', p. 4.

87 SPH, ELA Case Book, 8 January 1891-23 October 1892, Patrick B.

88 For examples, see SPH, ELA Letter Book Thomas Drapes to the Inspectors of Lunatics, 2 January 1885; 10 February 1886; 26 July 1887, 7 August 1888.

89 *Fourteenth Report of Lunacy Inspectors*, H. C. 1865 [3556] xxi, p. 132.

90 DPH, CLA Minute Book, 10 August 1883; 8 August 1890; 9 October 1891.

91 *Ibid.*, 12 August 1892.

92 *Ibid.*, 18 February 1888.

93 *Ibid.*, 10 January 1873.

94 *Ibid.*, CLA Minute Book, 21 November 1878.

95 M. Luddy, *Women and Philanthropy in Nineteenth-Century Ireland* (Cambridge: Cambridge University Press, 1995), pp. 21–67.

96 DPH, CLA Minute Book, September 1899–March 1900.

97 J. Conolly, *On the Construction and Government of Lunatic Asylums* (London: Churchill, 1847); Suzuki, 'The Politics and Ideology of Non-Restraint', 12.

98 SPH, ELA Letter Book, Joseph Edmundson to Inspectors of Lunatics, 12 April 1876; 20 January 1883.

99 DPH, CLA Minute Book, 11 September 1885.

100 *Fifty-first Report of Lunacy Inspectors*, H. C. 1902 [1265] xl, p. xxvi.

101 DPH, CLA Minute Book, 21 March 1884.

102 Bates, 'Keepers to Nurses?', pp. 13–23.

103 *Ibid.*, pp. 31–41.

104 Scull, *The Most Solitary of Afflictions*; Digby, *York Retreat*.

105 Digby, *York Retreat*.

106 Digby, 'Moral Treatment at the Retreat', p. 52.

107 *Ibid.*; Melling and Forsythe, *The Politics of Madness*, p. 49.

108 Digby, 'Moral Treatment at the Retreat, p. 53.

109 R. Porter, *Mind-Forg'd Manacles, A History of Madness in England from the Restoration to the Regency* (London: The Athlone Press, 1987), pp. 222–225.

110 Digby, 'Moral Treatment at the Retreat', p. 53. For some examples of the extensive literature on moral management see Digby, *York Retreat*, p. 33; Digby, 'Moral Treatment at the Retreat', pp. 52–72;. Digby, 'Changes in the Asylum', 218–239; M. Foucault, *Madness and Civilisation: A History of Insanity in the Age of Reason* (London: Tavistock, 1967), pp. 244–245; Porter, *Mind-Forg'd Manacles*, pp. 222–225; R. Porter, 'The Rage of Party: a Glorious Revolution in English Psychiatry?', *Medical History*, 27 (1983), 35–50; A. Scull, 'The Domestication of Madness', *Medical History*, 27 (1983), 233–248; A. Scull, 'Moral Treatment Reconsidered: Some Sociological Comments on an Episode in the History of British Psychiatry', in Scull (ed.), *Madhouses, Mad-Doctors and Madmen*, pp. 105–120; N. Tomes, 'The Great Restraint Controversy: a Comparative Perspective on Anglo-American Psychiatry in the Nineteenth Century', in Bynum, Porter and Shepherd (eds), *Anatomy of Madness III*, pp. 190–228.

111 Kelly, 'Dr William Saunders Hallaran', 79–84; C. S. Breathnach, 'Hallaran's Circulating Swing', *History of Psychiatry*, 21:1 (March, 2010), 79–84.

112 W. S. Hallaran, *An Enquiry into the Causes Producing the Extraordinary Addition to the Number of Insane together with Extended Observations on the Cure of Insanity with Hints as to the Better Management of Public Asylums for Insane Persons* (Cork, 1810).

The second edition was published as *Practical Observations on the Causes and Cure of Insanity* (Cork, 1818).

113 Hallaran, *Practical Observations on the Causes and Cure of Insanity*, p. 88.

114 M. Ignatieff, *A Just Measure of Pain: The Penitentiary in the Industrial Revolution, 1750–1850* (London and New York: Macmillan, 1978), pp. 143–173.

115 Suzuki, 'The Politics and Ideology of Non-Restraint', 1–17.

116 *Report of Prison Inspectors*, H. C. 1824 [294] xxii, p. 11.

117 *Sixth Report of Prison Inspectors*, H. C. 1828 [68] xii, p. 11.

118 Suzuki, 'The Politics and Ideology of Non-Restraint', 1–17.

119 *Twentieth Report of Prison Inspectors*, H. C. 1842 [377] xxii, p. 95.

120 *Eight Report of Prison Inspectors*, H. C. 1857 [22.53.II] xvii, p. 12.

121 For example, see SPH, ELA Case Book, 8 January 1891–23 October 1892 Mary C.; Case Book, 10 January 1893–17 November 1894 Mary J., Ellen C.

122 For example, see SPH, ELA Case Book, 23 January 1895–25 December 1896 Winifred K.

123 SPH, ELA Case Book, 8 January 1891–23 October 1892, and Case Book, 10 January 1893–17 November 1894, Mary C.

124 *Third Report of Lunacy Inspectors*, H. C. 1847 [820] xvii, pp. 30–33.

125 DPH, CLA General Register, 1857–76.

126 *Eight Report of Lunacy Inspectors*, H. C. 1857 session 2, [2253] xvii, p. 12; Digby, 'Moral Treatment at the Retreat', p. 65.

127 *Eighth Report of Lunacy Inspectors*, H. C. 1857 session 2, [2253] xvii, appendix G.

128 DPH, CLA General Register, 1857–76.

129 Digby, 'Moral Treatment at the Retreat', p. 65.

130 For example, see Cherry, *Mental Health Care in Modern England*, p. 44; Charlotte MacKenzie, *Psychiatry for the Rich. A History of Ticehurst Private Asylum* (London and New York: Routledge, 1992), pp. 184–185.

131 For example, see SPH, ELA Case Book, 8 January 1891–23 October 1892, Mary C; T. Drapes, 'Hyoscin in Insanity', *British Medical Journal*, 1:1478 (1889), 942.

132 MacKenzie, *Psychiatry for the Rich*, p. 185.

133 DPH, CLA General Register, 1857–76.

134 *Fourth Report of Lunacy Inspectors*, H. C. 1849 [1054] xxiii, p. 5.

135 *Ibid.*, p.184; DPH, CLA General Register of Patients, 1857–76.

136 *Eleventh Report of Lunacy Inspectors*, H. C. 1862 [2975] xxiii, p. 22.

137 Finnane, *Insanity and the Insane*, pp. 202–203.

138 *Fourteenth Report of Lunacy Inspectors*, H. C. 1865 [3556] xxi, pp.12–13.

139 *Second Report of Lunacy Inspectors*, 1846 [736] xxii, p. 20.

140 *Ibid.*

141 *Ibid.*, p. 57.

142 E. Maziere Courtenay, 'On Irish Asylum Dietary', *JMS*, 32:137 (1886), 16–22.

143 *Twelfth Report of Lunacy Inspectors*, 1863 [3209] xx, p. 88.

144 *Ibid.*

145 SPH, ELA Case Book, 4 January 1897–20 December 1898, James K.

146 *Thirtieth Report of Lunacy Inspectors*, 1881 [C.2933], xlviii, p. 78.

147 Courtenay, 'On Irish Asylum Dietary', 21.

148 *Ibid.*

149 *Ibid.*

150 SPH, ELA Case Book, 8 January 1891–23 October 1892, Mary S.; Case Book, 10 January 1893–17 November 1894, James K.

151 *Fortieth Report of Lunacy Inspectors*, H. C. 1890–91 [C. 6503] xxxvi, p. 120; *Forty-first Report of Lunacy Inspectors*, H. C. 1892 [6803] xl, p. 101

152 *Forty-Ninth Report of Lunacy Inspectors*, H. C. 1900 [Cd.312] xxxvii, p. 119.

153 *Forty-third Report of Lunacy Inspectors*, H. C. 1894 [C.7466] xliii, p. 103

154 *Forty-Ninth Report of Lunacy Inspectors*, H. C. 1900 [Cd. 312] xxxvii, p. 119.

155 *Sixteenth Report of Prison Inspectors*, H. C. 1837–38 [186] xxix, p. 10.

156 *Ibid.*, pp. 36–37.

157 Busfield, 'The Female Malady?', 259–277.

158 *Sixteenth Report of Prison Inspectors*, H. C. 1837-38 [186] xxix, p. 10.

159 *Fifteenth Report of Prison Inspectors*, H. C. 1837 [123] xxxi, p. 9.

160 *Ibid.*, p. 31.

161 *Twenty-fourth Report of Lunacy Inspectors*, H. C. 1875 [1293] xxxiii, p. 9.

162 *Twenty-first Report of Prison Inspectors*, H. C. 1843 [462] xxvii, p. 88.

163 DPH, CLA Minute Book, 4 August 1852, 22 December 1852; *Sixteenth Report of Lunacy Inspectors*, H. C. 1867 [3894] xviii, p. 6.

164 Cherry, *Mental Health Care in Modern England*, p. 67.

165 SPH, ELA Case Book, 23 January 1895–25 December 1896, Ellen C.

166 Digby, 'Moral Treatment at the Retreat', p. 63; N. Tranter, *Sport, Economy and Society in Britain 1750–1914* (Cambridge: Cambridge University Press, 1998), p. 57.

167 DPH, CLA Minute Book, 21 December 1842; 17 May 1843; 21 June 1843; 17 December 1860.

168 *Ibid.*, 18 April 1849.

169 *Ibid.*, 10 April 1891; 8 April 1881.

170 *Ibid.*, 17 February 1862.

171 H. Cameron Lyster, *An Irish Parish in Changing Days* (London: Griffiths, 1933), p. 91.

172 Porter, *Mind-Forg'd Manacles*, p. 268.

173 *Ibid.*

174 Walsh, 'Race, Religion and Insanity', p. 229; J. Donat, 'Medicine and Religion: On the Physical and Mental Disorders that Accompanied the Ulster Revival of 1859', in W. F. Bynum, R. Porter, and M. Shepherd (eds), *Anatomy of Madness: Essays in the History of Psychiatry*, III (London: Tavistock, 1987), pp. 125–150; Michael, *Care and Treatment of the Mentally Ill in North Wales*, p. 103.

175 *Report of Lunacy Inspectors*, H. C. 1845 [645] xxvi, pp. 19–21.

176 *Report of Lunacy Inspectors*, H. C. 1845 [645] xxvi, p. 59.

177 *Ibid.*

178 *Report of Lunacy Inspectors*, H. C. 1844 [567] xxx, pp. 1–7.

179 8&9 Vic. c.107, s.24 (1845).

180 *Report of Lunacy Inspectors*, H. C. 1845 [645] xxvi, p. 38.

181 NLI Larcom Papers, Ms 7775, Amendment to Privy Council Rules, 14 October 1853.

182 P. Prior and D. V. Griffins, 'The Chaplaincy Question: The Lord Lieutenant of Ireland versus the Belfast Lunatic Asylum, *Éire-Ireland*, 33:2&3 (1997), 137–152; Walsh, 'Race, Religion and Insanity', p. 228.

183 Ó Cathaoir, 'The Poor Law in County Carlow, 1838–1923', pp. 688–689.

184 DPH, CLA Minute Book, 20 August 1845.

185 *Ibid.*, 17 September 1845.

186 *Ibid.*

187 DPH, CLA Minute Book, 20 December 1843.

188 *Ibid.*, 15 August 1855.

189 Chapter two.

190 DPH, CLA Minute Book, 24 July 1871.

191 The analysis of patients' religion is limited by the defects of the admission registers. Members of the Church of Ireland, Presbyterians and Wesleyans were not always identified separately. Between 1846 and 1894, patients' religion was not recorded.

192 Malcolm, '"The House of Strident Shadows"', p. 179.

193 DPH, CLA Minute Book, 9 September 1892.

194 Sometimes the relevant doctor was absent and the assessment was carried out the following day, for example see SPH, ELA Case Book, 8 January 1891–23 October 1892, Mary C.

195 Dawson, 'Note of a New Case-book Form', 268; D. F. Rambaut, 'Case-taking in Large Asylums', *JMS*, 49: 203 (January, 1903), 45.

196 Dawson, 'Note of a New Case-book Form', 268.

197 For examples, see SPH, ELA Case Book 10 January 1893–17 November 1894; James K. Casebook, 23 January 1895–25 December 1896, Winfred K.

198 SPH, ELA Case Book, 8 January 1891–23 October 1892, Patrick B., Mary S.

199 SPH, ELA Case Book, 8 January 1891–23 October 1892, Bridget D., Mary C.; Case Book, 10 January 1893–17 November 1894, Julia T., Maryanne W.

200 SPH, ELA Case Book, 10 January 1893–17 November 1894, Anne B.

201 SPH, ELA Case Book, 23 January 1895–23 December 1896, Anne E.

202 Marland, *Dangerous Motherhood*, p. 97.

203 Showalter, *The Female Malady*, p. 86.

204 D. H. Tuke, 'Observations on the Treatment of Insanity when Food Refusal of Food is a Prominent Symptom', *JMS*, 4:23 (October, 1857), 29.

205 SPH, ELA Case Book, 8 January 1891–23 October 1892, Mary C.

206 DPH, CLA Case Book, January 1906–January 1908, John. N.

207 Tuke, 'On Forced Alimentation', *JMS* 4:24 (1858), 204.

208 DPH, CLA General Register, 1857–76.

209 Tuke, 'On Forced Alimentation', 221.

210 *Ibid.*, 205.

211 Tuke, 'Observations on the Treatment of Insanity', 40.

212 Tuke, 'On Forced Alimentation', 204.

213 National Archives of Scotland, HH35/5 Minutes of the Prison Commission of Scotland, March 1909 to December 1919, Memo by Professor Thomas R Fraser, Medical Officer to the Prison Commission of Scotland, December 1909.

214 A. Beveridge, 'Madness in Victorian Edinburgh: A Study of Patients Admitted to the Royal Edinburgh Asylum under Thomas Clouston, 1873–1908 Part 2', *History of Psychiatry*, 6 (1995), 133–156, 134.

215 Melling and Forsythe, *The Politics of Madness*, p. 71; MacKenzie, *Psychiatry for the Rich*, p. 184.

216 No cause was ascribed to 58 per cent (3205) of admissions.

217 I. Dowbiggin, 'Degeneration and Hereditarianism in French Mental Medicine, 1840–90: Psychiatric Theory as Ideological Adaptation', in W. F. Bynum, R. Porter and M. Shepherd (eds), *Anatomy of Madness: Essays in the History of Psychiatry*, I (London: Tavistock, 1985), pp. 189–223; G. Jones, 'Eugenics in Ireland: the Belfast Eugenics Society, 1911–15', *Irish Historical Studies*, 28 (1992), 81–95; Scull, MacKenzie and Hervey (eds), *Masters of Bedlam*, p. 253.

218 M. Levine-Clark, '"Embarrassed Circumstances": Gender, Poverty and Insanity in the West-Riding of England in the Early Victorian Years', in Andrews and Digby (eds), *Sex and Seclusion*, pp. 123–148; Wright, 'Delusions of Gender?'; M. S. Micale, 'Hysteria Male/Hysteria Female: Reflections on Comparative Gender Construction in Nineteenth-Century France and Britain', in M. Benjamin (ed.), *Science and Sensibility. Gender and Scientific Enquiry, 1780–1945* (Oxford: Oxford University Press, 1991), pp. 200–242.

219 Chapter two.

220 DPH, CLA Male Case Book, January 1906–January 1908, Thomas M.

221 *Ibid.*, John George C.

222 Wright, 'Delusions of Gender', p. 162.

223 DPH, CLA Male Case Book, January 1906–January 1908, John George C.

224 *Ibid.*

225 Micale, 'Hysteria Male/Hysteria Female', p. 208.

226 M. S. Thompson, 'The Wages of Sin: The Problem of Alcoholism and General Paralysis in Nineteenth-Century Edinburgh', in W. F. Bynum, R. Porter, and M. Shepherd (eds), *The Anatomy of Madness*, III (London: Tavistock, 1987), pp. 316–340.

227 M. Luddy, 'An Outcast Community: the "Wrens" of the Curragh', *Women's History Review*, 1 (1992), 341–355.

228 J. F. Duncan, 'Cases of Syphilitic Insanity and Epilepsy', *DJMS*, 35 (1863), 35–36; T. Reade, 'Tertiary Syphilis – Third Series; the Growth, Progress and Present State of Knowledge of Nervous Syphilitic Diseases' *DJMS*, 36 (1863), 324–338.

229 Drapes, 'On the Alleged Increase of Insanity in Ireland', 528.

230 Fleetwood Churchill, 'On the Mental Disorders of Pregnancy and Childbirth', *DQJMS*, 9 (1850), 39; Dr Lindsey, 'On Puerperal Conditions', *DQJMS*, 43 (1872), 80–82; F. V. McDowell, 'Epileptic Puerperal Convulsions and Puerperal Mania treated by Chloral Hydrate', *DQJMS*, 43 (1872), 464–465; D. H. Scott, 'Puerperal Mania: Beneficial Effects of Belladonna', *DQJMS*, 13 (1838), 442–446; NAI, CSO CRF Wexford 1860.

231 Marland, 'At Home with Puerperal Mania', pp. 45–65.

232 DPH, CLA Male Case Book, January 1906–January 1908, John O'C.

233 Andrews and Digby, 'Gender and Class in the Historiography of British and Irish Psychiatry', in Andrews and Digby (eds), *Sex and Seclusion, Class and Custody*, pp. 7–44.

234   DPH, CLA Male Case Book, January 1906–January 1908, James S.

235   NAI, CSO CRF, Wexford 1851.

236   DPH, CLA Discharge Registers, 1846–1900; A. Shepherd and D. Wright, 'Madness, Suicide and the Victorian Asylum: Attempted Self-Murder in the Age of Non-Restraint', *Medical History*, 46 (2002), 175–196.

237   DPH, CLA Male Case Book, January 1906–January 1908, John W. and Martin D.

238   G. E. Berrios, 'Delusions as 'Wrong Beliefs': A Conceptual History', *British Journal of Psychiatry*, 159 (supplement 14) (1991), 6–13, 6.

239   *Ibid.*, 10.

240   *Ibid.*

241   Beveridge, 'Madness in Victorian Edinburgh'.

242   R. Mojtabai, 'Delusions as Error: the History of a Metaphor', *History of Psychiatry*, 11 (2000), 3–14; I. Dowbiggan, 'Delusional Diagnosis? The History of Paranoia as a Disease Concept in the Modern Era', *History of Psychiatry*, 11 (2000), 37–69.

243   DPH, CLA Male Case Book, January 1906–January 1908; Berrios, 'Delusions as "Wrong Beliefs"', 6.

244   Wright, 'Delusions of Gender?', p. 153.

245   Houston, *Madness and Society in Eighteenth Century Scotland*; Suzuki, *Madness at Home*, p. 180.

246   SPH, ELA Case Book, 8 January 1891–23 October 1892, Bridget D.

247   J. Bourke, 'Effeminacy, Ethnicity and the End of Trauma: The Sufferings of "Shell-Shocked" Men in Great Britain and Ireland, 1914–39', *Journal of Contemporary History*, 35 (2000), 57–69.

248   *Twenty-fifth Report of Lunacy Inspectors*, H. C. 1876 [1496] xxxiii, p. 9.

249   M. Guyatt, 'A Semblance of Home: Mental Asylum Interiors, 1880–1914', in S. McKellar and P. Sparke (eds), *Interior Design and Identity* (Manchester: Manchester University Press, 2004), pp. 48–71.

250   *Tenth General Report of Lunacy Inspectors*, H. C. 1861 [2901] xxvii, p. 3.

251   DPH, CLA Minute Book, 14 April 1880, 13 May 1881.

252   *Ibid.*

253   *Thirteenth Report of Lunacy Inspectors*, H. C. 1864 [3369] xxiii, p. 18.

254   Chapter five.

255   *Twenty-fifth Report of Lunacy Inspectors*, H. C. 1876 [1496] xxxiii, p. 7.

256   Chapter five.

257   *Irish Times* (24 November 1866); WCA, WX/BG 87/1/3/1 Enniscorthy Dispensary Minute Book, November–December 1866.

258   *Twenty-first Report of Lunacy Inspectors*, H. C. 1872 [647] xxvii, p. 12.

259   *Ibid.*; *Report of Lunacy Inspectors*, H. C. 1876 [1496] xxxiii, p. 12.

260   G. Jones, *'Captain of all these men of death' The History of Tuberculosis in Nineteenth and Twentieth Century Ireland* (Amsterdam and New York: Rodolpi, 2001), pp. 1–28, p. 45.

261   DPH, CLA Minute Book, 13 April 1883.

262   *Ibid.*, 10 October 1884.

263   *Ibid.*, 10 September 1886.

264   *Ibid.*, 13 April, 14 September and 10 October 1888.

265   *Ibid.*, 9 November 1888.

266   *Ibid.*, 21 December 1888.

267   *Ibid.*, 11 January 1889.

268   *Ibid.*, 10 January 1890.

269   *Ibid.*, 12 September 1890.

270   *Fortieth Report of Lunacy Inspectors*, H. C. 1890–91 [6503] xxxvi, p. 119.

271   Chapter three.

272   *Sixty-seventh Report of Lunacy Inspectors*, H. C. 1919 [32] xxv, p. xii; T. S. McClaughry, 'Influenza as a Factor in the Increase of Insanity in Ireland', *DJMS*, 302 (1897), 108–114.

8

Conclusion

The introduction of a state-funded asylum system to Ireland in 1817 occurred in the context of increased state intervention in social, medical and welfare services following the 1800 Act of Union. Its introduction reflected medical, social and political support for the institutionalisation of the mentally ill. Nonetheless, the 'politics of insanity' and of institutional provision were complex.[1] Finnane's analysis of the high politics of asylum governance identified a centralised structure that reflected the ambivalent attitude within British government towards Irish landlords' capacity for local government. This study of one asylum district in the southeast of Ireland has largely supported such a characterisation of central policy. The comparative assessment of different powers invested in the Irish lunacy inspectors and the English and Scottish commissioners in lunacy, and of the degree of autonomy granted to asylum boards highlights the colonial nature of Irish asylum governance.

A key concern of this study has been to interrogate local protagonists' interactions with these centralised structures thereby assessing how civil society negotiated the institutionalisation of the mentally ill. What has emerged is the extent to which, in local contexts, protagonists – magistrates, poor law guardians, dispensary and asylum doctors, and families – resisted and manoeuvred around the boundaries of the formal, centralised asylum and workhouse systems and the associated legislative frameworks. The conflict over the renovation of Carlow asylum during the last three decades of the nineteenth century demonstrates that asylum governors regularly resisted the lunacy inspectors' requests and the board of control's demands for structural improvements to asylums. This resistance was founded on a desire to reduce costs to local ratepayers and upon resentment at the intrusion of central agents in local affairs. Asylum governors were relatively successful in delaying and obstructing, particularly when the inspectorate went into decline in the 1880s. In 1898, the Local Government Act restructured asylum management committees, putting in place a management system that was more representative of the local ratepayers. These committees were better positioned to delay renovation programmes and were even more effective in resisting expensive but necessary building programmes.

The politics of the family and its influence on asylum admissions and discharges is a central theme of this study. As recent literature has convincingly argued, the family identified mental illness. The population's access to different forms of care within the institutional marketplace was relatively limited and, for a significant number of the mentally ill, this resulted in institutionalisation in asylums. Families by no means enjoyed full autonomy when seeking institutional provision. They were obliged to negotiate with other actors, including police, magistrates and dispensary doctors, and to operate within specific legal frameworks. These frameworks were deficient in many respects. As a consequence of the difficulties faced in securing ordinary admissions into overcrowded asylums, protagonists engaged with the asylum through the petty session courts under the dangerous lunatic legislation. Families were sometimes advised by other agents to adopt this route. Moreover, the failure to remove 'destitution' as the criteria for admission into workhouses complicated the situation further. The mentally ill were not entitled to relief on the grounds of sickness and the admission criteria limited the integration of the two welfare systems. These factors contributed to the increase in dangerous lunatic certifications, particularly after the 1870s, when the asylums were increasingly overcrowded. Members of civil society used the dangerous lunatic acts to circumnavigate a series of legislative inadequacies and inconsistencies in the governance of the Irish poor law and lunacy throughout the period.

Certification of a relative in public courts was for many families a final and, sometimes, distressing resort. While dangerous behaviour was embellished to secure certification, the evidence indicates that households managed difficult relatives at home until especially problematic behaviour such as pyromania, suicide and violence, erupted. The circumstances surrounding certification varied between families, and were determined by internal family politics that were defined by gender, class and marital status. As Suzuki has argued, families operated simultaneously as economic and emotional units, and the certification of a relative was the point when a family's capacity to withstand the emotional, economic and social consequences of a relative's behaviour had been exceeded.[2] The social origins of individuals admitted into Carlow and Enniscorthy asylums indicate that most patients emerged from poor, although not necessarily destitute households. Nonetheless, a significant minority were alone (without family) and destitute and were moved between local asylums and workhouses. The admission of small numbers of paying patients did not fundamentally alter this profile. Anxieties around the threat a person's mental collapse presented to family property and security informed the decision to certify a relative. However, there is limited evidence to suggest that certification in the southeast was explicitly linked to changes in patterns of land inheritance or with outbreaks of agrarian violence, factors Walsh identified in her work on Ballinsaloe asylum in the west of Ireland. At Carlow and Enniscorthy asylums patients arrived in extremely poor physical condition, highlighting the level of poverty and distress in households. The evidence also points to a degree of neglect. Patients' occupational profiles also confirm the relative poverty of households.

The social profile of patients demonstrates that there emerged a gender bias in patterns of admissions during the second half of the nineteenth century. Scholars of Irish psychiatry have noted the greater vulnerability of men to institutionalisation and this study has revealed that this occurred in the latter half of the nineteenth century and was only partially a result of post-Famine demographic changes. Gender was important in determining the method of certification, and greater numbers of men were certified through the petty session hearings, reflecting an increased anxiety around male violence in later nineteenth-century Ireland. Inside the asylum, gender influenced the experiences of patients and staff. For both staff and patients, life inside asylums was heavily disciplined and regimented. Female staff and patients were obliged to maintain rules of domesticity and respectability in spite of their different status within asylums. Thus, life for attendants and nurses living in these asylums was difficult. Working in relatively modest-sized asylums such as Enniscorthy and Carlow asylums ensured staff did not struggle with huge number of charges. Nonetheless, crowded and insanitary conditions and disruptive building programmes made the task of managing patients more difficult and fraught with the potential for violence.

This study has also looked at the various mechanisms by which asylums became established within local contexts. As the conflicts surrounding the subsequent division of the original Carlow asylum district and over the location of new institutions, such as Enniscorthy asylum, demonstrated, the asylums themselves became symbols of progress and paternalism in local communities. Consequently, there continued to be local enthusiasm for asylum building in spite of the constant drain on local rates. Kildare grand jury's demand for a separate institution suggests that this continued into the late nineteenth century in a region with a sufficiently robust local tax base. It has also been argued that by putting 'insanity on display' during petty session hearings, society not only publicly disciplined individuals, but the process provided the public with a medical and legal framework in which to situate certain behaviour. Prior, Walsh, Malcolm and Finnane have argued that the dangerous lunatic legislation was 'misused' and made an explicit connection between criminality and insanity. It has been argued here that the certification procedure also assisted in the establishment of asylums and medicine within a social distance.

While the language of certification emphasised 'violence', the warrants from the period 1838 to 1868 indicate that both lay people and doctors reported environmental factors and changes to patients' physical and internal states as psychiatric aetiologies. There is evidence that families and dispensary doctors pathologised patients' internal life and emotional states. The sources reveal further evidence of the impact that emigration had on nineteenth-century life and on patterns of certification. While relatives remaining in Ireland could fall prey to mental illness due to the emotional consequence of the emigration of family members, asylum doctors also had to cope with problems associated with discharging recovered patients whose families had moved elsewhere. Emigration featured in late nineteenth-century debates on high rates of institutionalisation in Ireland. By the last third of the nineteenth century, asylum doctors and other alienists invoked theories of degeneracy and hereditary insanity to explain high certification rates. Factors that were regarded as peculiar to Ireland, including high levels of political agitation, extreme poverty and emigration, were seen as placing pressure upon minds already adversely affected through hereditary influences. This was reflected in the changes to the format of asylum casebooks and the construction of clinical histories. These sought to identify hereditary insanity and focused on patients' physical condition. The impact changing medical theories had on patients' treatment inside the asylums was less apparent. Work, discipline and diet continued to occupy a central position within asylum regimes that were shaped by the ideologies of moral management and focused on maintaining a well-ordered, regulated institution.

This book has revealed the ways in which mental illness collapsed and compromised professional, welfare and private boundaries. The private worlds of poorer households were brought into the public domain when mental illness in families was exposed and certification was sought in petty session courts. Legal, lay and medical jurisdictions were compromised and fought over in efforts to establish clearly defined limits to expertise and influence. The contestation of boundaries between destitution and poverty, danger and harmlessness and curable and chronic determined the specific functions of workhouses and asylums in the confinement of mental illness and the social status of individuals within these institutions.

Notes

1   Melling and Forsythe, *The Politics of Madness*, p. 206.
2   Suzuki, *Madness at Home*, p. 180.

Select bibliography

Manuscript sources

Carlow County Library, Archives
Carlow Board of Guardians Records: Minute Books, 1846–1899.

Kildare Local Authority Archives
Athy Board of Guardians Records: Indoor Relief Register, 1888–1890.
Athy Board of Guardians Records: Minute Books, 1888.
Naas Board of Guardians Records: Minute Books, 1839–1922.

National Archives of Ireland
Office of the Lunatic Asylum Records: Minute Book, 1856–1896?; Letter Books,
    1874–1899; Rough Letter Book, 1848–1920.
Chief Secretary Office, Registered Papers.
Criminal Reference Files: Wexford, Kildare, Carlow and Kilkenny, 1839–1870.
Convict Department, Criminal Lunatic Books, 1843–59.
Petty Session Order Books: County Carlow Petty Session Order Books, 1910–
    1922. Athy Court County Kildare Petty Sessions Order Books, 1918–1919.
Carlow District Court Circulars to Petty Sessions.
Rathangan Court Petty Sessions Order Books, 1869–1873.

St Dympna's Psychiatric Hospital, Carlow
Records of Carlow District Lunatic Asylum:
Minutes of the Board of Governors, 13 February 1832–10 June 1925 (19 vols).
Rough Proceedings of the Board of Governors, 13 February 1832–June 1900 (4 vols).
Inspectors' Letter Book, September 1892–5 February [1925?].
Registers of Patient Admissions, May 1832–December 1922 (3 vols).

Register of Discharges, Removals and Deaths, January 1847–June 1900.
General Register of Patients, November 1857–April 1876.
Application for Admission, April 1832–November 1848.
Male Case Book, January 1906–January 1908.

St Senan's Psychiatric Hospital, Enniscorthy
Records of Wexford District Lunatic Asylum:
Proceedings of the Governors and Directors of Wexford District Lunatic Asylum,
    1867–1882; 1883–1898; 1898–1915.
Letter Books, 22 January 1868–January 1888.
Case Books, 1891–1900 (5 vols).
File of miscellaneous letters.

Wexford County Archive Service
Enniscorthy Board of Guardians Records: Minute Books, 1840–1900.
Dispensary Minute Books, [28 November 1854] –13 April 1897; 31 October 1900–
    24 October 1901; 31 October 1901–16 October 1902.

National Library of Ireland, Dublin
Larcom Papers.

Newspapers and journals
Carlow Sentinel
Carlow Post
Cork Examiner
Dublin Gazette
Dublin Journal of Medical Science
Dublin Times
Express
Freeman's Journal
Irish Times
Irish Builder
Journal of Mental Science
Journal of the Statistical and Social Inquiry Society in Ireland
Leinster Leader
Leinster Express
Nation

Reference works
Burke's Peerage and Baronetage (London: Harrison and Sons).
Byrne, J. O., *Compendium of Irish Sanitary Law* (Dublin: William McGee, 1875).

Birmingham, C. L., *Handbook of Irish Sanitary Law* (Dublin: Browne and Nolan, 1905).

Connolly, S. J. (ed.), *The Oxford Companion to Irish History* (Oxford: Oxford University Press, 2nd edn., 2002).

Constabulary Manual; or Guide to the Discharge of Police Duties (Dublin: A. Thom, 1870).

County Kildare Gaol, Bye-laws, Rules and Regulations made by the Board of Superintendence (Naas, 1861).

Dictionary of Irish Architects, 1720–1940 (www.dia.ie).

District Directory and Almanac for 1888 for the counties of Carlow, Kildare and Queen's County and portions of Wicklow and Kilkenny (Carlow, 1888).

Instruction Book for the Government and Guidance of Dublin Metropolitan Police (Dublin: A. Thom, 1879).

Hansard Parliamentary Debates.

Kilkenny City and County Guide and Directory (Dublin: Sealy, Bryers and Walker, 1884).

Lewis, S., *A Topographical Dictionary of Ireland, I and II* (London: S. Lewis and Co., 1837).

McGuire, J. and Quinn, J. (eds), *Dictionary of Irish Biography* (Cambridge: Cambridge University Press, 2009).

Mooney, T. A., *Compendium of the Irish Poor Law* (Dublin: A. Thom, 1887).

Nationalist and Leinster Times; District Directory and Almanac for 1888 for the counties of Carlow, Kildare and Queen's County and portions of Wicklow and Kilkenny (Carlow, 1888).

Oxford Dictionary of National Biography (Oxford: Oxford University Press, 2004).

Reid, A. *The Irish Constable's Guide* (Dublin: A. Thom, 1880).

Rules for the Regulation and Guidance of Attendants and Servants and other Persons in the Service of Carlow District Asylum (Naas, 1898).

Slater's *National Commercial Directory of Ireland.*

Thom's *Irish Almanac and Official Directory of Ireland.*

Vaughan W. E. and Fitzpatrick A. J. (eds), *Irish Historical Statistics, Population 1821–1971* (Dublin: Royal Irish Academy, 1978).

Parliamentary papers

Annual Report of the Inspectors General of the Prisons of Ireland, 1826–44.

Annual Report of the Inspectors of Criminal, District and Private Lunatic Asylums in Ireland, 1844–1922.

Report from the Committee on Madhouses in England, 1814–15.

Report from the Select Committee on the Lunatic Poor in Ireland, with Minutes of Evidence, 1817.

Report from the Select Committee of the House of Lords appointed to Consider the State of the Lunatic Poor in Ireland, 1843.

Copy of Treasury Minute, dated 10 August 1855, Appointing a Commission for Inquiring into the Erection of District Lunatic Asylums in Ireland; of the Report of the said Commissioners, dated 14 December 1855; and of further Treasury Minute, dated 18 December 1855.

Report of the Royal Commissioners of Inquiry into the State of Lunatic Asylums and other Institutions for the Custody and Treatment of the Insane in Ireland, 1857–58.

Report and Minutes of Evidence of the Select Committee on Poor Law Union and Lunacy Inquiry (Ireland), 1878–79.

Report and Minutes of Evidence of the Select Committee on Lunacy Law, 1878.

First and Second Report of the Committee appointed by the Lord Lieutenant of Ireland on Lunacy Administration (Ireland), 1890–91.

Alleged Increasing Prevalence of Insanity in Ireland. Special Report from the Inspectors of Lunatics to the Chief Secretary, 1894.

Contemporary printed material

'Carlow District Lunatic Asylum', *Irish Builder*, 12:266 (15 October 1870).

'Insanity and Hospitals for the Insane', *Dublin Journal of Medical Science*, 12 (1851), 376–420.

'Lunatic Asylum, Enniscorthy', *Irish Builder*, 8:146 (15 January 1866).

'Lalor, J.' *Journal of Mental Science*, 32:139 (October, 1886), 462.

'Medical Superintendence of Insanity', *Dublin Journal of Medical Science*, 33 (1862), 259–267.

'Twentieth Annual Report by Dr White of the Carlow District Hospital of the Insane Poor for the year ending 31 March 1853', *Dublin Quarterly Journal of Medical Science*, 16 (Aug–Nov 1853), 391–393.

Annual Report of the Carlow Mechanic Institute (Carlow, 1853).

Comerford, M., *Collections Relating to the Diocese of Kildare and Leighlin* (Dublin: J. Duffy, 1886).

Conolly, J., *On the Construction and Government of Lunatic Asylums* (London: Churchill, 1847).

Corbett, W. J., 'The Increase of Insanity', *Fortnightly Review*, 61:362 (1897), 321–442.

Courtenay, E. Maziere, 'On Irish Asylum Dietary', *Journal of Mental Science*, 32:137 (1886), 16–22.

Dawson, W. R., 'Note on a New Case-book Form', *Journal of Mental Science*, 49:205 (April, 1903), 267–271.

Drapes, T., 'On the Alleged Increase of Insanity in Ireland', *Journal of Mental Science*, 40:171 (October, 1894), 519–548.

Drapes, T., 'Psychology in Ireland', *Dublin Journal of Medical Science*, 87 (1889), 109–116.

Drapes, T., 'Hyoscin in Insanity', *British Medical Journal*, 1:1478 (1889), 942.

Fogerty, W., 'On the Planning of Lunatic Asylums', *Irish Builder*, 9:172 (February 1867), 39–40.

Hallaran, W. S., *Practical Observations on the Causes and Cure of Insanity* (Cork, 1818).

Neilson Hancock, W., 'On the Report of the Irish Lunacy Inquiry Commissioners and the Policy of Extending the English Law for the Protection of Neglected Lunatics to Ireland', *Statistical and Social Inquiry Society of Ireland*, 7:6 (July 1879), 454–461.

Humphreys, N. A., 'The Alleged Increase of Insanity', *Journal of the Royal Statistical Society*, 70:2 (1907), 203–241.

J. C. B. 'Eighth Report of the Inspectors of Lunatic Asylums in Ireland', *Journal of Mental Science*, 24: 4 (January 1858), 257–276.

Kirkpatrick, T. P. C., *A Note on the History of the Care of the Insane in Ireland* (Dublin: University Press, 1931).

Lalor, J., 'Observations on the Size and Construction of Lunatic Asylums', *Journal of Mental Science*, 7:35 (October 1860).

Lalor, J., *Observations on the Offices of Resident and Visiting Physicians of District Lunatic Asylums in Ireland* (Dublin: J. M. O'Toole, 1860).

Lockhart Robertson, C., 'Further Notes on The Alleged Increase in Insanity', *Journal of Mental Science*, 16:76 (1871), 473–497.

Lockhart Robinson, C., 'The Alleged Increase in Insanity', *Journal of Mental Science*, 15:69 (April, 1869), 1–23.

Lyster, C., *An Irish Parish in Changing Days* (London: Griffiths, 1933).

MacCabe, F., 'On the Alleged Increase in Lunacy,' *Journal of Mental Science*, 15:71 (October, 1869), 363–366.

Rambaut, D. F., 'Case-taking in Large Asylums', *Journal of Mental Science*, 49:204 (January, 1903) 45–52.

Tuke, D. H., 'Observations on the Treatment of Insanity when Food Refusal of Food is a Prominent Symptom', *Journal of Mental Science*, 4:23 (October, 1857), 27–42.

Tuke, D. H., 'Alleged Increase in Insanity', *Journal of Mental Science*, 32:139 (October, 1886), 360–376.

Tuke, D. H., 'Alleged Increase of Insanity', *Journal of Mental Science*, 40:169 (April 1894), 219–231.

Tuke, D. H., 'Increase in Insanity in Ireland', *Journal of Mental Science*, 40:171 (October 1894), 549–561.

Secondary sources

Books

Andrews, J., 'They're in the Trade ... of Lunacy, they 'cannot interfere' – they say':
  *The Scottish Lunacy Commissioners and Lunacy Reform in Nineteenth-Century
  Scotland* (London: Wellcome Trust, 1998).

Bartlett, P., *The Poor Law of Lunacy: The Administration of Pauper Lunatics in
  Mid-Nineteenth-Century England* (London: Leicester University Press, 1999).

Bourke, A., *The Burning of Bridget Cleary. A True Story* (London: Pimlico, 1999).

Bourke, J., *Husbandry to Housewifery: Women, Economic Change and Housework in
  Ireland 1890–1914* (Oxford: Oxford University Press, 1993).

Burke, H., *The People and the Poor Law in Nineteenth-Century Ireland* (Dublin:
  Women's Education Bureau, 1987).

Burke, P., *Social History of Knowledge. From Gutenberg to Diderot* (Oxford: Polity,
  2000).

Busfield, J., *Men, Women and Madness: Understanding Gender and Mental Disorder*
  (Basingstoke: Macmillan Press, 1996).

Carroll-Burke, P., *Colonial Discipline, The Making of the Irish Convict System*
  (Dublin: Four Courts Press, 2000).

Cherry, S., *Mental Health Care in Modern England. The Norfolk Lunatic Asylum, St.
  Andrew's Hospital, 1810–1998* (Woodbridge: Boydell Press, 2003).

Clark, S., *Social Origins of the Irish Land War* (Princeton: Princeton University
  Press, 1978).

Coleborne, C., *Madness in the Family. Insanity and Institutions in the Australasian
  Colonial World, 1860–1914* (Houndmills: Palgrave Macmillan, 2010).

Connell, K. H., *Irish Peasant Society* (Oxford: Clarendon Press, 1968).

Connolly, S. J., *Religion and Society in Nineteenth Century Ireland* (Dundalk:
  Dundalgan Press, 1985).

Crossman, V., *Local Government in Nineteenth-Century Ireland* (Belfast: Institute of
  Irish Studies, 1994).

Crossman, V., *The Poor Law in Ireland 1838–1948* (Dundalk: Irish Economic and
  Social History Society, 2006).

Crossman, V., *Politics, Pauperism and Power in late Nineteenth-Century Ireland*
  (Manchester: Manchester University Press, 2006).

Crawford, E. M., *Counting the People. A Survey of Irish Censuses, 1813–1911*
  (Dublin: Four Courts Press, 2003).

Cullen, L., *Economic History of Ireland Since 1660* (London: Batsford, 2nd edn, 1972).

Curtis, L. P., *Apes and Angels. The Irishman in Victorian Caricature* (Washington and
  London: Smithsonian Institution Press, 1997).

Daly, M. E., *The Buffer State: The Historical Roots of the Department of the
  Environment* (Dublin: Institute of Public Administration, 1997).

Daly, M. E., *The Slow Failure: Population Decline and Independent Ireland, 1920–1973* (Madison: Wisconsin University Press, 2006).

Daly, M. E. and Dickson, D., *The Origins of Popular Literacy in Ireland: Language Changes and Educational Development 1700–1920* (Dublin: Department of Modern History, Trinity College Dublin and Department of Modern Irish History, University College Dublin, 1990).

Digby, A., *Madness, Morality and Medicine: A Study of the York Retreat, 1796–1914* (Cambridge: Cambridge University Press, 1985).

Dixon, T., *From Passions to Emotions: The Creation of a Secular Psychological Category* (Cambridge: Cambridge University Press, 2003).

Dowbiggan, I. R., *Inheriting Madness: Professionalisation and Psychiatric Knowledge in Nineteenth-Century France* (California and Oxford: University of California Press, 1991).

Driver, F., *Power and Pauperism: the Workhouse System* (Cambridge: Cambridge University Press, 1993).

Eigen, J. P., *Witnessing Insanity: Madness and Mad-Doctors in the English Court* (New Haven and London: Yale University Press, 1995).

Feingold, W., *The Revolt of the Tenantry: Local Government, 1872–1886* (Boston: Northeastern University Press, 1984).

Finnane, M., *Insanity and the Insane in Post-Famine Ireland* (London: Croom Helm, 1981).

Fissell, M. E., *Patient, Power and the Poor in Eighteenth Century Bristol* (Cambridge: Cambridge University Press, 1991).

Fitzpatrick, D., *Irish Emigration 1801–1921* (Dublin: Dundalgan Press, 1984).

Fitzpatrick, D., *Oceans of Consolation: Personal Accounts of Irish Migration to Australia* (Cork: Cork University Press, 1994).

Foster, R. F., *Modern Ireland 1600–1972* (London: Penguin Books, 1989).

Foucault, M., *Madness and Civilisation: A History of Insanity in the Age of Reason* (London: Tavistock, 1967).

Foucault, M., *The Birth of the Clinic: An Archaeology of Medical Perception*, trans. A. M. Sheridan (London: Tavistock, 1976).

Garton, S., *Medicine and Madness: A Social History of Insanity in New South Wales, 1880–1940* (Kensington: New South Wales University Press, 1988).

Geary, L. M., *Medicine and Charity in Ireland 1718–1851* (Dublin: University College Dublin Press, 2004).

Guinnane, T., *The Vanishing Irish: Households, Migration and the Rural Economy in Ireland, 1850–1914* (Princeton: Princeton University Press, 1997).

Hoppen, K. T., *Elections, Politics and Society in Ireland, 1832–85* (Oxford: Clarendon Press, 1984).

Howe, S., *Ireland and Empire: Colonial Legacies in Irish History and Culture* (Oxford: Oxford University Press, 2000).

Houston, R. A., *Madness and Society in Eighteenth Century Scotland* (Oxford: Oxford University Press, 2000).

Jones, C. and Porter, R. (eds), *Reassessing Foucault. Power, Medicine and the Body* (London and New York: Routledge, 1994).

Jones, G., *'Captain of all these men of death'. The History of Tuberculosis in Nineteenth- and Twentieth-Century Ireland* (Amsterdam and New York: Rodolpi, 2001).

Karsten, P., *Between Law and Custom. "High" and "Low" Legal Cultures in the Lands of the British Diaspora – The United States, Canada, Australia and New Zealand, 1600–1900* (Cambridge: Cambridge University Press, 2002).

Lee, J. J., *The Modernisation of Irish Society* (Dublin: Clarendon Press, 1989).

Legg, M. L., *Newspapers and Nationalism: The Irish Provincial Press* (Dublin: Four Courts Press, 1999).

Luddy, M., *Prostitution and Irish Society 1800–1940* (Cambridge: Cambridge University Press, 2007).

MacDonald, M., *Mystical Bedlam: Madness, Anxiety and Healing in the Seventeenth Century* (Cambridge: Cambridge University Press, 1981).

MacDonagh, O., *States of Mind: A Study in Anglo-Irish Conflict, 1780–1980* (London: George Allen and Unwin, 1983).

MacKenzie, C., *Psychiatry for the Rich. A History of Ticehurst Private Asylum* (London and New York: Routledge, 1992).

Malcolm, E., *Swift's Hospital: A History of St. Patrick's Hospital, Dublin, 1746–1989* (Dublin: Gill and Macmillan, 1989).

Malcolm, E., *'Ireland Sober, Ireland Free'. Drink and Temperance in Nineteenth-Century Ireland* (Dublin: Gill and Macmillan, 1986).

Malcolm, E., *The Irish Policeman 1822–1922: A Life* (Dublin: Four Courts Press, 2008).

Marland, H., *Medicine and Society in Wakefield and Huddersfield, 1780–1870* (Cambridge: Cambridge University Press, 1989).

Marland, H., *Dangerous Motherhood. Insanity and Childbirth in Victorian Britain* (Houndmills: Palgrave Macmillan, 2004).

Melling, J. and Forsythe, B., *The Politics of Insanity. The State, Insanity and Society in England, 1845–1914* (London and New York: Routledge, 2006).

Michael, P., *Care and Treatment of the Mentally Ill in North Wales 1800–2000* (Cardiff: University of Wales Press, 2003).

Miller, K., *Irish Immigrants in the Land of Canaan: Letters and Memoirs from Colonial and Revolutionary America, 1675–1815* (Oxford: Oxford University Press, 2003).

Moran, J. E., *Committed to the State Asylum. Insanity and Society in Nineteenth-Century Quebec and Ontario* (Montreal and Kingston: McGill-Queen's University Press, 2000).

Moykr, J., *Why Ireland Starved? A Quantitative and Analytical History of the Irish Economy, 1800–1850* (London: George Allen and Unwin, 1983).

Ó Cíosain, N., *Print and Popular Culture 1750–1850* (London: Macmillan Press, 1997).

Ó Gráda, C., *Ireland: A New Economic History 1780–1939* (Oxford: Oxford University Press, 1994).

Ó Gráda, C., *Black '47 and Beyond: the Great Irish Famine in History, Economy and Memory* (New Jersey: Princeton University Press, 1999).

Ó Gráda, C., *Ireland Before and After the Famine: Explorations in Economic History, 1808–1925* (Manchester: Manchester University Press, 1993).

O'Neill, K., *Family and Farm in Pre-Famine Ireland. The Parish of Killashandra* (Madison and London: University of Wisconsin Press, 1984).

Oppenheim, J., *'Shattered Nerves': Doctors, Patients, and Depression in Victorian England* (Oxford: Oxford University Press, 1990).

Parry-Jones, W. L. I., *The Trade in Lunacy: A Study of Private Madhouses in England in the Eighteenth and Nineteenth Centuries* (London: Routledge & Kegan Paul, 1972).

Pick, D., *Faces of Degeneracy. A European Disorder, c.1848–c.1918* (Cambridge: Cambridge University Press, 1989).

Porter, R., *Mind-Forg'd Manacles, A History of Madness in England from the Restoration to the Regency* (London: The Athlone Press, 1987).

Prior, P., *Madness and Murder. Gender, Crime and Mental Disorder in Nineteenth-Century Ireland* (Dublin: Irish Academic Press, 2008).

Reynolds, J., *Grangegorman: Psychiatric Care in Dublin since 1815* (Dublin: Institute of Public Administration, 1992).

Robins, J., *Fools and Mad: A History of the Insane in Ireland* (Dublin: Institute of Public Administration, 1986).

Scull, A., *Museums of Madness: the Social Organisation of Insanity in Nineteenth-Century England* (London: Allan Lane, 1979).

Scull, A., *The Most Solitary of Afflictions: Madness and Society in Britain, 1700–1900* (New Haven and London: Yale University Press, 1993).

Scull, A., MacKenzie C. and Hervey N. (eds), *Masters of Bedlam. The Transformation of the Mad-Doctoring Trade* (New Jersey: Princeton University Press, 1996).

Skultans, V., *Madness and Moral Ideas of Insanity in the Nineteenth Century* (London: Routledge, 1975).

Smith, L. D., *Cure, Comfort and Safe Custody: Public Asylums in Early Nineteenth-Century England* (Leicester: Leicester University Press, 1999).

Showalter, E., *The Female Malady: Women, Madness and English Culture, 1830–1980* (London: Virago Press, 1991).

Suzuki, A., *Madness at Home. The Psychiatrist, the Patient and the Family in England, 1820–1860* (California: University of California Press, 2006).

Tomes, N., *A Generous Confidence: Thomas Story Kirkbride and the Art of Asylum-Keeping, 1840–1883* (Cambridge: Cambridge University Press, 1984).

van Krieken, R., *Children and the State: Social Control and the Formation of Australian Child Welfare* (North Sydney: George Allen & Unwin, 1992).

Vaughan, M., *Curing their Ills: Colonial Power and African Illness* (Cambridge: Cambridge University Press, 1991).

Articles

Adair, R., Forsythe B. and Melling, J., 'A Danger to the Public? Disposing of Pauper Lunatics in Late-Victorian and Edwardian England: Plympton St Mary Union and the Devon County Asylum, 1867–1914', *Medical History*, 42:1 (1998), 1–25.

Adair, R., Forsythe, B. and Melling, J., 'Families, Communities and the Legal Regulation of Lunacy in Victorian England: Assessments of Crime, Violence and Welfare in Admissions to the Devon Asylum, 1845–1914', in P. Bartlett and D. Wright (eds), *Outside the Walls of the Asylum. The History of Care in the Community* (London: The Athlone Press, 1999), pp. 153–180.

Adair, R., Forsythe B. and Melling, J., 'Migration, Family Structure and Pauper Lunacy in Victorian England: Admissions to the Devon County Pauper Lunatic Asylum, 1845–1900', *Continuity and Change*, 12 (1997), 373–401.

Alderman, D. H., 'Integrating Space into a Reactive Theory of the Asylum: Evidence from post-Civil War Georgia', *Health and Place*, 3 (1997), 111–122.

Andrews, J., 'Raising the Tone of Asylumdom: Maintaining and Expelling Pauper Lunatics at the Glasgow Royal Asylum in the Nineteenth Century', in J. Melling and B. Forsythe (eds), *Insanity, Institutions and Society 1800–1914. Social History of Madness in Comparative Perspective* (London and New York: Routledge, 1999), pp. 200–222.

Andrews, J., 'Case Notes, Case Histories and the Patient's Experience of Insanity at Gartnavel Royal Asylum, Glasgow, in the Nineteenth Century', *Social History of Medicine*, 11:2 (1998), 255–281.

Andrews, J., 'The Boundaries of Her Majesty's Pleasure: Discharging Child-Murderers from Broadmoor and Perth Criminal Lunatic Department, c. 1860–1920', in M. Jackson (ed.), *Infanticide Historical Perspective on Child Murder and Concealment, 1550–2000* (Farnham and Burlington: Ashgate, 2002), pp. 216–248.

Bartlett, P., 'The Asylum and the Poor Law: The Productive Alliance', in J. Melling and B. Forsythe (eds), *Insanity, Institutions and Society, 1800–1914. Social History of Madness in Comparative Perspective* (London and New York: Routledge, 1999), pp. 48–67.

Bartlett, P., 'The Asylum, the Workhouse and the Voice of the Insane Poor in 19[th]C England', *International Journal of Law and Psychiatry*, 21:4 (1998), 421–432.

Bartlett, P., 'Legal Madness in the Nineteenth Century', *Social History of Medicine*, 14 (2001), 107–131.

Berrios, G. E., 'Obsessional Disorders during the Nineteenth Century: Terminology and Classification Issues', in W. F. Bynum, R. Porter and M. Shepherd (eds), *Anatomy of Madness: Essays in the History of Psychiatry,* I (London: Tavistock 1987), pp. 166–187.

Berrios, G.E., 'Delusions as "Wrong Beliefs": A Conceptual History', *British Journal of Psychiatry,* 159 (supplement 14) (1991), 6–13.

Beveridge, A., 'Life in the Asylum: Patient's Letters from Morningside, 1873–1908', *History of Psychiatry,* 9 (1998), 431–469.

Beveridge, A., 'Madness in Victorian Edinburgh: A Study of Patients Admitted to the Royal Edinburgh Asylum under Thomas Clouston, 1873–1908 Part 2', *History of Psychiatry,* 6 (1995), 133–156.

Bourke, J., '"The Best of all Home Rulers": The Economic Power of Women in Ireland, 1880–1914', *Irish Economic and Social History,* 13 (1991), 34–47.

Bourke, J., 'Effeminacy, Ethnicity and the End of Trauma: The Sufferings of "Shell-Shocked" Men in Great Britain and Ireland, 1914–39', *Journal of Contemporary History,* 35 (2000), 57–69.

Bowler, P., 'Race Theory and the Irish', in S. Ó Síocháin (ed.), *Social Thought on Ireland in the Nineteenth Century* (Dublin: University College Dublin, 2009), pp. 135–146.

Boyle, P. P. and Ó Gráda, C., 'Fertility Trends, Excess Mortality and the Great Irish Famine', *Demography,* 23:4 (1986), 543–562.

Breathnach, C. S., 'Hallaran's Circulating Swing', *History of Psychiatry,* 21:1 (March, 2010), 79–84.

Breen, R., 'Dowry Payments and the Irish Case', *Comparative Studies in Society and History,* 26:2 (1984), 280–296.

Bretherton, G., 'Irish Inebriate Reformatories, 1899–1902: An Experimentation in Coercion', in I. O'Donnell and F. McAuley (eds), *Criminal Justice History. Themes and Controversies from Pre-Independence Ireland* (Dublin: Four Courts Press, 2003), pp. 214–232.

Busfield, J., 'Sexism and Psychiatry', *Sociology,* 23 (1989), 343–364.

Busfield, J., 'The Female Malady? Men, Women and Madness in Nineteenth-Century Britain', *Sociology,* 28:1 (1994), 259–277.

Bynum, W. F., 'Rationales for Therapy in British Psychiatry 1780–1835', in A. Scull (ed.), *Madhouses, Mad-Doctors and Madmen: The Social History of Psychiatry in the Victorian Era* (Philadelphia: University of Pennsylvania Press, 1981), pp. 35–57.

Bynum, W. F., 'The Nervous Patient in Eighteenth- and Nineteenth-Century Britain: the Psychiatric Origins of British Neurology', in W. F. Bynum, R. Porter and M. Shepherd (eds), *Anatomy of Madness: Essays in the History of Psychiatry,* I (London: Oxford University Press, 1988), pp. 89–102.

Clark, M. J., 'The Rejection of Psychological Approaches to Mental Disorder in Late Nineteenth Century British Psychiatry', in A. Scull (ed.), *Madhouses, Mad-Doctors and Madmen: The Social History of Psychiatry in the Victorian Era* (Philadelphia: University of Pennsylvania Press, 1981) pp. 271–301.

Clondrau, F., 'The Patient's View Meets the Clinical Gaze', *Social History of Medicine*, 27:3 (2007), 525–540.

Coleborne, C., 'Passage to the Asylum: the Role of the Police in Committals of the Insane in Victoria, Australia, 1848–1900', in R. Porter and D. Wright (eds), *The Confinement of the Insane. International Perspectives, 1800–1965* (Cambridge: Cambridge University Press, 2003), pp. 129–148.

Coleborne, C., '"His Brain was Wrong, His Mind Astray": Families and the Language of Insanity in New South Wales, Queensland, and New Zealand, 1880s–1910', *Journal of Family History*, 31:1 (2006), 45–65.

Coleborne, C., 'Families, Patients and Emotions: Asylums for the Insane in Colonial Australia and New Zealand, c.1880–1910', *Social History of Medicine*, 19:3 (2006), 425–442.

Cooter, R., 'Phrenology and British Alienists, 1825–45', *Medical History*, 20:1&2 (1976), 1–21, 135–151.

Cronin, M., '"You'd be Disgraced!" Middle-Class Women and Respectability in Post-Famine Ireland', in F. Lane (ed), *Politics, Society and the Middle Class in Modern Ireland* (Houndmills: Palgrave Macmillan, 2010), pp. 107–129.

D'Arcy, F. A., 'The Decline and Fall of Donnybrook Fair: Moral Reform and Social Control in Nineteenth-Century Dublin', *Saothar*, 13 (1987), 7–21.

Davis, G., 'The Historiography of Public Health Records in Research: A Critique of Case Notes', online publications, University of Edinburgh (2002).

Digby, A., 'Moral Treatment at the Retreat, 1796–1846', in W. F. Bynum, R. Porter and M. Shepherd (eds), *Anatomy of Madness: Essays in the History of Psychiatry*, II (London: Tavistock, 1987), pp. 52–72.

Digby, A., 'Changes in the Asylum: The Case of York, 1777–1815', *Economic History Review*, 2nd series, 36:2 (1983), 218–239.

Digby, A., 'Women's Biological Straitjacket', in S. Mendus and J. Rendall (eds), *Sexuality and Subordination: Interdisciplinary Studies of Gender in the Nineteenth Century* (Cambridge: Cambridge University Press, 1994), pp. 192–220.

Dixon, T., 'Patients and Passions: Languages of Medicine and Emotion', in F. Bound Alberti (ed.), *Medicine, Emotion and Disease, 1700–1950* (Houndmills: Palgrave Macmillan, 2006), pp. 22–52.

Dowbiggin I., 'Degeneration and Hereditarianism in French Mental Medicine, 1840–90: Psychiatric Theory as Ideological Adaptation', in W. F. Bynum, R. Porter and M. Shepherd (eds), *Anatomy of Madness: Essays in the History of Psychiatry*, I (London: Tavistock, 1985), pp. 189–223.

Dowbiggan, I., '"Delusional Diagnosis?" The History of Paranoia as a Disease Concept in the Modern Era', *History of Psychiatry*, 11 (2000), 37–69.

Edginton, B.,'A Space for Moral Management. The York Retreat's Influence on Asylum Design', in L. Topp, J. E. Moran and J. Andrews (eds), *Madness, Architecture and the Built Environment. Psychiatric Spaces in Historical Context* (London: Routledge, 2007), pp. 85–104.

Ellis, R., 'The Asylum, the Poor Law and a Reassessment of the Four-Shilling Grant: Admissions to the County Asylums of Yorkshire in the Nineteenth Century', *Social History of Medicine*, 19:1 (2006), 55–73.

Ernst, W., 'European Madness and Gender in Nineteenth-Century British India', *Social History of Medicine*, 9:3 (1996), 357–382.

Ernst, W., 'Asylum Provision and the East India Company in the Nineteenth Century', *Medical History*, 42 (1998), 476–502.

Ernst, W., 'Out of Sight and Out of Mind: Insanity in Early-Nineteenth-Century British India', in J. Melling and B. Forsythe (eds), *Insanity, Institutions and Society 1800–1914. Social History of Madness in Comparative Perspective* (London and New York: Routledge, 1999), pp. 245–267.

Feingold, W. L., 'The Tenants' Movement to Capture the Irish Poor Law Boards, 1877-1886', *Albion*, 7:3 (1975), 216–231.

Finnane, M.,'Asylums, Families and the State', *History Workshop*, 20 (1985), 134–147.

Finnane, M., 'Irish Psychiatry. Part 1: The Formation of a Profession', in H. Freeman and G. E. Berrios (eds), *150 Years of British Psychiatry* (London: Tavistock, 1996), pp. 306–313.

Finnane, M., 'Irish Crime with the Outrage: the Statistics of Criminal Justice in the Later Nineteenth Century', in N. M. Dawson (ed.), *Reflections on Law and History* (Dublin: Four Courts Press, 2006), pp. 203–222.

Fissell, M. E., 'The Disappearance of the Patient's Narrative and the Invention of Hospital Medicine', in R. French and A. Wear (eds), *British Medicine in the Age of Reform* (London and New York: Routledge, 1991), pp. 92–109.

Fitzpatrick, D., 'Irish Farming Families before the First World War', *Comparative Studies in Society and History*, 25:2 (1983), 339–374.

Fitzpatrick, D., 'Marriage in post-Famine Ireland', in A. Cosgrave (ed.), *Marriage in Ireland* (Dublin: College Press, 1985), pp. 116–131.

Fitzpatrick, D., 'Divorce and Separation in Modern Irish History', *Past and Present*, 114:1 (1987), 172–196.

Fitzpatrick, D., 'Women and the Great Famine', in M. Kelleher and J. H. Murphy (eds), *Gender Perspectives in Nineteenth-Century Ireland: Public and Private Spheres* (Dublin: Irish Academic Press, 1997), pp. 50–69.

Forsythe, B., Melling, J. and Adair, R., 'The New Poor Law and the County Pauper Lunatic Asylum. The Devon Experience 1834–1884', *Social History of Medicine*, 9:3 (1996), 335–355.

Forsythe, B., Melling J. and Adair, R., 'Politics of Lunacy: Central State Regulation and the Devon Pauper Lunatic Asylum, 1845–1914', in J. Melling and B. Forsythe (eds), *Insanity, Institutions and Society, 1800–1914. Social History of Madness in Comparative Perspective* (London and New York: Routledge, 1999) pp. 68–92.

Foucault, M., 'About the Concept of the "Dangerous Individual" in 19th-Century Legal Psychiatry', *International Journal of Law and Psychiatry*, 1 (1978), 1–18.

Foucault, M., 'Madness and the Absence of Work', *Critical Inquiry*, 21 (1995), 290–298.

Garton, S., 'Policing the Dangerous Lunatic: Lunacy Incarceration in New South Wales, 1843–1914', in M. Finnane (ed.), *Policing in Australia: Historical Perspectives* (Kensington: New South Wales University Press, 1987), pp. 75–87.

Griffin, B., 'Prevention and Detection of Crime in Nineteenth-Century Ireland', in N. W. Dawson (ed.), *Reflections on Law and History. Irish Legal History Society Discourses and Other Papers, 2000–2005* (Dublin: Four Court Press, 2006), pp. 99–125.

Griffin, B., '"Such Varmint". The Dublin Police and the Public, 1838–1913', *Irish Studies Review*, 13:4 (1995/6), 21–25.

Guinnane, T. W. and Ó Gráda, C., 'Mortality in the North Dublin Union during the Great Famine', *Economic History Review*, 55:3 (2002), 487–506.

Healy, D., 'Irish Psychiatry. Part 2: Use of the Medico-Psychological Association by its Irish Members – Plus ça Change!', in H. Freeman and G. H. Berrios (eds), *150 Years of British Psychiatry* (London: The Athlone Press, 1996), pp. 314–320.

Hervey, N., 'A Slavish Bowing Down: the Lunacy Commission and the Psychiatric Profession 1845–60', in W. F. Bynum, R. Porter and M. Shepherd (eds), *The Anatomy of Madness: Essays in the History of Psychiatry, II* (London: Tavistock Press, 1985), pp. 98–131.

Hirst, D. and Michael, P., 'Family, Community and the Lunatic in Mid-Nineteenth-Century North Wales', in P. Bartlett and D. Wright (eds), *Outside the Walls of the Asylum: the History of Care in the Community 1750–2000* (London: The Athlone Press, 1999), pp. 66–85.

Hunter, J. M. and Shannon, G. W., 'Jarvis Revisited: Distance-Decay in Service Areas of mid-19th Century Asylums', *Professional Geographer*, 37:3 (1985), 296–302.

Jackson, A., 'The Survival of the Union', in J. Cleary and C. Connolly (eds), *The Cambridge Companion to Modern Irish Culture* (Cambridge: Cambridge University Press, 2005), pp. 25–41.

Jackson, M., '"It Begins with the Goose and Ends with the Goose": Medical Legal and Lay Understandings of Imbecility in *Ingram v Wyatt*, 1824–1832', *Social History of Medicine*, 11:3 (1998), 361–380.

Jewson, N. D., 'The Disappearance of the Sick-man from Medical Cosmology, 1770–1870', *Sociology*, 10 (1976), 225–244.

Jones, G., 'Eugenics in Ireland: the Belfast Eugenics Society, 1911–15', *Irish Historical Studies*, 28 (1992), 81–95.

Jones, G., '"Strike out Boldly for the Prizes that are Available to You": Medical Emigration from Ireland 1860–1905', *Medical History*, 54:1 (2010), 55–74.

Joyce, P., 'Postal Communication and the Making of the British Technostate', Centre for Research on Socio-Cultural Change, Working Paper Series, 54 (August 2008).

Kane, A. E., 'The Ritualization of Newspaper Reading and Political Consciousness: the Role of Newspapers in the Irish Land War', in L. W. McBride (ed.), *Reading Irish Histories: Texts, Contexts and Memory in Modern Ireland* (Dublin: Four Courts Press, 2003), pp. 40–62.

Kelly, B., 'Dr William Saunders Hallaran and Psychiatric Practice in Nineteenth-Century Ireland', *Irish Journal of Medical Science*, 177:1 (2008), 79–84.

Kelm, M. E., 'Women, Families and the Provincial Hospital for the Insane, British Columbia, 1905–15', *Journal of Family History*, 19 (1994), 177–193.

Kiely, K., 'Poverty and Famine in county Kildare, 1820–1850', in W. Nolan and T. McGrath (eds), *Kildare: History and Society. Interdisciplinary Essays on the History of an Irish County* (Dublin: Geography Publications, 2006), pp. 507–514.

Lee, J. J., 'Women and the Church since the Famine', in M. MacCurtain and D. O Corrain (eds), *Women in Society the Historical Dimension* (Dublin: Greenwood Press, 1978), pp. 37–45.

Legg, M. L., 'Kilkenny Circulating Library Society and the Growth of Reading Rooms in Nineteenth-Century Ireland', in B. Cunningham and M. Kennedy (eds), *The Experience of Reading: Irish Historical Perspectives* (Dublin: Economic and Social History Society of Ireland, 1999), pp. 109–123.

Levine-Clark, M., 'Dysfunctional Domesticity: Female Insanity and Family Relationships among the West Riding Poor in the Mid-Nineteenth Century', *Journal of Family History*, 25:3 (2000), 341–361.

Levine-Clark, M., '"Embarrassed Circumstances": Gender, Poverty and Insanity in the West-Riding of England in the Early Victorian Years', in J. Andrews and A. Digby (eds), *Sex and Seclusion, Class and Custody: Perspectives on Gender and Class in the History of British and Irish Psychiatry* (Amsterdam and New York: Rodopi, 2004), pp. 123–148.

MacDonald, M., 'Medicalization of Suicide in England: Laymen, Physicians and Cultural Change, 1500–1870' in C. E. Rosenberg and J. Golden (eds), *Framing Disease: Studies in Cultural History* (New Brunswick: Rutgers University Press, 1997), pp. 85–103.

MacDonald, M., 'Women and Madness in Tudor and Stuart England', *Social Research*, 53:2 (1986), 261–281.

MacDonald, M., 'Lunacy in Seventeenth- and Eighteenth-century England: Analysis of Quarter Sessions Records Part I', *History of Psychiatry*, 2:8 (1991), 437–456.

McCabe, D., 'Magistrates, Peasants and the Petty Sessions Courts: Mayo 1823–50', *Cáthair na Mart*, 5 (1985), 45–53.

McCabe, D., 'Open Court: Law and the Expansion of Magisterial Jurisdiction at Petty Sessions in Nineteenth-Century Ireland', in N. M. Dawson (ed.), *Reflections on Law and History. Irish Legal History Society Discourses and Other Papers, 2000–2005* (Dublin: Irish Academic Press, 2006), pp. 126–162.

McCandless, P., 'Liberty and Lunacy: the Victorians and Wrongful Confinement', in A. Scull (ed.), *Madhouses, Mad-doctors and Madmen. The Social History of Psychiatry in the Victorian era* (Philadelphia: University of Pennsylvania Press, 1981), pp. 339–362.

McConnel, J., 'John Redmond and Irish Catholic Loyalism', *English Historical Review*, 125:512 (2010), 83–111.

McLoughlin, D., 'Workhouses and Irish Female Paupers', in M. Luddy and C. Murphy (eds), *Women Surviving. Studies in Irish Women's History in the Nineteenth and Twentieth Centuries* (Dublin: Poolbeg Press, 1990), pp. 117–147.

McMahon, R., 'The Court of Petty Sessions and Society in pre-Famine Galway', in R. Gillespie (ed.), *The Remaking of Modern Ireland 1750–1950* (Dublin: Four Courts Press, 2004), pp. 101–137.

MacDonagh, O., 'Ideas and Institutions, 1830–45', in W. E. Vaughan (ed.), *A New History of Ireland V: Ireland Under the Union, 1801–1870* (Oxford: Clarendon Press, 1989), pp. 193–217.

Malcolm, E., '"The House of the Strident Shadows": the Asylum, the Family and Emigration in Post-Famine Rural Ireland', in E. Malcolm and G. Jones (eds), *Medicine, Disease and the State in Ireland, 1650–1940* (Cork: Cork University Press 1999), pp. 177–194.

Malcolm, E., 'Asylums and Other "Total Institutions" in Ireland: Recent Studies', *Éire-Ireland*, 22 (1987), 151–160.

Malcolm, E., 'The Reign of Terror in Carlow: the Politics of Policing Ireland in the late 1830s', *Irish Historical Studies*, 32:125 (2000), 59–74.

Malcolm, E., '"Ireland's Crowded Madhouses": the Institutional Confinement of the Insane in the Nineteenth-and Twentieth-Century Ireland', in R. Porter and D. Wright (eds), *The Confinement of the Insane. International Perspectives, 1800–1965* (Cambridge: Cambridge University Press, 2003), pp. 315–333.

Malcolm, E., '"What Would People Say if I Became a Policeman?": the Irish Policeman Abroad', in O. Walsh (ed.), *Ireland Abroad: Politics and Professions in the Nineteenth Century* (Dublin: Four Courts Press, 2003), pp. 95–107.

Malcolm, E., '"A Most Miserable Looking Object": The Irish in English Asylums, 1851–1901: Migration, Poverty and Prejudice', in J. Belchem and K. Tenfelde (eds), *Irish and Polish Migration in Comparative Perspective* (Essen: Klartext Verlag, 2003), pp. 115–123.

Malcolm, E., 'The Rise of the Pub: A Study in the Disciplining of Popular Culture', in J. S. Donnelly, Jr. and K. A. Miller (eds), *Irish Popular Culture* (Dublin: Irish Academic Press, 1998), pp. 50–77.

Malcolm, E. and Lowe W.J., 'The Domestication of the Royal Irish Constabulary, 1836–1922', *Irish Economic and Social History*, 19 (1992), 27–48.

Marks, S., '"Every Facility that Modern Science and Enlightened Humanity have Devised": Race and Progress in a Colonial Hospital, Valkenberg Mental Asylum, Cape Colony, 1894–1910', in J. Melling and B. Forsythe (eds), *Insanity, Institutions and Society 1800–1914. A Social History of Madness in Comparative Perspective* (London and New York: Routledge, 1999), pp. 268–291.

Marland, H., 'At Home with Puerperal Mania: the Domestic Treatment of the Insanity of Childbirth in the Nineteenth Century', in P. Bartlett and D. Wright (eds), *Outside the Walls of the Asylum: the History of Care in the Community 1750–2000* (London: The Athlone Press, 1999), pp. 45–65.

Marland, H., '"Destined to a Perfect Recovery": the Confinement of Puerperal Insanity in the Nineteenth Century', in J. Melling and B. Forsythe (eds), *Insanity, Institutions and Society 1800–1914. A Social History of Madness in Comparative Perspective* (London and New York: Routledge, 1999), pp. 137–156.

Marland, H., 'Languages and Landscapes of Emotion: Motherhood and Puerperal Insanity in the Nineteenth Century', in F. Bound Alberti (ed.), *Medicine, Emotion and Disease, 1700–1950* (Houndmills: Palgrave Macmillan, 2006), pp. 53–78.

Mellet, D. J., 'Bureaucracy and Mental Illness: The Commissioners in Lunacy 1845–90', *Medical History*, 25 (1981), 221–250.

Melling J. and Forsythe B., 'Accommodating Madness: New Research in the Social History of Insanity and Institutions', in J. Melling and B. Forsythe (eds), *Insanity, Institutions and Society, 1800–1914. A Social History of Madness in Comparative Perspective* (London and New York: Routledge, 1999), pp. 1–30.

Melling, J., Adair R. and Forsythe B., '"A Proper Lunatic for Two Years": Pauper Lunatic Children in Victorian and Edwardian England. Child Admissions to the Devon County Asylum, 1845–1914', *Journal of Social History*, 31 (1997), 371–405.

Melling, J., Adair R. and Forsythe B., 'Families, Communities and the Legal Regulations of Lunacy in Victorian England: Assessments in Admissions to the Devon Asylum, 1845–1914', in P. Bartlett and D. Wright (eds), *Outside the Walls of the Asylum: the History of Care in the Community 1750–2000* (London: The Athlone Press, 1999), pp. 153–180.

Melling, J. and Turner R., 'The Road to the Asylum: Institutions, Distance and the Administration of Pauper Lunacy in Devon, 1845–1914', *Journal of Historical Geography*, 25:3 (1999), 298–332.

Miller K. and Boling, B. D., '"Golden Street, Bitter Tears": the Irish Image of America during an era of Mass Migration', *Journal of American Ethnic History*, 10:1/2 (1990/91), 16–35.

Mojtabai, R., 'Delusions as Error: the History of a Metaphor', *History of Psychiatry*, 11 (2000), 3–14.

Moran, J. E., 'The Signal and the Noise: the Historical Epidemiology of Insanity in Ante-Bellum New Jersey', *History of Psychiatry*, 14 (2003), 281–301.

Murphy, E., 'The Lunacy Commissioners and the East London Guardians, 1845–1897', *Medical History*, 46:4 (2002), 495–524.

Murphy, E., 'The New Poor Law Guardians and the Administration of Insanity in East London, 1834–1844', *Bulletin of the History of Medicine*, 77:1 (2003), 45–74.

National Gallery of Ireland, *A Time and a Place. Two Centuries of Irish Social History* (Dublin: National Gallery of Ireland, 2007).

O'Brien, E., 'The Royal College of Surgeons in Ireland: A Bicentennial Tribute', *Journal of the Irish Colleges of Physicians and Surgeons*, 13:1 (January, 1984), 29–31.

Ó Cathaoir, E., 'The Poor Law in County Carlow, 1838-1923', in T. McGrath (ed.), *Carlow: History and Society. Interdisciplinary Essays on the History of an Irish County* (Dublin: Geography Publications, 2008), pp. 691–700.

O'Hanrahan, M., 'The Tithe War in County Kilkenny, 1830–1834', in W. Nolan, and K. Whelan (eds), *Kilkenny: History and Society. Interdisciplinary Essays on the History of an Irish County* (Dublin: Geography Publications: 1990), pp. 481–506.

O'Neill, T. P., 'Fever and Public Health in Pre-Famine Ireland', *Journal of the Royal Society of Antiquaries of Ireland*, 103 (1973), 1–34.

O'Shea, S., 'Carlow Poor Law Union: the Early Years', *Carloviana*, 52 (2003), 28.

Philo, C., 'Journey to Asylum: a Medical Geographical Idea in Historical Context', *Journal of Historical Geography*, 21 (1995), 148–168.

Philo, C., '"Fit Localities for an Asylum": the Historical Geography of the Nineteenth Century "Mad-Business" in England as viewed through the pages of the *Asylum Journal*', *Journal of Historical Geography*, 13 (1987), 398–415.

Porter, R., 'Introduction', in R. Porter and D. Wright (eds), *The Confinement of the Insane. International Perspectives, 1800–1965* (Cambridge: Cambridge University Press, 2003), pp. 1–19.

Porter, R., 'The Patient's View: Doing Medical History from Below', *Theory and Society*, 14:2 (1985), 175–198.

Prestwich, P., 'Family Strategies and Medical Power: Voluntary Committal in a Parisian Asylum, 1876–1914', *Journal of Social History*, 27 (1994), 799–818.

Prior, P. M., 'Women, Mental Disorder and Crime in Nineteenth Century Ireland', in A. Byrne and M. Leonard (eds), *Women and Irish Society* (Belfast: Beyond the Pale Publications, 1997), pp. 219–232.

Prior, P. M., 'Mad, Not Bad: Crime, Mental Disorder and Gender in Nineteenth-Century Ireland', History of Psychiatry, 8:32 (1997), 501–506.

Prior, P. M., 'Prisoner or Patient? The Official Debate on the Criminal Lunatic in Nineteenth-Century Ireland', History of Psychiatry, 15:2 (2004), 177–192.

Prior, P. M., 'Dangerous Lunacy: the Misuse of the Mental Health Law', Journal of Forensic Psychiatry and Psychology, 14:3 (2003), 525–541.

Prior, P. M. and Griffins, D., 'The Chaplaincy Question: The Lord Lieutenant of Ireland versus the Belfast Lunatic Asylum', Éire/Ireland, 33:2&3 (1997), 137–152.

Ray, L., 'Models of Madness in Victorian Asylum Practice', Archives of European Sociology, 22 (1981), 229–264.

Reuber, M., '"Moral Management and the Unseen Eye": Public Lunatic Asylums in Ireland, 1800–1845', in E. Malcolm and G. Jones (eds), Medicine, Disease and the State in Ireland, 1650–1940 (Cork: Cork University Press, 1999), pp. 208–233.

Risse, G. B. and Warner, J. H., 'Reconstructing Clinical Activities: Patient Records in Medical History', Social History of Medicine, 5 (1992), 183–205.

Rosenwein, B. H., 'Worrying about Emotions in History', American Historical Review, 107:3 (2002), 821–845.

Saunders, J., 'Quarantining the Weak-Minded: Psychiatric Definitions of Degeneracy at the Late-Victorian Asylum', in W. R. Bynum, R. Porter and M. Shepherd (eds), The Anatomy of Madness: Essays in the History of Psychiatry, III (London: Tavistock, 1987), pp. 273–296.

Scull, A., 'Moral Treatment Reconsidered: Some Sociological Comments on an Episode in the History of British Psychiatry', in A. Scull, Madhouses, Mad-Doctors, and Madmen: The Social History of Psychiatry in the Victorian Era (Philadelphia: University of Pennsylvania Press, 1981), pp. 105–120.

Scull, A., 'The Domestication of Madness', Medical History, 27 (1983), 233–248.

Scull, A., 'Madness and Segregative Control: The Rise of the Insane', Social Problems, 24:3 (1977), 337–351.

Scull, A., 'A Convenient Place to Get Rid of Inconvenient People', in A. D. King (ed.), Buildings and Society (London: Routledge and Kegan Paul, 1980), pp. 37–60.

Scull, A., 'A Victorian Alienist: John Conolly, FRCP, DCL (1794–1866)', in W. F. Bynum, R. Porter and M. Shepherd (eds), The Anatomy of Madness, Essays in the History of Psychiatry, I (London: Tavistock, 1985), 103–151.

Shephard, A. and Wright, D., 'Madness, Suicide and the Victorian Asylum: Attempted Self-Murder in the Age of Non-Restraint', Medical History, 46 (2002), 175–196.

Smith, C., 'Parsimony, Power and Prescriptive Legislation: the Politics of Pauper Lunacy in Northamptonshire, 1845–1876', Bulletin of the History of Medicine, 81:2 (2007), 359–385.

Smith, L. D., 'Behind Closed Doors: Lunatic Asylum Keepers, 1800–1860', *Social History of Medicine*, 1 (1988), 301–328.

Smith, L. D., 'Close Confinement in a Mighty Prison: Thomas Bakewell and his Campaign against Public Asylums, 1810–1830', *History of Psychiatry*, 5 (1994), 191–214.

Smith, L. D., 'The County Asylum and the Mixed Economy of Care', in J. Melling and B. Forsythe (eds), *Insanity, Institutions and Society 1800–1914. A Social History of Madness in Comparative Perspective* (London and New York: Routledge, 1999), pp. 33–47.

Steiner-Scott, E., '"To Bounce a Boot Off Her Now & Then..." Domestic Violence in Post-Famine Ireland', in M. Gialanella Valiulis and M. O'Dowd (eds), *Women and Irish History* (Dublin: Wolfhound Press, 1997), pp. 125–143.

Suzuki, A., 'Framing Psychiatric Subjectivity: Doctor, Patient and Record-Keeping at Bethlem in the Nineteenth century', in J. Melling and B. Forsythe (eds), *Insanity, Institutions and Society, 1800–1914: A Social History of Madness in Comparative Perspective* (London and New York: Routledge, 1999), pp. 115–136.

Suzuki, A., 'Lunacy in Seventeenth and Eighteenth-Century England: Analysis of Quarter Sessions Records Part I', *History of Psychiatry*, 1 (1991), 437–456.

Suzuki, A., 'Lunacy in Seventeenth and Eighteenth-Century England: Analysis of Quarter Sessions Records Part II', *History of Psychiatry*, 3 (1992), 29–44.

Suzuki, A., 'The Politics and Ideology of Non-Restraint: the Case of the Hanwell Asylum', *Medical History*, 39 (1995), 1–17.

Suzuki, A., 'Lunacy and Labouring Men: Narratives of Male Vulnerability in Mid-Victorian London', in R. Bivins and J. V. Pickstone (eds), *Medicine, Madness and Social History. Essays in Honour of Roy Porter* (Houndmills: Palgrave Macmillan, 2007), pp. 118–128.

Theriot, N. M., 'Negotiating Illness: Doctors, Patients, and Families in the Nineteenth Century', *Journal of the History of the Behavioural Sciences*, 37:4 (2001), 349–368.

Theriot, N. M., 'Women's Voices in Nineteenth Century Medical Discourse: A Step toward Deconstructing Science', *Signs*, 19 (1993), 1–31.

Thomas, E. G., 'The Old Poor Law and Medicine', *Medical History*, 24:1 (1980), 1–19.

Thompson, M. S., 'The Wages of Sin: the Problem of Alcoholism and General Paralysis in Nineteenth-Century Edinburgh', in W. R. Bynum, R. Porter and M. Shepherd (eds), *The Anatomy of Madness: Essays in the History of Psychiatry*, III (London: Tavistock, 1987), pp. 316–340.

Tomes, N., 'The Great Restraint Controversy: a Comparative Perspective on Anglo-American Psychiatry in the Nineteenth Century', in W. R. Bynum, R. Porter and M. Shepherd (eds), *The Anatomy of Madness: Essays in the History of Psychiatry*, III (London: Tavistock, 1985), pp. 190–228.

Townsend, P. A., 'Academies of Nationality': the Reading Room and Irish National Movements, 1838–1905', in L. W. McBride (ed.), *Reading Irish Histories: Texts, Contexts and Memory in Modern Ireland* (Dublin: Four Courts Press, 2003), pp. 19–39.

Walsh, O., '"A Lightness of Mind": Gender and Insanity in Nineteenth Century Ireland', in M. Kelleher and J. H. Murphy (eds), *Gender Perspectives in Nineteenth-Century Ireland* (Dublin: Four Courts Press, 1997), pp. 159–167.

Walsh, O., 'Lunatic and Criminal Alliances in Nineteenth-Century Ireland', in P. Barlett and D. Wright (eds), *Outside the Walls of the Asylum: the History of Care in the Community* (London: The Athlone Press, 1999), pp. 132–152.

Walsh, O., 'The Designs of Providence: Race, Religion and Irish Insanity', in J. Melling and B. Forsythe (eds), *Insanity, Institutions and Society, 1800–1914: A Social History of Madness in Comparative Perspective* (London and New York: Routledge, 1999), pp. 223–242.

Walsh, O., 'Gendering the Asylums: Ireland and Scotland, 1847–1877', in T. Brotherstone, D. Simonton and O. Walsh (eds), *The Gendering of Scottish History: An International Approach* (Glasgow: Cruithne Press, 1999), pp. 199–215.

Walsh, O., 'Gender and Insanity in Nineteenth-Century Ireland', in J. Andrews and A. Digby (eds), *Sex and Seclusion, Class and Custody: Perspectives on Gender and Class in the History of British and Irish Psychiatry* (Amsterdam and New York: Rodopi, 2004), pp. 69–94.

Walton, J. K., 'Lunacy in the Industrial Revolution: A Study of Asylum Admission in Lancashire, 1848–50', *Journal of Social History*, 13:1 (1979–80), 1–22.

Walton, J. K., 'Casting Out and Bringing Back in Victorian England: Pauper Lunatics, 1840–1870', in W. F. Bynum, R. Porter and M. Shepherd (eds), *The Anatomy of Madness. Essays in the History of Psychiatry, II* (London: Tavistock, 1985), pp. 132–146.

Williamson, A., 'The Beginnings of State Care of the Mentally Ill in Ireland', *Economic and Social Review*, 1 (1970), 281–290.

Wright, D., 'Getting Out of the Asylum: Understanding the Confinement of the Insane in the Nineteenth Century', *Social History of Medicine*, 10:1 (2001), 137–155.

Wright, D., 'The Certification of Insanity in Nineteenth-Century England and Wales', *History of Psychiatry*, 9 (1998), 267–290.

Wright, D., 'Family Strategies and the Institutional Confinement of "Idiot" Children in Victorian England', *Journal of Family History*, 23:2 (1998), 190–208.

Wright, D., 'The Discharge of Pauper Lunatics from County Asylums in Mid-Victorian England The Case of Buckinghamshire, 1853–1872', in J. Melling and B. Forsythe (eds), *Insanity, Institutions and Society, 1800–1914*.

A Social History of Madness in Comparative Perspective (London and New York: Routledge, 1999), pp. 93–112.

Wright, D., 'Delusion of Gender?: Lay Identification and Clinical Diagnosis of Insanity in Victorian England', in J. Andrews and A. Digby (eds), *Sex and Seclusion, Class and Custody. Perspectives on Gender and Class in the History of British and Irish Psychiatry* (Amsterdam and New York: Rodolpi, 2004), pp. 149–176.

Theses

Bates, D., 'Keepers to Nurses? A History of the Irish Asylum Workers' Trade Union 1917–1924' (MA dissertation, University College Dublin, 2010).

Durnin, D., 'Intertwining Institutions: the Relationship between the South Dublin Union workhouse and the Richmond Lunatic Asylum, 1880–1911' (MA dissertation, University College Dublin, 2010).

Mauger, A., '"Confinement of the Higher Orders"? The Significance of Private Lunatic Asylums in Ireland, 1820–1860' (MA dissertation, University College Dublin, 2009).

McCabe, D., 'Law, Conflict and Social Order in County Mayo, 1820–1845', vols 1&2 (PhD dissertation, University College Dublin, 1991).

Saunders, J. F., 'Institutionalised offenders: a study of the Victorian institution and its inmates, with special reference to late nineteenth century Warwickshire' (PhD dissertation, University of Warwick, 1983).

Williamson, A. P., 'The Origins of the Irish Mental Hospital Service, 1800–1843' (M.Litt dissertation, Trinity College Dublin, 1970).

Index